T0319540

The Physician's Perspective on Medical Law, Volume I

AANS Publications Committee
Howard H. Kaufman, MD, and
Jeff L. Lewin, JD, Editors

Neurosurgical Topics

The American Association of
Neurological Surgeons

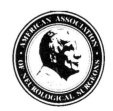

Library of Congress Catalog
ISBN: 1-879284-44-8

Neurosurgical Topics ISBN: 0-9624246-6-8

Warren R. Selman, MD, Chairman
AANS Publications Committee

Gay Palazzo, AANS Staff Editor

AANS1.4M897

Neurosurgical Topics SERIES

FORTHCOMING BOOKS

The Physician's Perspective on Medical Law, Volume II
Edited by Howard H. Kaufman, MD, and Jeff L. Lewin, JD

Advanced Techniques in Central Nervous System Metastases
Edited by Robert J. Maciunas, MD

Calvarial and Dural Reconstruction
Edited by Setti S. Rengachary, MD, and Edward C. Benzel, MD

DEDICATIONS

To Romaine Kaufman and my sons, Ezekiel and Zachary, at least one of whom may enter the legal profession.

H.H.K.

To Alison Williams Lewin and our children, Eleanor, Gregory, and Sylvia, for their tolerance during my immersion in this project and for the delightful exuberance with which they occasionally succeeded in distracting me from the task.

J.L.L.

To Joyce Herschberger whose hard work and persistence were essential to the completion of this project, and to Gay Palazzo for her patience while awaiting the manuscript and for her superb editorial refinements thereof.

H.H.K.
J.L.L.

CONTENTS

VOLUME II

PART III: THE PHYSICIAN AND PUBLIC HEALTH ISSUES

LIST OF CONTRIBUTORS

Volumes I and II

Alan M. Ducatman, MD, MS
Director
Institute of Occupational and
    Environmental Health
West Virginia School of Medicine
Morgantown, West Virginia

Mathis P. Frick, MD
Department of Radiology
Robert C. Byrd Health Sciences Center
West Virginia University
Morgantown, West Virginia

James L. Frost, MD
Deputy Chief Medical Examiner
Office of the Chief Medical Examiner
North Central Region
State of West Virginia
Morgantown, West Virginia

Mark Gibson, MD
Professor and Chairman
Department of Obstetrics and Gynecology
Robert C. Byrd Health Sciences Center
West Virginia University
Morgantown, West Virginia

Ellen E. Hrabovsky, MD
Professor and Chief
Section of Pediatric Surgery
Robert C. Byrd Health Sciences Center
West Virginia University
Morgantown, West Virginia

Howard H. Kaufman, MD
Department of Neurosurgery
Robert C. Byrd Health Sciences Center
West Virginia University
Morgantown, West Virginia

Robert W. Keefover, MD
Associate Professor
Departments of Neurology and
    BehavioralMedicine and Psychiatry
Robert C. Byrd Health Sciences Center
West Virginia University
Morgantown, West Virginia

Leroy J. Korb, MD
Department of Radiology
Robert C. Byrd Health Sciences Center
West Virginia University
Morgantown, West Virginia

Jeff L. Lewin, JD
Professor of Law
Widener University School of Law
Wilmington, Delaware

Joyce McConnell, JD, LLM
Associate Professor
College of Law
West Virginia University
Morgantown, West Virginia

Robert F. Munzner, PhD
Chief, Neurological Devices Branch,
Device Evaluation
US Food and Drug Administration
Center for Devices and Radiological Health
Rockville, Maryland

G. Robert Nugent, MD
Professor of Neurosurgery
Robert C. Byrd Health Sciences Center
West Virginia University
Morgantown, West Virginia

Perry Oxley, JD
Waters, Warren & Harris
Clarksburg, West Virginia

Conrad J. Pesyna, BS
Director of Medical Records
West Virginia Hospitals, Inc.
Morgantown, West Virginia

Sandra A. Price, JD
Risk Manager
Robert C. Byrd Health Sciences Center
West Virginia University
Morgantown, West Virginia

Mark A. Reynolds, MD
Interim Director,
Jon Michael Moore Trauma Center
Interim Chief, Section of Trauma and Surgery
Assistant Professor
Department of Surgery
West Virginia University
Morgantown, West Virginia

Carolyn B. Reynolds, MD
Department of Emergency Medicine
Preston Memorial Hospital
Kingwood, West Virginia

Cheng B. Saw, PhD
Division of Radiation Oncology
University of Iowa Hospital and Clinics
200 Hawkins Drive W189Z-GH
Iowa City, Iowa

Raymond A. Smego, Jr., MD, MPH, FACP, DTM&H
Professor of Medicine
Section of Infectious Diseases
Director, International Health Program
Robert C. Byrd Health Sciences Center
West Virginia University
Morgantown, West Virginia

James M. Stevenson, MD
Professor and Chairman
Behavioral Medicine and Psychiatry
West Virginia University
Morgantown, West Virginia

Daniel R. Sullivan, MD, JD
Adjunct Professor
Department of Anesthesiology
Robert C. Byrd Health Sciences Center
West Virginia University
Morgantown, West Virginia

Gregory A. Timberlake, MD, FACS
Director of Trauma Services
Department of Neurosurgery
Health Sciences Center
Morgantown, West Virginia

Janie R. Vale, MD, MSPH
Columbia Occupational Medicine
Columbia, Missouri

Grace J. Wigal, JD
Director of Legal Research and
    Writing Program
West Virginia University College of Law
Morgantown, West Virginia

Janet M. Williams, MD, FACEP
Assistant Professor
Department of Emergency Medicine
West Virginia University
Morgantown, West Virginia

AANS Publications Committee

Warren R. Selman, MD, *Chair*
Michael L.J. Apuzzo, MD
Julian E. Bailes, Jr., MD
Daniel L. Barrow, MD
Joshua B. Bederson, MD
Edward C. Benzel, MD
T. Forcht Dagi, MD

John G. Golfinos, MD
Howard H. Kaufman, MD
Christopher M. Loftus, MD
Robert J. Maciunas, MD
Ian E. McCutcheon, MD
Setti S. Rengachary, MD
John A. Jane, MD, *ex officio*

The American Association of Neurological Surgeons is accredited by the Accreditation Council for Continuing Medical Education (CME) to sponsor continuing medical education for physicians.

The American Association of Neurological Surgeons designates the continuing medical education activity as 15 credit hours in Category I of the Physician's Recognition Award of the American Medical Association.

Preface

The professional activities of most physicians lead to numerous contacts with the legal system, either in relation to patients or to public health issues about which physicians have unique experience and knowledge. In our experience many physicians feel that they are neither informed about nor comfortable with the legal rules that affect their relations with patients and with society. This monograph has been prepared to provide information about these rules and about the legal and social context in which they arise.

Physicians have an ethical and legal responsibility to participate in the legal system, both as advocates for patients and as good citizens. In order for physicians to carry out these responsibilities and comport themselves appropriately, they should become familiar with the legal system and the legal rules that govern their participation in judicial proceedings.

Physicians must understand the legal rules governing their relations with patients. In addition to familiarity with the general rules about the physician-patient relationship and the handling of confidential patient information, physicians face special problems in making medical decisions at the end of life, evaluating patients who may lack mental competence, and protecting vulnerable patients such as children, spouses, and the elderly.

Beyond caring for their patients, physicians as citizens ought to take an active role in public health issues that cause the greatest problems in our society, especially violence, accidents, firearms, alcohol, tobacco and infectious disease. They also should be aware of problems arising from exposure to such potential public health hazards as radiation, toxic substances, and regulated drugs and devices.

Physicians must also be prepared to protect both themselves and their patients in interactions with the health care system. For themselves, physicians need to negotiate their way through the systems that control their licensure and privileges. Physicians need to assist their patients and also protect their own monetary interests in relation to various private and public payors; the newly evolving systems encompassed in the term "managed care" pose special challenges. Physicians should understand their role in determining patient eligibility for public benefits from the federal Social Security program and state workers' compensation systems. Finally, physicians confront the risk of medical malpractice claims by their patients and the problems posed by this aspect of the law.

We note that a book on this subject necessarily must be considered a work in progress. Many of the chapters involve areas of law that are evolving rapidly in response to medical advances and emerging social developments. The issue of assisted suicide is being considered by the United States Supreme Court as this book is going to press. The proliferation of medical information transmission via the Internet has generated proposals for protecting confidentiality in computerized medical records. Turning to public health issues, there has been a recent decrease in the amount of violent crime, but the reason is not certain. Competing interest groups are seeking to tighten or ease restrictions on accessibility of guns. With regard to efforts to curtail the use of tobacco, the Food and Drug Administration has begun to institute new regulations of nicotine, while newspapers report important developments in lawsuits by states and individuals against tobacco companies. Responding to concern about abuses by managed care organizations in exacting large profits while limiting patient care, courts and legislatures are developing new rules to control these entities and protect patient rights. Accordingly, the editors and authors plan on regularly revising this book and possibly converting it to a looseleaf format to better accommodate anticipated changes in the law which are certain to occur at irregular and unpredictable intervals.

We hope this book will prove useful in presenting information that can help physicians, as well as lawyers and others, understand the legal aspects of physicians' activities. Although this book is primarily about law, most of the chapters are written by non-lawyers. Frequently, the authors convey physician perspectives on controversial medical and social issues. No consensus exists on many of these issues, either within the medical or legal professions or among the editors and authors of this book. The views expressed in any particular chapter are not necessarily shared by the editors or by authors of other chapters. We hope the book provides both a stimulus to and a foundation for informed debate on these important topics.

Howard H. Kaufman, M.D.
Morgantown, West Virginia

Jeff L. Lewin, J.D.
Wilmington, Delaware

June 1997

CHAPTER 1

BACKGROUND: THE AMERICAN LEGAL SYSTEM

JEFF L. LEWIN, JD

This chapter provides a general overview of the American legal system as a background for the more detailed analysis of particular medicolegal issues presented in the remainder of the book. In the interests of clarity and brevity, this chapter necessarily must present a simplified description of a topic that warrants book-length treatment.[13,28,53]

The American legal system is difficult to describe because it is not a unitary institution, but instead consists of a complex interrelationship among various law-making institutions that trace their lineage to feudal England and reflect the American experience of two centuries of political, economic, and social change. The evolution of the American legal system is itself the subject of several important books.[33,38-40]

Much of the complexity of the American legal system reflects inherent tensions among the system's conflicting values and goals. For example, the goal of achieving "justice" in dispute resolution encompasses two incompatible values: consistency in the universal application of general rules, and fairness in the individualized evaluation of each case on its unique facts. The law seeks to accomplish both of these incompatible goals, thereby creating a sense of injustice whenever strict application of a general rule seems unduly harsh or whenever a special exception to a general rule raises the specter of bias or prejudice. A similar tension exists between our desires for the legal system to provide stability and predictability but also flexibility and adaptability. The Constitution of the United States itself reflects a contradiction between our high regard for democracy and our distrust of majorities.[17,19,26]

More fundamentally, because of the absence of shared values in our pluralistic society, we must rely upon formal rules to organize social behavior, yet because of the limitations of language, the interpretation of those rules is impossible without reference to the underlying values they seek to accomplish.[19,24,25,48,54] Thus, in the absence of shared values, every act of legal interpretation—whether of a constitution, statute, regulation, or judicial decision—represents a potential source of controversy and conflict.

The foregoing tensions are intrinsic to each of the fundamental aspects of the American legal system, which include: 1) the predominance of the "common law" as both a source of law and a mode of analysis; 2) the dual sovereignty of federal and state governments; 3) the separation of powers among the legislative, executive, and judicial branches of government; 4) judicial review of the constitutionality of legislation and executive action; 5) a hierarchy of authority among the diverse sources of American law, with the courts having ultimate interpretative authority; and 6) the adversary system of justice for civil and criminal litigation.

THE COMMON LAW SYSTEM

What does it mean to say that the American legal system is a common law system? The term "common law" has various meanings, depending on the context.[28] Originally, the term described the law of England that was common to the entire nation rather than local. Prior to widespread legislation, the law of England was expressed primarily through judicial opinions, so the term common law also refers to judge-made law or "case law," as opposed to statutory law. The phrase "at common law" sometimes is used to mean the legal rules that existed in medieval England, but it often is used to refer to any legal rule that was applied by the courts prior to legislation on a particular subject. For purposes of this book, the "common law method" or mode of analysis refers to the process by which the law is discovered and applied by the common law courts.

The term is used in a broader sense to characterize the legal systems of "common law countries," which are derived from the English legal system and rely heavily upon judge-made law, in contrast to the "civil law countries" of continental Europe, whose legal systems are derived from a Roman law tradition and rely primarily on legislative codes. (Forty-nine of the American states have common law legal systems, but Louisiana retains a civil law code-based legal system resulting from its history as a Spanish and French colony.) The term also is used more narrowly to distinguish the rules applied by common law courts from those applied in special courts of equity or admiralty.

One distinctive feature of the American legal system is its reliance on the common law method or mode of analysis. The medieval English jurists conceived of law as "natural law," a higher law, inherent in human nature, that applied universally to all human societies. The task of the medieval jurist was to discover this law by studying existing customs and practices. In fashioning various local customs into a single body of general principles, judges placed great reliance on previous judicial decisions in similar cases, thereby giving rise to the doctrine of judicial precedent.[13] If a previous court had adjudicated a matter on similar facts, then the prior decision served as precedent for applying the same rule of law in the current case. If the current case presented unique facts, the judge would attempt to derive the applicable legal rule through the process of reasoning by analogy from previous cases.

Under the common law system, a judicial decision serves two functions.[13,28] First, it resolves the dispute between the two parties with finality under the doctrine of *res judicata* ("the thing has been adjudicated"), precluding the parties from relitigating the issues. Second, it serves as precedent for future decisions under the doctrine of *stare decisis* (from *stare decisis et non quieta movere*, "let the decision stand and do not disturb what is settled"). The doctrine of *stare decisis* binds a court to follow its own decisions in subsequent cases, as well as binding subordinate courts in the same jurisdiction.

Eventually, the natural law viewpoint gave way to the positivist view that law was a human creation and that judges made law rather than discovering it.[28] The transformation from a naturalist to a positivist orientation did not, however, undermine the use of precedent, for the doctrine of *stare decisis* continued to serve important social interests: uniformity and predictability for members of society; justice for those whose expectations were based on actions in reliance on prior precedent; justice insofar as like cases are treated equally; and efficiency for judges in providing a ready source of legal rules.

The doctrine of precedent provides flexibility insofar as no two cases are identical, so that judges may be able to apply a different rule in a novel situation by demonstrating that the facts are "distinguishable" from those in prior cases so that the judges are not bound by the principle expressed in those cases. A court may apply precedent broadly to various analogous situations or apply it narrowly only to cases with essentially identical facts. (Much of the first year of study in most American law schools is devoted to teaching the common law mode of analysis in interpreting, applying, and distinguishing judicial precedent.) American courts have achieved additional flexibility by employing a relaxed doctrine of *stare decisis* in which the jurisdiction's highest court is not absolutely bound by prior precedent but has the power to overrule its own past decisions if it concludes they were poorly reasoned or maladaptive to changed social or economic conditions.[13,24,25,53] The common law at any given time thus consists of the accumulation of judicial opinions, and it constantly evolves as courts confront new situations or overrule past decisions.

Our common law system thus magnifies the difficulties of interpretation that exist within any system of legal rules.[42,48,54,60] All such systems must confront both factual indeterminacy resulting from the fallibility of human witnesses and the imprecision of language[31,32] and legal indeterminacy resulting from imprecision of language and the likelihood of gaps or inconsistencies within any human-created system of rules.[42,60] The ad hoc evolution of common law doctrine exacerbates these problems because of the added difficulty of extracting general legal rules from particularized decisions, the increased likelihood of gaps or inconsistencies in the rules resulting from such decisions, and the ever-present possibility that existing precedent may be limited by new distinctions or overruled altogether.[49] As a result, persons seeking legal advice frequently are frustrated by the inability of even the best attorneys to tell them with certainty what rule will apply to their particular situation.

DUAL SOVEREIGNTY

Our legal system recognizes the dual sovereignty of the federal and state governments. That is, each American is both a citizen of the United States and of a particular state (or territory), and the 50 state governments exist and exercise authority over their citizens independently of the federal government. The original 13 American colonies adopted their constitutions prior to 1780, during the struggle for independence from Britain, and they functioned as independent sovereigns under the Articles of Confederation of 1781, finally ceding a portion of their sovereignty to the United States upon ratification of the Constitution in 1788.[28]

The Constitution of the United States established the supremacy of the federal government, but it created a federal government of limited enumerated powers: to control foreign affairs; provide for national defense; regulate interstate commerce; impose taxes; establish a national currency, post office, and roads; and make uniform laws for bankruptcy, patents, and copyrights. Although the Constitution forbade any state interference with foreign affairs or interstate commerce, it left the states with full power to regulate their own internal affairs under what is known as the "police power"—the right to legislate for the health, safety, morals, and general welfare of the community. The Tenth Amendment to the Constitution, ratified as part of the Bill of Rights, effective in December 1791, made this assumption explicit: "The powers not delegated to the United States by the Constitution, nor prohibited by it to the States, are reserved to the States respectively, or to the people." This division of authority between federal and state government "was the unique contribution of the Framers to political science and political theory."[62]

Each state has authorized the creation of various subordinate local governmental units (e.g., counties, cities, and towns). These local governments are not sovereign but derive all of their powers from an express grant of state authority.

The conflict between advocates of broad federal authority and champions of "states' rights" is a recurrent theme in American political and constitutional history. The federal government's power was dramatically expanded by Chief Justice John Marshall's (1755-1835) opinion for the Supreme Court in *McCulloch v. Maryland*,[52] which declared that the Constitution's express grant of specific powers necessarily included the "implied powers" required for their implementation; in particular, the Court ruled that the powers to establish a currency and raise taxes implied the power to charter a national bank that would be immune from state taxation. The scope of federal authority was further broadened in the 20th century when the power to regulate interstate commerce was interpreted as including the power to regulate discrete local activities that either individually or through cumulative aggregate impact have a "substantial economic effect" on interstate commerce.[59]

The expansion of federal regulation in the 20th century has substantially diminished the regulatory authority of the states. Under the pre-emption doctrine, federal legislation on a subject precludes inconsistent state legislation, but in many instances it may even preclude all state legislation because the federal law is said to occupy the field.[59] Nevertheless, the federal government has no power to regulate purely intrastate activity that does not substantially affect interstate commerce,[61] and state law continues to play a fundamental role in ordering the day-to-day lives of American citizens.

Separation of Powers

The Constitutions of the United States and of the individual states establish a tripartite governing structure, with a legislative body (Congress or the state legislatures or assemblies), an executive (the president or state governors and their administrative agencies), and a judicial system. The traditional description of the separation of powers—that the legislature makes the law, the executive carries out the law, and the judiciary applies the law to resolve disputes—is overly simplistic. In fact, all three branches of government participate in "making" the law.

The Legislature

Article I of the U.S. Constitution vests the legislative power in a bicameral Congress composed of a House of Representatives and a Senate. The House of Representatives, which currently has 435 representatives elected for two-year terms from Congressional Districts established on the basis of current census figures, gives each state representation in proportion to its population. The Senate, with two senators from each state, gives the states equal representation in recognition of their partial relinquishment of independent sovereignty in order to create the United States. Senators are elected to six-year terms, which are staggered so that roughly one-third of the seats are contested in each biennial election.

Each state has its own legislature or general assembly. Virtually all of these bodies (except Nebraska) are bicameral. Under the principle of one person/one vote, the U.S. Supreme Court has mandated that both houses in state legislatures be apportioned according to population.[15]

The process by which Congress enacts federal legislation is beyond the scope of this chapter; it is ably described elsewhere.[28] State legislative procedures are similar to the federal process, but their effectiveness is impaired by the fact that members of most state legislatures do not devote full time to their duties.[28]

Executive and Administrative Agencies

Federal and state constitutions give the executive very little power to make law. Indeed, the general grant of executive power in Article II of the U.S. Constitution is so vague that it does not seem to justify the vast power exercised by the American Presidency.[59] Apart from the power to make treaties (with the advice and consent of the Senate) and the constitutional role as Commander in Chief of the armed forces, the primary constitutional duties of the President are to appoint ambassadors, judges, and executive officers and to "take Care that the Laws be faithfully executed."

Presidents and governors can issue executive orders to their subordinates without legislative involvement, but such orders do not have the force of law upon ordinary citizens. While presidents and governors can propose the enactment of legislation, they have no formal role in the legislative process prior to passage in both houses, and then only through the veto power. For federal legislation, the President has 10 days in which to veto the legislation; if this power is exercised, a bill still can become law if the veto is overridden by a two-thirds majority in both houses. Similar veto provisions exist in most state constitutions.

The executive's most significant participation in law-making is through the action of executive or administrative agencies.[13,53] Many federal and state laws are enforced by specialized executive agencies, of which there are two main types: executive agencies and semi-independent administrative agencies.

Traditional executive agencies or departments report directly to the chief executive (president or governor) and function as extensions of the power of the chief executive in carrying out the law. At the federal level, relevant executive agencies include the Food and Drug Administration (FDA), the Occupational Safety and Health Administration (OSHA), and the Social Security Administration (SSA). Traditional executive agencies at the state and local level include police, prosecutors, and public health inspectors.

"Administrative agencies" or "independent agencies" are semi-independent of the chief executive insofar as: 1) they can function without direct interference by the chief executive, and 2) their members generally are removable only for cause. Examples of semi-independent administrative agencies include the Federal Trade Commission (FTC), the National Labor Relations Board (NLRB), and the Securities and Exchange Commission (SEC) at the federal level; medical licensure boards and worker's compensation commissions at the state level; and municipal zoning boards at the local level.

Although formally an extension of the executive branch, executive and administrative agencies also perform functions that are usually thought of as legislative or judicial. That is, in addition to carrying out or enforcing the law, agencies also participate in creating the law and in deciding how to apply it in individual cases.

Agencies perform a quasi-legislative or "rule-making" function when they promulgate regulations to implement regulatory statutes. Legislatures frequently draft regulatory statutes in the form of broad general directives to protect public health, safety, and welfare, delegating to executive or administrative agencies the task of writing more detailed regulations to establish precise standards. For example, Congress enacted the Food and Drug Act to prohibit the marketing of unsafe drugs, but the regulations that require successive trials on animal and human populations were promulgated by the FDA.

Agencies perform a quasi-judicial or adjudicatory function when they make an individualized decision whether to grant a benefit (e.g., Social Security or worker's compensation benefits), to issue a permit (e.g., a new drug approval, a medical license, or a building permit), or to impose a penalty for violation of a statute or regulation. The federal system employs more than 1,200 "administrative law judges," including 700 in the Social Security Administration alone, to take testimony and render decisions or recommendations in adjudicatory matters.[13] While adjudicatory agency decisions generally are subject to judicial review, in many cases the reviewing court does not receive new evidence on the merits of the case but instead limits its consideration to whether the agency correctly followed its procedures and took into account all of the appropriate factors.

In response to the proliferation of federal executive and administrative agencies and the expansion of their powers, Congress enacted the federal Administrative Procedure Act[1] in 1946 to assure that these agencies employed uniform and fair procedures in carrying out their rule-making and adjudicatory functions. Each state has equivalent statute-setting guidelines for the procedures of its agencies. These procedures often require public notice and public hearings prior to promulgation of new rules, and they often mandate formal or informal hearings with an opportunity to present evidence for participants in individual adjudications.

The Judicial System

The federal government and each state government has its own separate judicial system. The federal and state judicial systems generally are independent, except that the U.S. Supreme Court has the power to review state judicial decisions that may conflict with the Constitution or statutes of the United States, and lower federal courts may in narrowly defined circumstances intervene in state court proceedings to prevent violation of federally created rights.

The federal and state judicial systems consist of trial courts and one or more levels of appellate courts. In the trial courts, the "fact finder" (usually a jury but sometimes a judge) hears the evidence to determine the facts and then applies the law to the facts to decide the case. The appellate courts generally must accept the facts as determined by the trial courts and review the case to see whether the law was correctly applied.

Most appellate court decisions and a limited number of trial court opinions are embodied in written opinions that are published in chronological order for each court system. These published decisions constitute the source of common law precedent.

Each state establishes its own judicial system. The 50 state court systems vary greatly in structure and in the terminology used to describe them.[13,14,28] The trial courts of "general jurisdiction" in most states are organized on a county-by-county basis and may be variously referred to as district, circuit, or superior courts or courts of common pleas. These county courts have jurisdiction over most civil lawsuits and criminal prosecutions. Most states also employ a variety of lower trial courts (e.g., justices of the peace, magistrates, municipal courts, police courts, and traffic courts) that have limited jurisdiction over small claims, traffic offenses, and other minor criminal offenses.

Roughly half of the states have one or more levels of intermediate appellate courts that hear appeals from the county trial courts. Some states have separate courts for criminal and civil appeals, and others divide their intermediate appellate courts into two or more districts. In virtually all states having an intermediate appellate court, disappointed litigants have an absolute right to take an appeal to this level. Cases typically are heard by panels of three judges.[14,28]

Every state has a supreme court consisting of five to nine judges or justices. In states having an intermediate appellate court, the supreme court generally has discretion regarding whether to entertain a further appeal, whereas in states without an intermediate appellate court, the supreme court (except in West Virginia) must consider all appeals.[14,28]

In the federal system, the trial courts are known as "district courts." Each state and federal territory contains one or more federal judicial districts.[3] (The most populous states—California, New York, and Texas—each have four districts.) The federal district courts have jurisdiction over three categories of cases.[28] First, they have jurisdiction over all cases in which the United States is a party, including all federal criminal prosecutions and all enforcement actions by federal regulatory agencies.[28] Second, under their "federal question jurisdiction," the

district courts have the power to decide "all civil actions arising under the Constitution, laws, or treaties of the United States."[9] Finally, the district courts have jurisdiction over civil suits in which there is a "diversity" of citizenship (suits between citizens of different states or between a citizen and foreign states or their citizens) in order to protect out-of-state parties from the fear that they might not get a fair hearing in state courts.[10] In such suits, the district court is to apply the law of the state in which it sits,[27] including that state's "choice of law" rules for determining whether to apply the law of another state.[45] Diversity jurisdiction is currently limited to suits in which the amount in controversy exceeds $50,000.[10]

The intermediate appellate courts in the federal system are known as circuit courts of appeal. There currently are 13 federal judicial circuits: 11 numbered circuits accept cases from regional groupings of three or more states and territories; a District of Columbia Circuit accepts cases from the District Court for the District of Columbia; and a Federal Circuit accepts appeals involving a miscellaneous group of specialized statutes, including patents, trademarks, international trade, and claims against the United States as a defendant.[2,8]

In virtually all civil and criminal cases, the losing party has an absolute right to take an appeal from a final decision of the district court to the appropriate circuit court of appeals.[7] Each appeal is decided by a panel of three judges. As a result of the burgeoning federal appellate caseload, many cases are decided on the basis of written briefs, without oral argument, and in a growing number of cases the decision is set forth in a memorandum order without a written opinion explaining the basis for the decision.

The Supreme Court of the United States is the highest federal appellate court. The Supreme Court's appellate caseload is now almost entirely discretionary.[14] It has the option to grant a "writ of certiorari" to review important cases from the federal circuit courts of appeal[5] and final decisions of state courts that are claimed to conflict with federal law.[6] The Supreme Court denies between 85% and 90% of the more than 5,000 petitions for certiorari filed each year; of the cases the Court accepts, many are disposed of summarily without an opinion, so that it decides only about 200 cases per year with full opinions.[14,28]

Although the Supreme Court primarily functions as an appellate court, Section 2 of Article III of the Constitution gives the Supreme Court original jurisdiction over cases affecting ambassadors and other public ministers and cases in which a state is a party. While the parties in most of these situations have the option of proceeding in state courts, the Supreme Court has exclusive jurisdiction in controversies between two or more states.[4] The Court's original jurisdiction was severely curtailed by the Eleventh Amendment to the U.S. Constitution, which prohibits suit against a state in federal court without its consent. In its history the Court has decided fewer than 200 cases under its original jurisdiction, most of which involved suits between adjacent states arising from disputes over boundaries or water rights.[14] For fact-finding in these cases, the Court usually refers the dispute to a special master for a hearing and a factual report.[14]

Section 2 of Article II of the Constitution empowers the President to appoint federal judges, "with the Advice and Consent of the Senate," and it grants judges tenure during "good behavior," which is essentially a lifetime appointment. State practices for staffing their courts vary and include partisan election, nonpartisan election, gubernatorial appointment, legislative appointment, merit selection, and selection by sitting judges.[14] In the past 50 years, nearly half of the states have adopted the "Missouri Plan," under which judges are appointed by the governor from a list recommended by a nonpartisan nominating commission and thereafter must run in periodic retention elections.

JUDICIAL REVIEW

One fundamental aspect of the American legal system is the power of the judiciary to review the constitutional validity of actions of the legislature and the executive. The power of judicial review was not mentioned in the Constitution, but was established in Chief Justice John Marshall's 1803 opinion for the Supreme Court in *Marbury v. Madison.*[50] Marshall asserted that the power of judicial review was implicit in the structure of the Constitution, which declared the supremacy of the Constitution and mandated that courts apply the law to decide particular cases. As of 1992, the Supreme Court had invalidated all or part of 141 federal laws, including 71 enacted between 1864 and 1937 and 59 between 1953 and 1986.[14] In addition to constitutional review of legislation, the federal judiciary has the power to invalidate unconstitutional actions of the President or of federal executive or administrative agencies. For example, in *Youngstown Sheet & Tube Co. v. Sawyer,*[63] the Court ruled that President Truman acted beyond his constitutional authority in ordering the seizure of steel mills to avert a strike.

Early in the 19th century, the Supreme Court under John Marshall also established its power of judicial review to invalidate state legislation that was inconsistent with the Constitution of the United States,[30] including legislation inconsistent with the federal government's supreme authority over interstate commerce.[35] The Supreme Court also has the power to invalidate state legislation that is inconsistent with federal statutes or with duly ratified treaties that have the force of law. As of 1992, the Supreme Court had invalidated roughly 1,200 state statutes or constitutional provisions that were deemed inconsistent with federal law.[14]

Under Marshall, the Supreme Court also established the power to review decisions of state courts that were inconsistent with the Constitution of the United States.[22,51] In the exercise of this power, the Supreme Court has overturned the convictions of prisoners or reversed judgments in civil cases because of the unconstitutionality of the underlying criminal or civil law or because pretrial or trial procedures were constitutionally deficient. As is true of judicial review of state legislation, judicial review of state court decisions is not limited to constitutional questions but includes the power to reverse decisions that are inconsistent with federal legislation or treaties.

The power of judicial review of legislation is not the exclusive province of the Supreme Court of the United States. All of the lower federal courts and all state courts have the power to treat as invalid any federal or state legislation that is inconsistent with the Constitution or the laws and treaties of the United States.[14] In addition, the state courts exercise the power of judicial review with respect to their own state constitutions, so they can invalidate state legislation or executive action on state as well as federal constitutional grounds.

While judicial review is fundamental to the American legal system, it is also a source of controversy, both in theory and in application.[13,17,19,24-26,48,53,57] In terms of legal theory, controversy exists over how to interpret the words of a constitution or statute. Does one mechanically apply the words according to their current meaning, or according to the meaning at the time they were written, or with reference to the underlying concepts or values of the authors, or with reference to current concepts or values that have emerged historically through legal and political evolution of the framers' general conceptions?[24,25,48,49,57] In terms of political theory, some question whether judicial review by an appointed judiciary is undemocratic.[17,19,26] At a practical level, judicial review creates a public conflict between different branches or levels of government, frequently in cases with substantial political or economic significance, thereby highlighting the tensions inherent in the American legal system.

SOURCES OF LAW

The law governing the rights of American citizens emanates from various levels of government—federal, state, and local—and from various sources within each level. Federal law is established by the U.S. Constitution, by treaty (not discussed here), by federal legislation, and by agency regulation, all of which are subject to definitive interpretation by the federal judiciary. Similarly, state law arises from state constitutions, legislation, agency regulations, and judicial interpretation thereof, but the common law continues to furnish much of the substance of state law. Agreements among the states, known as interstate compacts, provide yet another source of domestic law.

A hierarchy exists among the various sources of law, which the courts enforce through judicial review. The Constitution of the United States is "the supreme Law of the Land," to which all other laws are subordinate. The

statutes and treaties of the United States have equal status and are subordinate only to the federal Constitution. Federal executive orders and agency regulations are valid only if consistent with the Constitution and federal statutes, but they are superior to all state law. Within each state, this hierarchy is repeated, with the state constitution at the top, followed by state statutes, and then by state administrative rules and regulations, but all subject to federal law. Finally, county and municipal governments can exercise only those powers delegated to them by the state. Local legislation, commonly called ordinances, and the rules and regulations of local administrative bodies apply only within the particular county or city.

Through the power of judicial review, the courts would seem to have ultimate legal authority. The system of checks and balances, however, precludes any branch of government from having the last word on a topic. Indeed, in one sense the judiciary comes at the bottom of the foregoing legal hierarchy, because any common law rule can be superseded by legislation. Thus, the legislature can, with the executive's concurrence, nullify any objectionable common law rule by enacting legislation on the topic. Similarly, the legislature can negate an objectionable judicial interpretation of a statute by amending the statute. Finally, an objectionable judicial interpretation of a constitution can be overridden through amendment of the constitution itself. On at least two occasions, for example, the U.S. Constitution has been amended in direct response to a controversial decision of the Supreme Court. The Eleventh Amendment (1798), which deprived the federal courts of jurisdiction in suits by citizens against the states, followed quickly after a judicial victory by a creditor against the State of Georgia in a federal court.[21] The Sixteenth Amendment (1913), which allowed the federal government to impose an income tax on individuals without apportionment among the states on a per capita basis, was enacted in response to the Supreme Court's invalidation of the first federal income tax in 1895.[56]

The discussion below summarizes key aspects of the principle sources of American law: constitutions, legislation, agency regulations, and the common law.

Constitutions

The Constitution of the United States establishes the tripartite structure of the federal government and the federal system of dual sovereignty. The first three articles of the Constitution establish the composition and enumerated duties of the legislative, executive, and judicial branches. Article IV addresses the role of the states within a federal system, including the requirement that they give "Full Faith and Credit" to the laws and judicial proceedings of other states, the mandate that citizens of each state "be entitled to all Privileges and Immunities of Citizens in the several States," a provision for the admission of new states, and a federal guarantee of a republican form of government and a protection against invasion. The final three articles of the constitution address details of the creation of the new government: the process of amendment (Article V), the assumption by the United States of the debts and obligations of the old government under the Articles of Confederation (Article VI), and ratification by the states (Article VII). Article VI also declares that the Constitution, laws and treaties of the United States "shall be the supreme Law of the Land."

In addition to establishing the structure of federal government and the extent of its powers relative to the states, the Constitution of the United States, especially through its various amendments, establishes the fundamental individual rights of American citizens. The first 10 amendments, known as the Bill of Rights, were ratified shortly after the Constitution itself. These amendments establish many of the freedoms that we now associate with American democracy:

- The First Amendment prohibits Congress from making any law to establish a religion or interfere with the free exercise of a religion, and it prohibits any abridgement of freedom of speech, freedom of the press, the right of peaceable assembly, and the right to petition the government for redress of grievances.

- The Fifth Amendment provides that "No person shall . . . be deprived of life, liberty, or property, without due process of law; nor shall private property be taken for public use without just compensation."

- The Seventh Amendment protects the right to trial by jury in suits at common law.

Several of the amendments in the Bill of Rights protect the rights of potential defendants in criminal cases:

- The Fourth Amendment protects citizens against unreasonable searches and seizures and requires that warrants for search or arrest be issued only upon "probable cause."

- The Fifth Amendment requires indictment by grand jury, forbids a second prosecution ("double jeopardy") for the same offense, protects against compulsory self-incrimination, and requires due process before any deprivation of life, liberty and property.

- The Sixth Amendment provides the right to a speedy and public trial by an impartial jury, the right to be informed of the nature of the charges, the right to confront opposing witnesses, the right to compulsory process for defense witnesses, and the right to assistance of counsel.

- The Eighth Amendment prohibits excessive bail, excessive fines, and the infliction of "cruel and unusual punishments."

In 1833, the Supreme Court declared that the Bill of Rights protected citizens only against actions of the federal government and did not give citizens any protection against state governments.[16] Consequently, at the conclusion of the Civil War, the Constitution offered no protection against the "Black Codes" enacted in former confederate states to deny newly freed black Americans such fundamental freedoms as the rights to move, vote, own land, make contracts, bring suit, or testify in court. Congress reacted by passing the Thirteenth, Fourteenth and Fifteenth Amendments to the Constitution (the "Civil War Amendments") and the Civil Rights Act of 1866.[11]

- The Thirteenth Amendment (1865) abolishes the institution of slavery within the United States, making permanent and binding upon the states Abraham Lincoln's Emancipation Proclamation of 1863, which was a wartime measure that applied only to slaves in Confederate territory.

- The Civil Rights Act of 1866 provides that

"All persons born in the United States . . . are hereby declared to be citizens of the United States; and such citizens, of every race and color . . . shall have the right . . . to full and equal benefit of all laws and proceedings for the security of person and property, as is enjoyed by white citizens, and shall be subject to like punishment, pains, and penalties, and to none other."[11]

- The Fourteenth Amendment (enacted in 1866, ratified in 1868) constitutionalizes the Civil Rights Act of 1866, defining citizenship and prohibiting states from depriving American citizens of due process of law or equal protection of the laws: "All persons born or naturalized in the United States . . . are citizens of the United States and of the State wherein they reside. No State shall make or enforce any law which shall abridge the privileges or immunities of citizens of the United States; nor shall any State deprive any person of life, liberty, or property, without due process of law; nor deny any person within its jurisdiction the equal protection of the laws."

- The Fifteenth Amendment (1870) declares that "The right of citizens of the United States to vote shall not be denied or abridged by the United States or by any State on account of race, color, or previous condition of servitude."

Privileges and Immunities

The impact of the Fourteenth Amendment (and of the Civil Rights Act of 1866) was substantially limited by the Supreme Court's 1873 decision in the *Slaughter-House Cases*,[58] which interpreted the "Privileges and Immunities" clause of the Fourteenth Amendment as forbidding state abridgment only of rights conferred by federal law and as affording no protection with respect to rights arising under state law; the Bill of Rights continued to be viewed as a limitation on the federal government and not as a source of rights protected against state governments.[13,59]

Due Process

Eventually, the Supreme Court interpreted the "Due Process" clause of the Fourteenth Amendment as protecting citizens against state infringement of certain provisions of the Bill of Rights that are "fundamental to the American scheme of justice."[23] As a result, almost all of the protections of the Bill of Rights currently are applicable against state governments under the Due Process clause of the Fourteenth Amendment.[13,53,59]

Due Process has two aspects, procedural and substantive. Procedural Due Process is the right to fair procedures in judicial and quasi-judicial proceedings, both civil and criminal. Examples include the right to notice of the claims or charges one faces, the right to confront and cross-examine opposing witnesses, the right to compel attendance of witnesses on one's own behalf, and the right to counsel.

Substantive Due Process is a more nebulous concept.[59] In addition to the selective incorporation of many provisions of the Bill of Rights, the Supreme Court uses a Substantive Due Process analysis to accord constitutional protection to other preferred interests that are viewed as fundamental. Between 1897 and 1938, the Supreme Court used it to invalidate nearly 200 federal and state statutes regulating labor-management relations, employment conditions, minimum wages, and entry into business that were held to unreasonably interfere with the natural rights of property and contract because they supposedly did not promote the public interest but benefited some persons at the expense of others.[59] In the face of pressure for the enactment of New Deal legislation during the 1930s, the Supreme Court eventually retreated from its aggressive use of Substantive Due Process analysis to invalidate regulatory statutes. In recent years, Substantive Due Process analysis has protected fundamental personal rights not explicitly mentioned in the Constitution, such as the right to privacy and personal autonomy exemplified in the right to educate one's children by sending them to private school, the right to liberty of conscience in refusing to salute the flag, and the right to reproductive freedom through access to birth control and abortion.[59]

Equal Protection

The Equal Protection clause of the Fourteenth Amendment had little impact as long as the courts allowed state-enforced segregation under the doctrine of "separate but equal."[55] Since that doctrine was repudiated in *Brown v. Board of Education*,[20] the federal courts have taken a more active role in invalidating legislation and regulations that discriminated on the basis of race.

The Equal Protection clause does not require that all citizens be treated identically, but only that there be a "rational basis" for any legislative classifications. Thus, laws that impose special licensing requirements on physicians, hospitals, or pharmaceutical companies are permissible if there is a legitimate reason for singling them out. In most cases, the courts presume that the legislature had a rational basis for its classification, but this deference is not warranted when a law provides unequal treatment based on race or other "suspect classifications," such as color, national origin, religion, and age, which frequently are the objects of prejudice and discrimination. When a statute or regulation provides unequal treatment on the basis of a suspect classification, the courts apply "strict scrutiny" and demand a more exacting fit between the state's purpose and the challenged law, presuming the law to be invalid unless the state can demonstrate the unequal treatment is reasonably related to a legitimate purpose that could not reasonably be accomplished through other means.[59] Classifications according to sex are treated separately, receiving an intermediate level of scrutiny, apparently because of the view that some gender differences may justify unequal treatment; the Supreme Court sometimes upholds "a legal distinction between the sexes [which] is made to appear natural, inevitable or otherwise necessary because it is enmeshed in the legal and social legacy of female subordination to men."[59]

Enforcement of Constitutional Rights

The provisions of the U.S. Constitution are not self-executing. Congressional action often is necessary to vindicate federal constitutional rights, and several constitutional amendments expressly empower Congress "to enforce this article by appropriate legislation."

Ultimately, however, enforcement of constitutional rights requires the availability of a judicial forum in which those rights can be vindicated. In many cases these rights can be protected by a judicial declaration that the challenged governmental action is unconstitutional or an injunction forbidding its continuation, but in some cases citizens also have the right to recover money damages as compensation for violation of their constitutional rights by agents of the federal or state government.[12]

Legislation

Within the limits established by the federal and state constitutions, the federal and state legislative bodies have broad powers to enact legislation on a broad variety of topics. Some of this legislation represents a modernization of traditional common law rules, but much of it has extended the power of government to regulate economic and social behavior of individuals and business enterprises far beyond the traditional scope of the common law.

The codification movement of the mid-19th century viewed common law precedent as haphazard and incomplete and sought to replace the common law with comprehensive and unified statutory codes.[13,28] Although this movement was not entirely successful, it eventually resulted in the codification of several important areas of law. In most states, virtually the entire body of common law crimes has been replaced by a criminal code. Likewise, each state has replaced its archaic common law rules of pleading in criminal and civil cases with detailed codes of criminal and civil procedure. In an effort to harmonize the laws of various states to facilitate interstate commerce, the American Bar Association established the National Conference of Commissioners on Uniform State Laws to draft statutory codes for state adoption.[13,28] The Conference has drafted dozens of uniform acts, many of which have been adopted in whole or in part by large numbers of states. Most prominently, the Uniform Commercial Code, a version of which has been adopted in every state except Louisiana, has supplanted the common law rules governing contracts for the sale of goods, secured transactions, and negotiable instruments.

In addition to reforming common law rules, federal and state legislation has been enacted to regulate a variety of economic activities that previously were subject to only minimal restrictions at common law. For example, at common law the sale of new drugs and devices was limited only indirectly by the threat of liability for breach of contract, fraud, or negligence, whereas federal legislation now imposes detailed prerequisites and affirmative obligations. Federal and state regulation of the issuance and sale of stock in public corporations goes well beyond the requirements imposed by the common law rules about contracts and fraud. Comprehensive and detailed environmental regulations regarding air and water pollution and solid and hazardous wastes bear little resemblance to the restrictions previously imposed by the common law of nuisance.

As federal and state statutes are enacted, they are published sequentially. The permanent official publication of federal legislation is known as the U.S. Statutes at Large; each state maintains an equivalent official legislative record. With the proliferation of legislation, it became both more important and more difficult to locate the applicable laws on a particular topic. To facilitate accessibility, all federal and state legislation is now compiled into comprehensive codes, organized according to subject matter, and updated on a regular basis.[13] The compilation of federal statutes is the *United States Code.*

Although legislation has largely supplanted the common law in many fields, these statutes ultimately must be enforced in judicial proceedings. As a result, the judiciary is responsible for the interpretation of federal and state statutes, and in doing so the courts continue to employ the common law mode of analysis. Thus, previous interpretations of a statute serve as precedent under the doctrine of *stare decisis.* Moreover, employing the common law method, courts have developed a system of general principles to guide the process of statutory interpretation, often called "statutory construction." As is true of constitutional interpretation, these principles of statutory construction are not entirely consistent, and their application often is controversial.[13,28,49,53]

Regulations

As described earlier, many regulatory statutes delegate to executive and administrative agencies the responsibility to write detailed regula-tions to implement a general legislative directive. All federal regulations are compiled in the Code of Federal Regulations, and notice of proposed regulations are published in the *Federal Digest.* Each state has an equivalent compilation of agency regulations.

Enforcement of these regulations, like the enforcement of statutes, requires the participation of the judiciary.[28] Some agencies lack independent power to impose sanctions and must bring any enforcement actions to the courts. Other agencies have the authority to undertake enforcement through internal adjudicatory proceedings; these proceedings are subject to judicial review. Regardless of whether the courts are involved in direct enforcement actions or indirect judicial review of agency enforcement actions, the courts ultimately have the authority to interpret the applicable regulations and determine whether they were violated.

In addition to interpreting the language of the regulations, the courts must determine whether the regulations are consistent with the legislative mandate. Courts can invalidate regulations that are inconsistent with the legislative mandate, and they also can invalidate statutes that are so vague that they fail to provide adequate guidance to the agency.

The Common Law

After the states achieved independence, they generally "received" or adopted, by constitution or by statute, much of the substance of the common law of England as it existed in 1776 or some relevant date, such as the adoption of the state constitution.[28] Because of the scarcity of published legal materials in post-Revolutionary America, lawyers had little direct access to the case law and relied primarily on treatises, especially Blackstone's *Commentaries on the Laws of England,* which was published in an American edition in 1803.[28] In the early 19th century, states began creating their own reporter systems to publish the decisions of their appellate courts, so by the middle of the 19th century, a substantial body of published American judicial opinions had accumulated as precedent. In the late 19th century, the West Publishing Company established a comprehensive *National Reporter System,* consisting of seven regional volumes for state decisions and five sets of federal reporters, publishing virtually all appellate opinions and selected opinions from the trial courts in chronological order. Relevant cases can be found with the use of a comprehensive digest system, a citation index, and various legal encyclopedias, treatises, and other secondary sources. The case law as well as a great deal of secondary material is now available on-line through two computer databases, LEXIS and WESTLAW.[13,28]

Despite the incursion of codes and regulatory statutes, the common law remains an important source of individual rights and responsibilities. This is especially so at the state level, particularly in such areas as the law of property, contract, and torts (redress for personal injuries and damage to property from wrongful acts). Although important statutes regulate various aspects of the law of property, contract, and torts, the fundamental rules and principles still derive from the common law. Thus, many of the day-to-day interactions of American citizens—as owners and renters, employers and employees, manufacturers and distributors, retailers and consumers, careless drivers and their victims, and doctors and patients—still are governed primarily by common law rules.

Moreover, while much of the substance of the common law has been supplanted by federal and state codes or regulatory statutes, the common law mode of analysis remains important whenever courts are called upon to interpret and enforce those statutes and the implementing regulations. The common law method also is employed whenever the courts confront questions of constitutional interpretation in exercising the power of judicial review. Annotated versions of the federal and state codes are available to help locate relevant judicial opinions interpreting their constitutions and statutes.

THE ADVERSARY SYSTEM OF DISPUTE RESOLUTION

The Adversary System

A distinctive feature of the American legal system is its reliance on the adversary system to resolve disputes through civil and criminal litigation.[28,46] Under our adversary system of justice, the parties to a dispute are responsible for informing the fact finder (judge or jury) of their version of the facts. The parties, through their attorneys, decide what issues to raise, what witnesses to call, what questions to ask, and what other evidence to introduce. Although the trial judge has the right to ask questions of the parties' witnesses and to require the testimony of additional witnesses, the judge primarily functions as an impartial umpire, controlling the conduct of the pretrial and trial process in accordance with rules of procedure and rules governing the admissibility of evidence.[13,28]

The adversary system differs dramatically from the inquisitorial system employed by the civil law countries of continental Europe and Latin America.[13,47] Under the inquisitorial system, the court acts as an investigative body, much like an American legislative committee. The judges decide what issues to pursue, which witnesses to call, and what questions to ask. Attorneys play a secondary role in suggesting what issues and evidence to pursue and in arguing to persuade the court of their significance. A trial under the inquisitorial system is not a unitary event but a series of hearings as the court decides to seek additional evidence in its investigation.

Commentators have long debated the relative merits of the adversarial and inquisitorial methods of dispute resolution.[13,36,46,47,53] Critics of the adversary system point out that the proceedings are not geared to seeking the "truth" but rather a choice between two partisan presentations, and they emphasize the waste and duplication in pretrial and trial proceedings, the tendency of each party to slant its evidentiary presentation, and the likelihood that the prevailing party will be the one with greater legal resources. Proponents of the adversary system, on the other hand, note the traditional American distrust of centralized authority and the risk that a unitary judicial investigation may prematurely jump to conclusions, thereby overlooking important issues and evidence. The adversary system increases the likelihood that all relevant issues and evidence will be explored. The extensive pretrial proceedings, though expensive and time-consuming, serve to narrow the issues and expedite trials, frequently resulting in settlements that avoid trial entirely. Finally, an adversary trial has intrinsic value to the participants and to society by allowing each party to present its own version of the facts in a public forum.

Classification of American Law

The American system of law can be classified into various categories. Although these categories do not reflect a comprehensive plan of codification, the distinctions often are employed by lawyers and are helpful for purposes of orientation and analysis.[28] Among the relevant distinctions are public and private law, criminal and civil law, and substance and procedure.

Public and Private Law

Lawyers frequently make a distinction between public law and private law. Public law addresses the functioning of government and the relations between individuals and the government, while private law addresses the rights of individuals among themselves.[28] Examples of public law include constitutional law, administrative law, tax law, environmental law and criminal law. Private law, which is also known in most civil law countries as "civil law," includes the fundamental rules of property, contract and tort (redress for injury to persons or property from wrongful acts), family law, commercial law (sales, secured transactions, negotiable instruments), and business law (agency, partnerships, corporations). The boundaries between public and private law are not at all clear.[18,34,37,43,44] Many regulatory statutes affect the rights of private citizens among each other, such as environmental laws that give private citizens a right to bring suit against polluters. Conversely, many areas of private law (e.g., labor-management relations or the issuance and exchange of corporate securities) have so great an impact on the economy and are so heavily regulated that these topics frequently are listed as examples of public law.

Criminal and Civil Cases

All cases in American courts are classified either as criminal or civil. Criminal cases are those in which the government is seeking to punish socially intolerable conduct through money fines or incarceration. Civil cases are all other lawsuits, including both actions under private law (e.g., for tort or breach of contract) and actions under public law seeking enforcement of statutory or constitutional rights. Criminal and civil cases differ in many respects.

Criminal prosecutions are brought by the federal, state, or local government.[28] A convicted defendant may be punished by a fine or imprisonment. The criminal law recognizes two major classes of crimes: a "felony" is a serious offense, punishable by incarceration for more than one year; a "misdemeanor" is any less serious offense. Because the stakes are higher in criminal cases, criminal defendants have certain constitutional protections (e.g., a right to appointed counsel, the right against self-incrimination), and the standard of proof is higher: conviction in a criminal case requires proof "beyond a reasonable doubt," whereas in civil cases the "preponderance of the evidence" standard requires only that the jury believe a proposition is "more probably true than not true."

Civil cases may be initiated by private parties or by the government. Private parties may bring civil actions to enforce contract rights or to redress or prevent invasions of their personal or property rights. The government may bring civil actions to enforce its regulatory statutes. Plaintiffs in civil actions may seek a court order ("injunction") to prevent further violation of their rights or they may seek monetary compensation ("damages") for injuries previously suffered. The scope of compensatory damages may include reimbursement for actual economic loss ("special damages"), such as property damage, medical bills, and lost earnings or profits, and an award for intangible non-pecuniary losses ("general damages"), such as emotional distress, pain and suffering, grief, or loss of enjoyment of life. If the defendant's conduct was reckless or malicious, the defendant may be ordered to pay "punitive damages" which are not based on the harm to the plaintiff but are intended to punish the defendant and deter others from engaging in similar outrageous acts.

Substance and Procedure

Substantive law refers to legal rights and obligations, whereas procedural law determines how the courts will adjudicate legal disputes. The following chapters of this book discuss the substance of public and private law applicable to various topics of concern to physicians.

Procedural law applies more generally whenever the government or private parties seek to enforce their substantive rights in the courts. A federal or state court will always apply its own rules of procedure, even when the substantive rights of the parties are determined by the law of another jurisdiction. Each state has its own "choice of law rules" for determining when a lawsuit brought in its courts should be resolved according to the law of another state. Also, suits under federal law can be brought in a state court, in which case the court would apply federal substantive law and state procedural rules. Conversely, when a lawsuit is heard in federal court based on the diversity of citizenship of the parties, the federal court must apply the relevant substantive rules of state law,[27] but it would follow federal rules of procedure.

Rules of Procedure

The conduct of litigation in the trial courts is governed by rules of procedure and rules of evidence. Throughout the entire period of English common law development, procedural and substantive rules were inextricably linked through the highly technical and arcane rules of common law pleading. Each legal right could be enforced only through one or more particular "forms of action," and these could be invoked only through written pleadings containing precise verbal formulations. The codification movement in the 19th century led to the enactment of more general rules of pleading for criminal and civil actions. Although the rules differ in each jurisdiction, most states model their rules after the Federal Rules of Civil Procedure and the Federal Rules of Criminal Procedure.

Civil Procedure

A civil trial is commenced by the plaintiff, who files a complaint in court and serves it on the defendant.[13,28] The defendant must file an answer. The parties then engage in "discovery," during which they can obtain information about the opponent's claims or defenses by use of requests for production of documents, written questions or "interrogatories," "depositions" at which oral questions are directed to the parties or witnesses, requests for "admission" of undisputed facts, and physical or mental examinations of the parties. Pretrial motions may be filed to narrow the issues for trial or even dispose of the case entirely if, based on the undisputed facts, one of the parties is entitled to prevail as a matter of law. The vast majority of all civil litigation is resolved without a full trial, either through negotiated settlements or pretrial motions that result in judgment for one of the parties.

Criminal Procedure

Under the Fifth Amendment, all federal criminal cases must be initiated by a grand jury indictment. State criminal procedures vary.[13,28] While many state prosecutions start with a grand jury indictment, most are initiated by an arrest, either by a police officer who has witnessed a crime or upon a warrant issued by a magistrate based on 1) a "complaint" filed by a police officer or a civilian complainant (usually the victim), or 2) an "information" filed by the prosecutor. After arrest, the defendant is brought before a judge for "arraignment," at which time the defendant is informed of the charges, enters a plea, and posts bond for release pending further proceedings. A "preliminary hearing" may be held to determine whether there is "probable cause" (i.e., whether there is sufficient evidence of the defendant's guilt, if not rebutted or otherwise explained away, to obtain a conviction at trial).

Pretrial and trial procedure in criminal cases is governed to a large extent by constitutional protections afforded by the Bill of Rights. The most important of these are the Fourth Amendment protections against unreasonable searches and seizure, the Fifth Amendment rights to indictment by grand jury and due process of law and against self-incrimination or double jeopardy, and the Sixth Amendment rights to counsel, to a speedy trial, and to subpoena witnesses for testimony at trial.

Except for the right to cross-examine witnesses at a preliminary hearing, the defendant has only a limited right to "discovery" of the prosecution's evidence. The prosecution has an obligation to make available any exculpatory evidence and certain witness statements. The defendant has no obligation to reveal information to the prosecution except the identity of alibi witnesses. Most criminal prosecutions are resolved without a trial on the basis of a guilty plea by the defendant, usually obtained through "plea bargaining" negotiations in which the prosecutor agrees to accept a plea to a less serious crime or to recommend a less severe penalty.

Trial Procedure

Trial procedures in civil and criminal cases are essentially the same.[13,28] Unless the parties waive their right to trial by jury, a trial begins with selection of the jury. The attorneys then make opening statements, often in the form of a story, to summarize the evidence they will introduce at trial. The evidence consists of the testimony of witnesses and exhibits, such as weapons, clothing, specimens, documents, diagrams, or charts. The side with the burden of proof (the plaintiff or the prosecution) presents its "case-in-chief" by calling witnesses and asking them questions on "direct examination"; each witness may be interrogated by the defense attorney on "cross-examination." After the plaintiff or prosecution rests, the defense calls witnesses for direct examination who are then subject to cross-examination by the plaintiff or prosecution. The plaintiff or prosecution may call rebuttal witnesses to contradict any new evidence introduced by the defense. After all witness testimony is complete, the attorneys for both sides make closing arguments to explain why the jury should believe their version of the facts and decide the case in their favor. Either before or after the closing arguments, the jury receives instructions from the judge about the applicable law, including the burden of proof, and about how to apply the law to the facts.

The losing party can file a post-trial motion requesting that the trial judge enter "judgment notwithstanding the verdict" and overrule the decision of the jury if its verdict is not supported by substantial evidence. If unsuccessful with post-trial motions, the losing party can appeal the judgment.

Rules of Evidence

The rules governing the admissibility of evidence at trial are themselves a product of the common law system and have evolved over several centuries. In 1975, however, Congress adopted the Federal Rules of Evidence,[29] a comprehensive system of evidentiary rules for the federal courts that represented a substantial revision of the common law rules. Roughly 35 states have adopted modern evidence codes modeled in whole or in part on the Federal Rules of Evidence.[41] Accordingly, even though state evidence rules may vary, the Federal Rules will be cited here as representative of both federal and state practice.

Rules of evidence serve several related purposes, all of which seek to assist the jury in evaluating the evidence. One is to avoid introduction of irrelevant material that wastes time and risks confusing the jury. Another is to exclude unreliable evidence to which a jury might give too much credence, such as hearsay testimony about an out-of-court statement by another person, which cannot be tested under cross examination to determine its accuracy. A third purpose is to exclude emotionally-charged evidence that might prejudice a jury's consideration of the evidence as a whole.

The Federal Rules of Evidence distinguish between two types of witnesses: occurrence witnesses and expert witnesses.

Occurrence Witnesses

The rules of evidence generally limit the witnesses to an event to testifying about their own firsthand observations based on "personal knowledge" (Rule 601). Occurrence witnesses ordinarily are not permitted to testify about "hearsay" (facts which they learned from others) (Rule 802), although numerous exceptions exist that allow introduction of hearsay testimony if certain requirements are met to assure its reliability (Rules 803 and 804). Nor may occurrence witnesses go beyond their observations to testify about their inferences, opinions, or conclusions. The boundary between observation and opinion is never entirely clear, however, and occurrence witnesses are permitted to testify to opinions that are "rationally based on perception" (Rule 701), such as the sobriety of a pedestrian or the speed of a vehicle.

Expert Witnesses

The law recognizes a special category of witness, the "expert witness," to whom special rules apply (Rules 701-706). An expert witness is anyone qualified "by knowledge, skill, experience, training, or education" whose "scientific, technical, or other specialized knowledge will assist the trier of fact to understand the evidence or to determine a fact in issue" (Rule 702). Unlike ordinary witnesses, an expert witness can testify in the form of an opinion (Rule 702). Also, unlike lay witnesses, an expert's testimony may be based on hearsay so long as it is "of a type reasonably relied upon by experts in the particular field" (Rule 702), such as notations in a patient's chart by members of the medical staff.

The law frequently requires that proof of certain essential facts be established by expert testimony. For example, a jury ordinarily will not be permitted to find for the plaintiff in a claim for professional malpractice unless a member of the profession testifies that the defendant's conduct failed to measure up to the profession's standard of care. In personal injury cases, expert testimony often is needed to establish that the accident or event was a substantial contributing cause of the plaintiff's injuries or that the plaintiff's injuries are permanent.

The Physician as Witness

When physicians testify, they frequently serve as both occurrence witnesses and expert witnesses. A physician who was a treating or consulting physician may testify as an ordinary occurrence witness with respect to any direct observations. The physician is an expert witness, however, whenever the testimony consists of opinions about the diagnosis of a condition, its cause, its prognosis, etc. A physician who has no direct involvement in a case may be retained to testify as an expert witness for either side. The testimony of a retained expert may be based on a review of the patient's medical records or an examination of the patient or both. Although expert witnesses ordinarily are retained by the parties, the judge has the power to appoint an impartial expert who agrees to serve for reasonable compensation (Rule 706).

Situations in which physicians are likely to become involved as occurrence or expert witnesses are discussed in Chapter 2. Physicians' participation as occurrence and expert witnesses in pretrial and trial proceedings receive more detailed treatment in Chapters 3 and 4.

REFERENCES

1. 5 USC §§551 et seq
2. 28 USC §41
3. 28 USC §81-133
4. 28 USC §1251
5. 28 USC §1254
6. 28 USC §1257
7. 28 USC §1291
8. 28 USC §1295
9. 28 USC §1331
10. 28 USC §1332
11. 42 USC §1981
12. 42 USC §1983
13. Abadinsky H: **Law and Justice: An Introduction to the American Legal System.** 3rd ed. Chicago, Ill: Nelson-Hall, 1995, 446 pp
14. Abraham HJ: **The Judicial Process: An Introductory Analysis of the Courts of the United States, England, and France.** 6th ed. New York, NY: Oxford University Press, 1993, 415 pp
15. *Baker v Carr*, 369 US 186 (1962)
16. *Barron v Baltimore*, 32 US (7 Pet) 243 (1833)
17. Bickel A: **The Least Dangerous Branch.** Indianapolis, Ind: Bobbs-Merrill, 1962, 303 pp
18. Brest P: State action and liberal theory: a casenote on *Flagg Brothers v. Brooks.* **U Pa Law Rev 130:** 1296-1330, 1982
19. Brest P: Who decides? **S Calif Law Rev 58:**661-681, 1985
20. *Brown v Board of Education*, 347 US 483 (1954)
21. *Chisholm v Georgia*, 2 US (2 Dall) 419 (1793)
22. *Cohens v Virginia*, 19 US (6 Wheat) 264 (1821)
23. *Duncan v Louisiana*, 391 US 145 (1968)
24. Dworkin R: **Taking Rights Seriously.** Cambridge, Mass: Harvard University Press, 1977, 293 pp
25. Dworkin RM: **Law's Empire.** Cambridge, Mass: Belknap Press, 1986, 470 pp
26. Ely JH: **Democracy and Distrust: A Theory of Judicial Review.** Cambridge, Mass: Harvard University Press, 1980, 268 pp
27. *Erie RR v Tompkins*, 304 US 64 (1938)
28. Farnsworth EA: **An Introduction to the Legal System of the United States.** 2nd ed. New York, NY: Oceana Publications, 1983, 172 pp
29. Federal Rules of Evidence, 28 USC
30. *Fletcher v Peck*, 10 US (6 Cranch) 87 (1810)
31. Frank J: Are judges human? **U Pa Law Rev 80:**17-53, 1931
32. Frank J: **Law and the Modern Mind.** New York, NY: Brentano's, 1930, 362 pp
33. Friedman LM: **A History of American Law.** 2nd ed. New York, NY: Simon & Schuster, 1985, 781 pp

34. Gavison R: Feminism and the public/private distinction. **Stanford Law Rev 45:**1-45, 1982
35. *Gibbons v Ogden*, 22 US (9 Wheat) 1 (1824)
36. Gross SR: The American advantage: the value of inefficient litigation. **Mich Law Rev 85:**734-757, 1987
37. Horwitz MJ: The history of the public/private distinction. **U Pa Law Rev 130:**1423-1428, 1982
38. Horwitz MJ: **The Transformation of American Law, 1780-1860.** Cambridge, Mass: Harvard University Press, 1977, 356 pp
39. Horwitz MJ: **The Transformation of American Law, 1870-1980: The Crisis of Legal Orthodoxy.** New York, NY: Oxford University Press, 1992, 361 pp
40. Hurst JW: **The Growth of American Law: The Law Makers.** Boston, Mass: Little, Brown, & Co, 1950, 502 pp
41. Joseph GP, Saltzburg SA: **Evidence in America: The Federal Rules in the States.** Charlottesville, Va: The Michie Company, 1987, 4 vols
42. Kelman M: **A Guide to Critical Legal Studies.** Cambridge, Mass: Harvard University Press, 1987, 360 pp
43. Kennedy D: The stages of the decline of the public/private distinction. **U Pa Law Rev 130:**1349-1357, 1982
44. Klare K: The public/private distinction in labor law. **U Pa Law Rev 130:**1358-1422, 1982
45. *Klaxon v Stentor Electric Mfg Co*, 313 US 487 (1941)
46. Landsman S: **The Adversary System: A Description and Defense.** Washington, DC: American Enterprise Institute, 1984, 55 pp
47. Langbein JH: The German advantage in civil procedure. **U Chic Law Rev 52:**823-866, 1985
48. Levinson S: Law as literature. **Texas Law Rev 60:** 373-403, 1982
49. Llewellyn K: Remarks on the theory of appellate decision and the rules or canons about how statutes are to be construed. **Vand Law Rev 3:**395-406, 1950
50. *Marbury v Madison*, 5 US (1 Cranch) 137 (1803)
51. *Martin v Hunter's Lessee*, 14 US (1 Wheat) 304 (1816)
52. *McCulloch v Maryland*, 17 US (4 Wheat) 316 (1819)
53. Mermin S: **Law and the Legal System: An Introduction.** 2nd ed. Boston, Mass: Little, Brown, & Co, 1982, 462 pp
54. Peller G: The metaphysics of American law. **Calif Law Rev 73:**1151-1290, 1985
55. *Plessy v Ferguson*, 163 US 537 (1896)
56. *Pollock v Farmer's Loan and Trust Co*, 157 US 429 (1895)
57. Simon LG: The authority of the framers of the Constitution: can originalist interpretation be justified? **Calif Law Rev 73:**1482-1539, 1985
58. *Slaughter-House Cases*, 83 US (16 Wall) 36 (1873)
59. Tribe LH: **American Constitutional Law.** 2nd ed. Mineola, NY: The Foundation Press, 1988, 1778 pp
60. Tushnet M: Following the rules laid down: a critique of interpretivism and neutral principles. **Harvard Law Rev 96:**781-827, 1983
61. *United States v Lopez*, 115 SCt 1624 (1995)
62. *United States v Lopez*, 115 SCt 1624, 1634, 1638 (1995) (Kennedy J, concurring)
63. *Youngstown Sheet & Tube Co v Sawyer*, 343 US 579 (1952)

CHAPTER 2

THE PHYSICIAN AND THE LEGAL SYSTEM

JEFF L. LEWIN, JD

This chapter provides an overview of "medicolegal relations,"[16] the complex relationship between medicine and law, or more concretely, between physicians and the legal system. Physicians regularly confront medicolegal issues in the course of evaluating and treating their patients. It is important that physicians recognize these issues and know how to respond to them appropriately.

The interaction between physicians and the legal system is bi-directional, involving both physician input to the legal system and the impact of the legal system on medical practice. The long-established field of forensic medicine addresses medical input to the legal system with respect to the investigation, preservation, preparation, and presentation of evidence and medical opinion in courts and other legal settings.[16] The newer fields of medical law, health law, and public health law encompass legal regulation of medicine, other health fields, and public health programs, respectively,[16] which have come to dominate the practice of medicine. The growing body of medicolegal literature includes a comprehensive text by the American College of Legal Medicine on "legal medicine," the academic study of medicolegal relations;[3] a loose-leaf treatise providing legal guidance to physicians;[47]

and a two-volume legal treatise on health law.[20]

This chapter focuses on fundamental medicolegal issues that directly affect relations between physicians and their patients in the daily practice of their profession. (Medicolegal issues that pertain to physician input to the legal system are addressed in Chapters 3 and 4, and in other chapters.)

This chapter identifies and summarizes the fundamental medicolegal issues in a physician's practice, many of which are explored more comprehensively in other chapters. The first section of this chapter surveys the legal rules pertaining to the physician's relationship with individual patients. It provides an overview of topics that are addressed at length in other chapters, especially those in Part II (Patients and the Law). The second section identifies situations in a physician's practice that raise medicolegal issues and are likely to involve the physician with the legal system. It surveys the types of disputes in which physicians are likely to be called upon to provide testimony as occurrence or expert witnesses in legal proceedings. The next section explores the extent of the physician's ethical and legal duty to participate and cooperate in legal proceedings involving their patients. The final three sections explore the legal obligations of physicians with respect to information obtained from their patients, including: 1) whether physicians have an ethical or legal duty to preserve and record evidence beyond that necessary for medical treatment of their patients; 2) the physician's duty of disclosure under statutory and non-statutory reporting requirements; and 3) the limits of confidentiality and of the physician-patient privilege in legal proceedings.

LEGAL DUTIES OF PHYSICIANS TO THEIR PATIENTS

Physicians' duties to their patients involve both ethical and legal obligations. Physicians presumably are familiar with their ethical obligations, so these are not explored systematically here. Most of these ethical obligations are reflected in corresponding legal obligations, however. Legal obligations exist insofar as courts will enforce these duties against physicians by issuing injunctions to compel performance or by awarding damages for nonperformance.

The Physician-Patient Relationship

The initial medicolegal issue concerning obligations to patients concerns the creation of the physician-patient relationship[26] (see Chapter 5). The physician-patient relationship is consensual, and physicians are not compelled to accept or treat strangers. Nevertheless, various state licensure statutes circumscribe a physician's right to refuse patients based on such criteria as Medicare or Medicaid coverage or HIV infection, while federal civil rights laws forbid discrimination on the basis of race, gender, religion, national origin, or disability.[26]

The physician-patient relationship arises in most cases from mutual agreement, but physicians may be held to have accepted these duties in the absence of an express agreement with the patient. Whether a physician-patient relationship legally exists is a factual determination. Courts will imply the existence of a relationship, and thus subject the physician to potential malpractice liability, if the physician undertook to render treatment or the circumstances caused the patient to have a reasonable expectation of treatment.[26] Questions regarding the existence and scope of the relationship may arise in a variety of other special situations: gratuitous advice in a nonmedical setting; "second-opinion" referrals; examinations by physicians at the request of employers, insurers, or adverse parties to litigation; services by pathologists or radiologists whose sole contact is with a treating physician; treatment by substitute and covering physicians, house staff, emergency room physicians, or clinical faculty; and telephone contacts.[26] (For further discussion of the creation of the physician-patient relationship and the legal and ethical issues this entails, see Chapter 5. Special issues concerning the existence and scope of the physician-patient relationship in the treatment of incompetent patients, pregnant women, and vulnerable populations are explored in various chapters, including Chapters 6, 8, and 11.)

Consent to Treatment

Once the physician-patient relationship has been established, questions frequently arise about consent to particular treatment. The law recognizes a patient's rights to autonomy, privacy, and bodily integrity, and it enforces the ethical requirement that treatment only be rendered with the consent of the patient. Physicians who render treatment without the patient's informed consent may be subject to criminal prosecution for battery and are liable for damages in civil suits under various legal theories, including assault, battery, negligence, malpractice, or the tort of lack of informed consent.[8] The necessity of patient consent to treatment is reflected in the corresponding right of competent adult patients to refuse medical treatment. (The topic of informed consent receives extensive treatment in Chapters 5 and 6. The topic is discussed in many other chapters, including Chapters 7 and 27.)

Exercise of Reasonable Skill and Care

The law imposes a duty on the physician, consistent with medical ethics, to possess and exercise that degree of skill and knowledge that would be expected of a reasonable physician under similar circumstances.[25] A physician who fails to fulfill this duty is considered to be negligent and is subject to liability in damages for medical malpractice. (The physician's duty of care is discussed in Chapter 27.) An issue warranting special attention is the risk of improper assessment or inadequate follow-up associated with the dramatic increase in reliance on the telephone for all phases of medical care, with telephone contacts accounting for between 11% and 50% of all medical encounters.[53]

Medical Records and Confidentiality

Complete and accurate medical records are essential to appropriate treatment of patients over time and by multiple doctors, and records also play a key evidentiary role whenever medical testimony is relevant to a legal dispute.[24] There are two types of medical records: 1) hospital medical records, and 2) physicians' private office records. Standards governing contents of hospital medical records are established by the Joint Commission on Accreditation of Hospitals, and they are legally imposed by various state hospital licensing and accreditation regulations as well as by federal regulations applicable to participants in Medicare reimbursement. Physicians' private office records are subject to fewer statutory or regulatory rules, but standards have been established by professional organizations and are enforced by the courts.[24] Failure to maintain complete, timely, and accurate records can constitute medical malpractice.[20] In addition, failure to maintain the confidentiality of medical records may subject a physician or hospital to liability for malpractice or invasion of privacy.[23] (The general principle of confidentiality as to all patient disclosures receives comprehensive treatment in Chapter 5. The rules governing the maintenance of medical records and the protection of their confidentiality are covered in Chapter 22. The duty to maintain confidentiality during litigation is discussed below.)

CASES WITH MEDICOLEGAL IMPLICATIONS

Physicians frequently are called upon to serve as witnesses in legal proceedings involving their patients, which may involve criminal prosecutions, civil suits, or various federal and state administrative adjudications of claims for government benefits. It is important to understand the two distinct capacities in which a physician can testify, as an occurrence witness or as an expert witness. Special rules govern the participation of physicians as occurrence and expert witnesses in pretrial and trial proceedings (see Chapters 3 and 4).

When physicians testify, they frequently serve as both occurrence witnesses and expert witnesses. A physician who was a treating or consulting physician may testify as an ordinary occurrence witness with respect to any direct observations. The physician is also considered an expert witness, however, whenever the testimony consists of opinions about the diagnosis of a condition, its cause, or its prognosis. Thus, whenever a physician is called to testify in a case involving a patient, the physician will be giving testimony as both an occurrence witness and an expert witness. A physician who has no direct involvement with a patient's care also can be retained to testify as an expert witness. The testimony of a retained expert may be based on a review of the patient's medical records or an examination of the patient or both.

Physicians can become witnesses in five general categories of cases: 1) criminal cases; 2) civil personal injury litigation; 3) other civil litigation involving patients; 4) administrative adjudication of patient claims for government benefits; and 5) civil litigation involving business aspects of practice.

Criminal Cases

Physicians, especially emergency department physicians, frequently become witnesses in criminal prosecutions of the persons responsible for patient injuries. Many of these cases are also the subject of mandatory reporting requirements (see below). Criminal prosecutions are especially likely in reportable cases involving deaths or traumatic injuries from gunshots, stabbings or other violent acts, and cases involving abuse of vulnerable populations (i.e., children, the elderly, or spouses). In most of these cases, the physician's patient is the victim, and the physician is called by the prosecution to describe the wounds and give opinion testimony on such matters as the etiology of the injury, the amount of force used, and whether the injury could have been accidental or self-inflicted (see Chapters 11 and 12).

Criminal cases sometimes require physician testimony on the issues of whether the defendant was insane at the time of the crime or whether the defendant is currently competent to stand trial. Indigent defendants whose sanity or competence is called into question have the right to request that the court retain the services of a psychiatrist to evaluate, report on, and testify about the defendant's mental and emotional status (see Chapter 7). Physicians other than psychiatrists, such as neurologists or neurosurgeons, may be called upon for evaluation and testimony if there is evidence that the defendant's mental or emotional impairment is the result of organic disease.

Civil Personal Injury Litigation

Physicians frequently are asked by their patients to serve as witnesses in civil cases in which patients seek to recover money damages from the persons alleged to have injured them. In theory, every reportable injury to a patient could result in a civil lawsuit as well as a criminal prosecution, but in reality most victims of crime do not pursue a civil remedy because criminal defendants generally lack the resources to pay a substantial judgment. Patients are more likely to sue for injuries that are the result of accidents, rather than intentional criminal misconduct, for the defendants are more likely to have substantial resources and/or liability insurance coverage. The three situations in which patients (or their families) are most likely to bring suit for their injuries are those arising from automobile accidents, allegedly defective products, and unsatisfactory medical treatment (i.e., malpractice claims) (see Chapters 10 and 27).

Claims for personal injury account for more than half of all civil jury trials in the United States. Roughly 98% of all personal injury lawsuits are settled prior to trial, and a large percentage of all potential claims are resolved by private negotiation without a lawsuit being filed. Physicians play an important role in the resolution of all such claims, providing information that enables the parties to evaluate the likelihood the plaintiff would prevail and the cause and extent of the plaintiff's injuries. In order for parties to resolve a claim without a lawsuit, they usually call upon the physician to produce the patient's medical records and prepare a report. In lawsuits that are dismissed prior to trial, treating physicians frequently are involved in pretrial proceedings, especially preparation of reports and participation in depositions (see Chapter 3). Defendants in personal injury cases routinely retain the services of one or more physicians to examine the plaintiff and prepare a report evaluating the plaintiff's injuries. The plaintiff may also retain one or more physicians to examine and evaluate the plaintiff's injuries to supplement the testimony of the treating physician.

Malpractice claims differ from other civil litigation in that physicians are parties to the litigation as well as witnesses. In addition to the malpractice defendant, other physicians who witnessed relevant events are potential occurrence witnesses. In order to determine whether the defendant complied with the applicable standard of care, both the plaintiff and defendant can be expected to retain one or more nontreating physicians as expert witnesses. Indeed, in most cases the plaintiff is legally required to present expert testimony from a physician on the issue of malpractice (see Chapter 27).

Other Civil Litigation Involving Patients

Physicians may be called to testify in other civil cases involving their patients that do not involve claims for personal injury. Many of these cases are discussed in greater detail in other chapters of this book. For example, suits may be brought seeking judicial guidance with respect to treatment of minors or incompetent patients (Chapter 5) or with respect to termination of life support in terminally ill or incompetent patients (Chapter 6). For patients suffering from mental or emotional impairment (Chapter 7), lawsuits may be brought to appoint guardians for incompetents or to civilly commit patients who present a danger to themselves and others, and ordinary lawsuits may raise issues as to the competency of a person to perform a particular function, such as capacity to contract, capacity to make a will, or competency to testify in court.

Administrative Benefit Claims

Physicians frequently become involved in proceedings in which their patients seek to obtain federal Social Security disability benefits or state workers' compensation benefits. (These topics receive extensive treatment in Chapters 25 and 26; to the extent that a disability involves mental or emotional incompetence, relevant discussion also may be found in Chapter 7). Many of these claims are handled in administrative proceedings, and they frequently are resolved on the basis of written reports without depositions or live testimony. On the other hand, claims that are not resolved on the basis of the written record can culminate in formal hearings before an administrative tribunal or a regular trial court in which the proceedings resemble those in ordinary civil litigation.

Civil Litigation Involving Business Aspects of Practice

Physicians may become involved in civil litigation arising out of disputes over the denial or revocation of medical licenses. Since the 19th century, physicians have been licensed by the state. The right to practice one's profession is a property right, protected against federal and state infringement by the Fifth and Fourteenth Amendments to the United States Constitution. Hence, the procedures applicable to the grant and revocation of medical licenses are subject to constitutional due process requirements. (The legal issues in suits regarding denial or revocation of medical licenses are discussed in Chapter 20.)

As physicians have become more dependent on hospital affiliation for their practices, a new body of law has developed concerning the grant, denial, and revocation of hospital staff privileges. Physicians have challenged denial of staff privileges on a variety of legal grounds, including suits against hospitals and members of peer review committees under the anti-trust laws. Special rules and requirements have been enacted with respect to reporting impaired physicians to licensing board and hospital peer review committees. Most significantly, the Health Care Quality Improvement Act of 1986 established a National Practitioner Data Bank for the exchange of information concerning state disciplinary actions, actions affecting institutional staff privileges, and malpractice actions; persons or organizations participating in peer review activities who comply with statutory requirements obtain immunity from certain types of legal liability. (All of these important topics receive comprehensive coverage in Chapters 20 and 21.)

The practice of physicians is also substantially affected by the rising cost of medical care, the dominance of private health insurance, and more recently by the emergence of managed care organizations. Disputes often arise between physicians and private or governmental institutions involved in health care finance (e.g., private medical insurers, Medicare, or Medicaid) or managed health care (e.g., health maintenance organizations or preferred provider organizations). (Issues pertaining to health care finance and disputes with private or governmental institutions involved in health care finance are discussed in Chapters 23 and 24.)

Physicians may also become involved in civil litigation involving other business aspects of their medical practice, including disputes arising from the break-up of a group practice or ordinary contractual disputes with patients, employees, vendors, landlords, or others. These topics generally are beyond the scope of this book; more extensive discussions can be found in other texts and treatises.[3,20,47]

THE DUTY TO COOPERATE OR PARTICIPATE IN LEGAL PROCEEDINGS

Participation as a witness in legal proceedings can be time-consuming and is sometimes unpleasant. Nevertheless, physicians have both an ethical and a legal obligation to participate in legal proceedings when they have direct first-hand knowledge of relevant facts.

The physician's ethical duty to participate in legal proceedings is reflected in the American

Medical Association (AMA) statement that physicians have an ethical obligation to assist in the administration of justice: "As a citizen and as a professional with special training and experience, the physician has an ethical obligation to assist in the administration of justice."[4(No.9.07)] The AMA recognizes a further duty to participate when patients request help in protecting their rights: "If a patient who has a legal claim requests the physician's assistance, the physician should furnish medical evidence, with the patient's consent, in order to secure the patient's legal rights."[4(No.9.07)] Some courts describe the physician's obligation to assist a patient in litigation as the "doctor's duty of total care."[21,22]

The legal obligation to appear as a witness in judicial proceedings is an important aspect of the due process rights of parties to criminal and civil litigation to compel the attendance of witnesses. In criminal cases, the Seventh Amendment to the U.S. Constitution gives every criminal defendant the right to compel the attendance of witnesses, and this power is available to prosecutors in criminal cases, to all parties in civil cases, and to parties in many administrative adjudicatory proceedings. Parties can compel the attendance of witnesses by serving them with a subpoena, an order issued by the court to attend proceedings (either a trial or a deposition) at a stated time and place. Disobedience of a subpoena is contempt of court, which can be punished by a fine or imprisonment. In addition, a court has the power to enforce its subpoena by arresting the witness to assure that he or she will appear at the next appointed time.

Moreover, a physician can be held civilly liable for damages suffered by a patient as a result of the physician's failure to cooperate in legal proceedings.[5] In one case, a treating physician failed to appear at a trial, and without his crucial testimony the patient's attorney had to settle the lawsuit on unfavorable terms; the physician was held liable for the plaintiff's losses.[45] In another case, a patient settled a lawsuit on unfavorable terms after a treating physician threatened not to appear as a witness or cooperate in pretrial proceedings; the physician escaped liability for the patient's losses because the patient's attorney could have used a subpoena to compel the physician's attendance at a pretrial deposition or at trial.[21] Although the appeals court upheld the decision in favor of the defendant physician in that case, it emphasized that the physician had an ethical as well as a legal duty to cooperate in the proceedings, quoting with approval the following statement by a judge in another case:

> [M]embers of a profession, especially the medical profession, stand in a confidential or fiduciary capacity as to their patients. They owe their patients more than just medical care for which payment is exacted; there is a duty of total care; that includes and comprehends a duty to aid the patient in litigation, to render reports when necessary and to attend court when needed.[21]

Conceivably, the court could have decided the case in the plaintiff's favor based on the dilemma necessarily posed for the plaintiff by the physician's threat of noncooperation in light of the obvious difficulty of obtaining convincing testimony from a treating physician who was attending under compulsion. Even though the ruling in this case favored the physician, a physician in another state or in a slightly different factual context might well be required to compensate a patient who felt compelled to settle a lawsuit on unfavorable terms because of the physician's threat of noncooperation.

IS THERE A DUTY TO PRESERVE AND RECORD EVIDENCE?

Physicians are likely to have an opportunity to observe and record a great deal of evidence that will be important in subsequent criminal and civil proceedings but is not necessarily relevant to medical treatment. This evidence can be grouped into three categories: physical characteristics of wounds and adjacent clothing; patients' personal effects; and statements by patients and their associates.

Beyond recording the medically relevant information, there is some question about the extent to which a physician has an affirmative duty to preserve and record potential evidence. Preservation of such evidence may be of no direct medical benefit to the patient, but it may promote the patient's welfare whenever the patient is the victim of a crime or wrongful act and would desire retribution or compensation from the wrongdoer. On the other hand, if the patient is suspected of wrongdoing, the patient might prefer that such evidence be ignored or destroyed.

Apart from the interests of the patient, society's interest in the preservation of such evidence may impose ethical or legal duties on the physician. The intentional destruction of evidence is obstruction of justice, a serious crime. In treating a patient, however, the physician necessarily must destroy much of the physical evidence: clothing is cut away from the wound; the superficial skin is altered or excised in the process of operating on a wound; and foreign objects are removed. None of the necessary medical procedures of a physician would constitute criminal acts.

The question is whether the physician has any ethical or legal duty to make special efforts to preserve such evidence in the course of these procedures, such as by physically retaining certain items, taking photographs, or making written notes or diagrams that could later serve to refresh the physician's memory when called as a witness. (For a discussion of what evidence to preserve or record and an explanation of how to do so, see especially Chapters 11 and 12.)

With regard to medical ethics, an affirmative answer is suggested by an opinion of the AMA Council on Ethical and Judicial Affairs, which declares that "the physician has an ethical obligation to assist in the administration of justice."[4(No.9.07)] To assist in the administration of justice, a physician should make reasonable efforts to preserve and record potential evidence that would assist in identifying the perpetrators of criminal conduct. Likewise, the physician's duty to advance the interests of the patient suggests an ethical obligation to preserve any evidence that would assist the patient in obtaining redress through criminal prosecution or a civil suit for damages. Thus, the physician's ethical duty to assist in the administration of justice and protect patient interests may be interpreted as imposing an ethical obligation to preserve evidence of wound characteristics that might assist in a criminal prosecution, exonerate the patient in a criminal investigation, or help the patient to obtain recovery in a civil lawsuit. Likewise, physicians may have an ethical duty to preserve significant patient statements by writing them down so that the document would be available to refresh the memory of witnesses in subsequent criminal, civil, or administrative proceedings.

Physicians and hospital staff also have a legal duty to preserve certain forms of evidence, and they may be subject to a civil suit by patients who suffer losses because of its destruction. Corresponding to criminal liability for obstruction of justice is the potential civil liability to patients for the tort known as "spoliation of evidence." In some states, a person can recover money damages for spoliation of evidence if the person suffered a loss in a criminal or civil proceeding because the defendant intentionally or negligently lost or destroyed important evidence.[12,18,20,38,39]

Most states do not yet recognize such a tort, however, and those that do so generally impose liability only on persons who are legally or contractually bound to retain such evidence. In *Smith v. Superior Court,*[43] for example, the court held that the defendant's car dealership could be held liable because it had expressly agreed to retain certain automotive parts so that experts could determine the cause of a wheel assembly failure, evidence that was essential to the plaintiff's civil action. The tort of spoliation of evidence may be used to enforce an existing contractual or legal duty to preserve evidence, but it does not itself give rise to any independent duty to preserve or record relevant information. Courts in other cases have refused to allow plaintiffs to pursue a claim for spoliation of evidence when the defendant had no duty to preserve it.

As applied to the physician-patient relationship, the physician can be held liable for spoliation of evidence only insofar as there is a duty to preserve the particular evidence. Such a duty would exist with respect to any of the patient's personal effects, which would be held by the physician's associates as a "bailment," a contractual relationship under which they would have the duty to take reasonable care for the property's safekeeping. Thus, physicians or their associates could be held liable for spoliation of evidence whenever they failed to perform their legal duties to protect the patient's personal possessions. Insofar as there is a legal duty to maintain accurate medical records, physicians could be held liable for spoliation of evidence if they lost or destroyed patient medical records, either intentionally or through negligence.[10,19,20] Liability probably could be imposed as well for failure to enter relevant information into a patient's medical records. Even without the tort of spoliation of evidence, however, the loss or destruction of patient records may be actionable as medical malpractice.[11,20]

Apart from protecting patients' personal effects and retaining accurate information relevant to patients' medical treatment, it would not appear that physicians have any legal duty to preserve or record potential evidence that may be useful to the authorities or to patients in criminal or civil proceedings. Thus, whatever the physician's ethical obligations, it does not appear that the law will impose liability for failure to retain relevant evidence of wound characteristics or marks on adjacent clothing. Likewise, except for patient statements that are relevant to medical treatment, it does not appear that physicians have any legal obligation to document patient statements that may have significance in criminal, civil, or administrative proceedings.

REPORTING REQUIREMENTS

Many cases seen by physicians are the subject of legal reporting requirements.[29] Most of these reporting requirements are statutory, but in recent years several state courts have imposed reporting requirements based on common law principles.

Statutory Reporting Requirements

Acting under the police power to protect public health, safety, and welfare, every state has enacted statutes mandating that physicians report certain events to public authorities. (The federal government has no comparable general reporting statutes applicable to physicians.) While state statutes vary, the four primary categories of reportable events under state law are deaths under suspicious circumstances, injuries with suspicious etiology (injuries from weapons or violent acts), injuries to members of vulnerable groups, and infectious diseases. All such reportable events have the potential of leading to criminal prosecutions, civil lawsuits, or administrative benefit claims.

Suspicious Deaths

The attending physician is legally required to report the fact of a patient's death under suspicious, unusual, or unnatural circumstances. While the standards vary from state to state, they generally require reporting of deaths when:[29,32,51]

- there is evidence of violence or suicide;
- the decedent was an inmate of a public institution;
- a patient dies within 24 hours of hospital admission or surgery;
- a person apparently in good health dies suddenly and unexpectedly; or
- there is no attending physician to certify the cause of death.

It has been estimated that 20% of all deaths meet these criteria and warrant a medicolegal investigation.[51] The forensic investigation of these deaths, which would be carried out by a coroner or medical examiner,[29,50,51] may lead to criminal prosecutions for intentional or negligent homicide, as well as civil lawsuits by the families of the victims against those responsible for causing or failing to prevent the death. (The particular observations that physicians should make and record in these cases are discussed further in Chapters 11 and 12.) Reporting also is required of any death from an infectious disease that might constitute a threat to public health (see below).

Injuries with Suspicious Etiology

Each state has its own list of reportable injuries from violent acts, the purpose of which is to alert the authorities to potential criminal violations. Many states require reporting of all gunshot wounds, and some require reporting of stabbing, poisoning, or other categories of traumatic injuries.[29] For example, Pennsylvania has a broad statute that requires a physician who treats a person injured by any deadly weapon to report the injury and the name of the injured person to the police.[1] In addition to criminal prosecutions by the state, these reportable injuries may lead to civil lawsuits by the victims. (The incidence and nature of reportable traumatic injuries from violent acts are discussed further in Chapters 11 and 12.)

Injuries to Vulnerable Populations

The other category of reportable acts focuses on the identity of the victims rather than the etiology of injury, requiring reporting of traumatic injuries to members of vulnerable groups, including children, the elderly, and spouses.[9,20,29] Some states also require reporting of industrial accidents.[20]

Virtually all states require physicians and other health care professionals to report evidence of suspected child abuse,[9,29,31,37] which may set in motion proceedings to protect the child from further abuse as well as leading to criminal prosecution of the perpetrators. Estimates of child abuse range from one to four million incidents per year.[37] Every health care practitioner should be aware of the AMA diagnostic and treatment guidelines for child abuse as well as the specific criteria and requirements of the state statute[9] (see Chapter 11A).

The elderly represent another vulnerable group that is frequently subject to abuse by frustrated caregivers, and a growing number of states have elder abuse reporting statutes.[9,28] It has been estimated that between 1.5 and 2 million older adults are abused or neglected each year in the United States[28] (see Chapter 11C).

Spouses represent a third group that is vulnerable to abuse (see Chapters 11B and 12C). While most states have recognized the alarming incidence of spouse abuse and have enacted statutes to provide protection and remedies to the victims, very few states have reporting requirements for physicians.[9] The absence of reporting requirements for spouse abuse may reflect certain characteristics of this problem that differ from situations involving abuse of children and the elderly. Unlike abuse of children and of many seniors, spouse abuse generally occurs within a consensual relationship between two legally competent adults. It therefore may be appropriate to presume that victims of spouse abuse are capable of reporting such abuse themselves, without relying upon physicians. Moreover, a physician's report to the authorities of suspected spouse abuse could adversely affect the relationship between the parties, resulting in recriminations and further violence. On the other hand, many victims of spouse abuse also suffer from emotional problems that may affect their capacity to act appropriately for their own protection, which would warrant reporting of spouse abuse by physicians and other health care personnel.

Infectious Diseases

For infectious diseases, each state has its own reporting procedures and specifies the reportable diseases, which generally include contagious diseases such as tuberculosis and sexually transmitted diseases such as syphilis, gonorrhea, and acquired immunodeficiency syndrome (AIDS) (see Chapter 16).[20,29] Some require reporting of patients by name, while others allow anonymous reporting. For example, as of early 1994, all states required physicians to report AIDS cases to public health authorities, and 35 states required them to report cases of asymptomatic human immunodeficiency virus (HIV) infections (of which 10 allowed anonymous reporting).[20,41]

Immunity for Reporting

Reporting statutes usually protect physicians and other health care professionals who submit these reports by providing them with immunity from civil liability. That is, physicians who submit reports of infectious diseases or traumatic injuries pursuant to these statutes cannot be sued by their patients or others if the reports prove to be incorrect, even if the physician was negligent, provided that the report was submitted in good faith.[9,28,29,37] For example, on the basis of statutory immunity, a court dismissed the parents' lawsuit against a physician who had notified the authorities of suspected child abuse after erroneously ruling out a congenital anomaly (osteogenesis imperfecta, "brittle bone disease") that proved to be the true cause of the child's many broken bones, because the physician, although he may have been negligent, had acted in good faith.[2,9] No immunity exists, however, if the physician fails to comply with the statutory procedure and discloses suspected abuse to the wrong persons.[14,37,42]

Liability for Failure to Report Abuse

Physicians who neglect to detect or report cases of abuse run the risk of criminal prosecution and malpractice liability to the victims and their families.[25,37] In at least 42 states, failure to report child abuse can result in criminal prosecution.[37] With regard to civil liability, the California Supreme Court ruled that suit could be brought against a physician who negligently failed to report a suspected case of child abuse.[30] Thereafter, however, courts in Georgia,[13] Minnesota,[49] and Michigan[35] refused to impose civil liability for failure to report suspected child abuse.[37] Although there are too few cases to predict how the courts will rule in other states, the potential for liability here is greater than it is with nonstatutory reporting requirements (discussed below) because of the existence of a statute that makes reporting mandatory and provides immunity from liability for disclosure.

Nonstatutory Reporting Requirements

Even in the absence of reporting statutes, courts applying common law principles have declared that physicians have a legal duty to report certain events or conditions to third parties in order to warn them of a risk of violence, contagious disease, or some other danger.[17,20,23,26,29,40,44,47] The confidentiality of the physician-patient relationship generally militates against disclosure, but courts in several states have ruled that this concern is outweighed by the physician's obligation to protect third parties from hazards created by their patients.

The "duty to warn" most frequently arises in the practice of psychiatrists, psychologists, and other psychotherapists, whose mentally ill patients may present a danger to themselves or others. The first case in which a court ruled that there is a duty to warn potential victims, *Tarasoff v. Board of Regents,*[48] involved the failure of a psychiatrist to take appropriate steps to protect a young woman who was the object of a patient's obsession. The court declared:

> [W]hen a therapist determines, or pursuant to the standards of his profession should have determined, that his patient presents a serious danger of violence to another, he incurs an obligation to use reasonable care to protect the intended victim against such danger. . . .[The discharge of this duty] may call for [the therapist] to warn the intended victim of the danger, to notify the police, or take whatever other steps are reasonably necessary under the circumstances.[48]

The state courts have differed in their views as to what circumstances trigger a duty to warn potential victims.[17,20,23,40,44] At one end of the spectrum, courts in several cases have ruled that a duty to warn only exists where there have been specific threats against identifiable individuals. Some courts take an intermediate position and impose a duty to warn foreseeable victims even in the absence of specific threats. For example, one court allowed a lawsuit to proceed even though there had been no specific threats or expression of violent feelings against the victim, based on evidence that the patient was dangerous and had once fired a BB gun at a car in which the patient had thought the victim and her boyfriend were riding.[36] In the broadest expansion of the duty to protect, one court declared that the Veterans Administration could be held liable for failure to commit a patient who subsequently fired a shotgun into a crowded nightclub, despite the absence of either specific threats of violence or a specific target of the patient's anger.[33] At least a dozen states—Alaska, California, Colorado, Florida, Indiana, Kansas, Kentucky, Louisiana, Minnesota, Montana, New Hampshire, and Utah—have enacted statutes concerning the duty to warn.[40,44] While these statutes vary in scope and content, most of them require reporting only in instances of threats of violence against specific or reasonably identifiable victims.[40,44] Several of these statutes immunize physicians against liability for failure to predict or prevent violent behavior in the absence of explicit threats by the patient.[40,44]

Although patients are most likely to voice threats of violence to their psychiatrists, psychologists, or psychotherapists, such threats may also be expressed to primary care physicians and practitioners in unrelated specialized practices. Since virtually all physicians could be confronted with explicit or implicit threats of violence by their patients against third parties, all physicians ought to be familiar with the applicable state standards so that they are prepared to comply with both their legal and ethical obligations in evaluating the seriousness of the danger and balancing concern for the welfare of others against patient confidentiality.

Contagious diseases present another situation in which physicians have a duty to disclose confidential information to third parties.[20,23,29] It is well established that physicians can be held liable for failing to warn the family, neighbors or other specifically identifiable third parties of patients with infectious diseases such as scarlet fever or smallpox.[7,20,21] Warnings also may be necessary for family, friends, or associates of patients with diseases that may impair the patient's control of his or her activities, such as diabetes mellitus, cerebrocardiovascular disease, epilepsy, or other convulsive disorders.[23]

The AIDS epidemic presents unique challenges to physicians in fulfilling their conflicting duties to keep patient confidences and warn third parties of serious risks.[20] Several characteristics of AIDS exacerbate the conflict between patient confidentiality and the duty to warn third parties. First, concerns about privacy are amplified by the widespread fear and ignorance of AIDS and the history of prejudice and discrimination against gay men among whom AIDS has been most common. Second, the need for disclosure may be less pressing insofar as HIV cannot be transmitted through casual contact. On the other hand, disclosure may be more valuable insofar as sexual partners who are not yet infected may benefit from prompt disclosure. Finally, the fact that AIDS is currently incurable and almost invariably fatal makes prevention essential. (The positive response of patients to certain new treatments does not represent a cure, and it is too soon to evaluate the impact on long-term mortality rates.)

Beyond the statutes requiring disclosure to public health authorities, several states have enacted laws that permit but do not require physician disclosure of HIV test results to persons at risk from sexual or needle-sharing contacts with the infected person; these statutes provide immunity from liability whether the physician chooses to disclose the information or maintain confidentiality.[20] For example, California has a statute that immunizes physicians from liability for disclosure or nondisclosure;[52] this statute supersedes any common law obliga-

tion to warn third parties based on the *Tarasoff* decision.[20]

The physician's first resort should be to counsel the patient to inform any sexual or needle-sharing partners and to take special precautions. When patients indicate they will not do so, the physician's obligation to warn others depends on the law of the particular state. In the absence of definitive guidance from the state courts, it frequently is not clear whether the physician has any legal duty beyond reporting the disease to the patient and to public authorities.[20,23,41,47] The AMA takes the position that warning is appropriate if the patient cannot be persuaded to cease endangering identifiable third parties:

> Where there is no statute that mandates or prohibits reporting of seropositive individuals to public health authorities and it is clear that the seropositive individual is endangering an identified third party, the physician should 1) attempt to persuade the infected individual to cease endangering the third party; 2) if persuasion fails, notify authorities; and 3) if authorities take no action, notify and counsel the endangered third party.[20(§4-34,n.44)]

As AIDS victims are prone to various infections and tumors, physicians who practice in a wide array of fields can anticipate having to confront this issue. Hospitals and other health care institutions face similar tensions in deciding whether to warn patients about exposure to HIV-infected staff.[20] Another issue is whether patients infected with AIDS after a blood transfusion have a right to ascertain the identity of the donor.[20,23] Because the law concerning HIV-infected patients is changing rapidly, physicians are strongly encouraged to keep themselves informed of the current status of state statutes and court decisions that affect their legal obligations.

CONFIDENTIALITY AND TESTIMONIAL PRIVILEGE IN LITIGATION

Confidentiality

Confidentiality is a basic ethical aspect of medical practice and is essential to promote a free flow of information from patient to physician.[20,23] The Hippocratic Oath includes a promise not to divulge patient confidences. The AMA Council on Ethical and Judicial Affairs provides the following explanation of the duty of confidentiality:

> Confidentiality. The information disclosed to a physician during the course of the relationship between physician and patient is confidential to the greatest possible degree. The patient should feel free to make a full disclosure of information to the physician in order that the physician may most effectively provide needed services. The patient should be able to make this disclosure with the knowledge that the physician will respect the confidential nature of the communication. The physician should not reveal confidential communications or information without the express consent of the patient unless required to do so by law.[4(No.5.05)]

The confidentiality of information about patients, and especially physician-patient communications, has long been recognized by the courts applying common law principles.[20,23] Physicians can be held liable for compensatory damages if a patient suffers financial or emotional loss as a result of unauthorized disclosure of confidential information. Recovery in such cases may be based on a variety of legal theories, including the tort of invasion of privacy, breach of a fiduciary duty to maintain confidentiality, breach of an implied promise to maintain confidentiality, or breach of a duty of confidentiality defined by an applicable statute[20,23] (see Chapters 5 and 27).

A patient may consent to the disclosure of confidential information, however. Patients may implicitly consent to disclosure of medical records to other treating physicians, and they routinely consent to the release of information to third-party payers. A patient who seeks damages for personal injury must consent to the release of pertinent medical information as part of the pretrial discovery process (see Chapter 3).

Testimonial Privilege

In addition to the general duty of confidentiality, most states recognize a "testimonial privilege" that protects against disclosure of confidential medically-related patient information in legal proceedings, both during pretrial discovery and at trial. Although 43 states recognize some form of physician-patient privilege, the privilege plays a very limited role in protecting confidential patient information.[20,23] First, in many of these states the privilege is applicable only to psychiatrists. Second, the privilege applies only in legal proceedings and does not impose a general obligation of confidentiality in other contexts. Third, the testimonial privilege is subject to many exceptions, so that, depending on state law, it may be inapplicable in certain categories of cases: civil commitment proceedings; child custody disputes; will contests; and legal actions between physician and patient (e.g., claims for malpractice or for unpaid bills). Finally, and most importantly, the testimonial privilege may be waived by the patient. Under the "patient litigation exception," the testimonial privilege is deemed to be waived when a patient places his or her physical or mental status at issue in litigation. In most states, the waiver is limited to the specific subject matter or area relevant to the lawsuit, but in some states, the mere filing of a lawsuit with respect to an injury waives the right to assert the privilege as to any treating physician.[20,23]

Contact with the Patient's Opponent in Litigation

Both consent to release of confidential information and waiver of the testimonial privilege are the patient's prerogative. Physicians must take care not to misinterpret the extent of any consent or waiver by the plaintiff. Even when a patient has authorized disclosure of medical records in litigation, a physician can be held liable for unwarranted disclosure of information that was not relevant to the litigation.

At depositions or at trial, the patient's attorney is present and can object to any inquiry by the opponent into matters not covered by the consent or waiver. The greatest risk of physician error arises in *ex parte* communications between the physician and the patient's opponent (i.e., communications made outside the presence of the patient's attorney). To protect against inadvertent disclosure of confidential information, the courts in several states have forbidden attorneys from initiating *ex parte* contacts with the opposing party's treating physicians and have imposed liability on physicians for unauthorized disclosure of confidential patient information in such circumstances.[6,15,27,34] Most states, however, permit such *ex parte* contacts.[6,15,27,34,46]

To avoid inadvertent disclosures of confidential patient information, physicians should not communicate information about a patient with anyone other than the patient or the patient's attorney. When responding to subpoenas or other requests for medical records and reports from other parties, even if accompanied by a release signed by the patient, physicians should consider delivering patient records to the patient's attorney for transmittal to the opposing attorney so that any questions about the validity and scope of the waiver of confidentiality can be resolved prior to disclosure.

REFERENCES

1. 42 Purdon's Pa Cons Stat Ann §8334
2. *Ackerman v TriCounty Orthopedic Group, PO,* 373 NW2d 204 (Mich App 1985)
3. American College of Legal Medicine (ed): **Legal Medicine: Legal Dynamics of Medical Encounters.** 3rd ed. St. Louis, Mo: Mosby-Year Book, 1995, 754 pp
4. American Medical Association, Council of Ethical and Judicial Affairs: **Current Opinions.** Chicago, Ill: American Medical Association, 1989, 54 pp
5. Annotation, tort or statutory liability for failure or refusal of witness to give testimony. **ALR 3d 61:**1297, 1975
6. Asher JM, Glaser RA, Erard BH: *Ex parte* interview with plaintiff's treating physicians—the offensive use of the physician-patient privilege. **U Det Law Rev 67:** 501, 1990
7. Bateman TA: Annotation: liability of doctor of other health practitioner to third party contracting contagious disease from doctor's patient. **ALR 5th 3:**370, 1992
8. Bianco EA, Hirsh HL: Consent to and refusal of medical treatment, in American College of Legal Medicine (ed): **Legal Medicine: Legal Dynamics of Medical Encounters.** 3rd ed. St Louis, Mo: Mosby-Year Book, 1995, pp 274-296
9. Bisbing SB, McMenamin JP, Granville RL: Competency, capacity, and immunity, in American College of Legal Medicine (ed): **Legal Medicine: Legal Dynamics of Medical Encounters.** 3rd ed. St Louis, Mo: Mosby-Year Book, 1995, pp 27-45
10. *Bondu v Gurvich,* 473 So2d 1307 (Fla App 1984)
11. *Brown v Hamid,* 856 SW2d 51 (Mo 1993)
12. Casamassima AC: Spoliation of evidence and medical malpractice. **Pace Law Rev** 14:235-299, 1994
13. *Cechman v Tavis,* 414 SE2d 282 (Ga Ct App 1991)
14. *Comstock v Walsh,* 848 SW2d 7 (Mo 1993)
15. Corboy PH: Ex parte contacts between plaintiff's physician and defense attorneys: protecting the patient-litigant's right to a fair trial. **Loyola Univ Chic Law J 21:**1001, 1990
16. Curran WJ: Titles in the medicolegal field: a proposal for reform. **Am J Legal Med 1:**1, 1975
17. Firestone MR: Psychiatric patients and forensic psychiatry, in American College of Legal Medicine (ed): **Legal Medicine: Legal Dynamics of Medical Encounters.** 3rd ed. St Louis, Mo: Mosby-Year Book, 1995, pp 585-616
18. Fischer TG: Annotation, intentional spoliation of evidence, interfering with prospective civil action, as actionable. **ALR 4th 70:**984, 1989
19. *Fox v Cohen,* 406 NE2d 178 (Ill App 1980)
20. Furrow BR, Greaney TL, Johnson SH, et al: **Health Law.** St Paul, Minn: West Publishing, 1995, Vol 1: 772 pp, Vol 2: 752 pp
21. *Green v Otenasek,* 296 A2d 597 (Md 1972)
22. *Hammonds v Aetna Casualty & Surety Co,* 243 F Supp 793 (ND Ohio 1965)
23. Hirsch HL: Disclosure about patients, in American College of Legal Medicine (ed): **Legal Medicine: Legal Dynamics of Medical Encounters.** 3rd ed. St Louis, Mo: Mosby-Year Book, 1995, pp 312-342
24. Hirsch HL: Medical records, in American College of Legal Medicine (ed): **Legal Medicine: Legal Dynamics of Medical Encounters.** 3rd ed. St Louis, Mo: Mosby-Year Book, 1995, pp 297-311
25. Hoffman AC: Medical malpractice, in American College of Legal Medicine (ed): **Legal Medicine: Legal Dynamics of Medical Encounters.** 3rd ed. St Louis, Mo: Mosby-Year Book, 1995, pp 129-140
26. Howard ML, Vogt LB: Physician-patient relationship, in American College of Legal Medicine (ed): **Legal Medicine: Legal Dynamics of Medical Encounters.** 3rd ed. St Louis, Mo: Mosby-Year Book, 1995, pp 265-273
27. Jennings J: Note, the physician-patient relationship: the permissibility of ex parte communications between plaintiff's treating physicians and defense counsel. **Mo Law Rev 59:**441, 1994
28. Kapp MB: Geriatric patients, in American College of Legal Medicine (ed): **Legal Medicine: Legal Dynamics of Medical Encounters.** 3rd ed. St Louis, Mo: Mosby-Year Book, 1995, pp 488-493
29. Kaufman HH, Lewin J, Munzner R, et al: Ethical and legal responsibilities of the neurosurgeon: selected topics. **Neurosurgery 28:**918-923, 1991
30. *Landeros v Flood,* 551 P2d 389 (Cal 1976)
31. Leestma JE: Neuropathology of child abuse, in Leestma JE (ed): **Forensic Neuropathology.** New York, NY: Raven Press, 1988, pp 333-356
32. Leestma JE, Magee DJ: Pathology and neuropathology in the forensic setting, in Leestma JE (ed): **Forensic Neuropathology.** New York, NY: Raven Press, 1988, pp 1-23
33. *Lipari v Sears, Roebuck and Co,* 497 F Supp 185 (D Neb 1980)
34. Maloney WJ: Note, ex parte communication between physicians and attorneys: a change of course. **UMKC Law Rev 62:**405, 1993
35. *Marcelletti v Bathani,* 500 NW2d 124 (Mich Ct App 1993)
36. *McIntosh v Milano,* 403 A2d 500 (NJ Super 1979)
37. McMenamin JP, Garland LB: Children as patients, in American College of Legal Medicine (ed): **Legal

Medicine: Legal Dynamics of Medical Encounters. 3rd ed. St Louis, Mo: Mosby-Year Book, 1995, pp 456-487

38. Nesson CR: Incentives to spoliate evidence in civil litigation: the need for vigorous judicial action. Cardozo Law Rev 13:793, 1991

39. Nolte S: The spoliation tort: an approach to underlying principles. St Marys Law J 26:351, 1995

40. Robb B, Smith JT, Polizzotto S: Medical Malpractice in Psychiatric Care. 1996 Supplement. New York, NY: John Wiley & Sons, 322 pp

41. Royal MA: Patients with human immunodeficiency virus (HIV) infection and acquired immunodeficiency syndrome (AIDS), in American College of Legal Medicine (ed): Legal Medicine: Legal Dynamics of Medical Encounters. 3rd ed. St Louis, Mo: Mosby-Year Book, 1995, pp 516-530

42. *Searcy v Auerbach,* 980 F2d 609 (9th Cir 1992)

43. *Smith v Superior Court,* 198 Cal Rptr 829 (Cal App 1984)

44. Smith JT: Medical Malpractice in Psychiatric Care. Colorado Springs, Colo: Shepard's/McGraw Hill, 1986, 633 pp

45. *Spaulding v Hussain,* 551 A2d 1022 (NJ Super 1988)

46. *Steinberg v Jensen,* 534 NW2d 361 (Wis 1995)

47. Taraska JM: Legal Guide for Physicians. White Plains, NY: AHAB Press, 1997

48. *Tarasoff v Board of Regents,* 529 P2d 334, *modified,* 551 P2d 334 (Cal 1976)

49. *Valtakis v Putnam,* 504 NW2d 264 (Minn Ct App 1993)

50. Wecht CH: Forensic pathology, in American College of Legal Medicine (ed): Legal Medicine: Legal Dynamics of Medical Encounters. 3rd ed. St Louis, Mo: Mosby-Year Book, 1995, pp 567-584

51. Wecht CH: Forensic use of medical information, in American College of Legal Medicine (ed): Legal Medicine: Legal Dynamics of Medical Encounters. 3rd ed. St Louis, Mo: Mosby-Year Book, 1995, pp 558-566

52. West's Ann Cal Health & Safety Code §199.25(c)

53. Wick WR, Katz H: Telephone contacts and counseling, in American College of Legal Medicine (ed): Legal Medicine: Legal Dynamics of Medical Encounters. 3rd ed. St Louis, Mo: Mosby-Year Book, 1995, pp 343-350

CHAPTER 3

INTERFACE WITH THE LEGAL SYSTEM
BEFORE TRIAL

JEFF L. LEWIN, JD

This chapter describes the activities of physicians in the preparation for trial of civil disputes and criminal prosecutions. Formal pretrial proceedings are governed by rules of civil and criminal procedure, which vary from state to state. This chapter describes pretrial proceedings under the Federal Rules of Civil Procedure (Fed.R.Civ.P.)[15] and Federal Rules of Criminal Procedure (Fed.R.Crim.P.),[16] which govern proceedings in federal courts and serve as the models for modern procedural rules in many states.

OCCURRENCE WITNESS, EXPERT WITNESS, OR EXPERT CONSULTANT

Depending upon choice and circumstances, a physician might play one or more of the following roles in litigation: 1) an occurrence witness; 2) an expert witness; or 3) an expert consultant.[13]

A person having direct firsthand knowledge of relevant facts is an "occurrence witness." A physician might become an occurrence witness either in a nonprofessional context as an eyewitness to a crime or accident or through professional activity as the treating or consulting physician of a patient who is involved in litigation. As an occurrence witness in a nonprofessional setting, the physician will be subject to the rules for discovery of information from lay witnesses. As an occurrence witness in the context of a professional relationship, however, a physician usually will be asked to express "opinions" that go beyond the observed "facts" of the patient's history, symptoms, and test results. In particular, the physician is likely to be asked about: 1) the diagnosis, which is a conclusion based on professional evaluation of the observed facts; 2) the cause of the condition; or 3) the patient's prognosis (i.e., whether the condition is permanent or can be expected to improve or worsen). Because treating or examining physicians usually will be capable of stating opinions about diagnosis, causation, or prognosis, for many purposes they will be treated as "expert witnesses" and will be subject to special rules and procedures (see below).

A physician who was not a witness to any of the events giving rise to a dispute can later become involved in the proceedings as an expert witness or as an expert consultant. As an "expert witness," the physician would be retained by one of the parties or by the court to develop an expert opinion on a disputed issue with a view toward expressing that opinion at trial. As an "expert consultant," the physician would be retained by one of the parties to assist the attorneys in preparing their case for trial.

A retained expert can serve in both capacities, as a witness and as a consultant.[13,23,31,38] Indeed, one authority advises attorneys to initially retain all experts as consultants and decide later in the litigation whether to designate them as expert witnesses.[22] On the other hand, insofar as an expert witness initially was retained as a consultant, the opposing attorney can use this fact on cross-examination to undermine the expert's credibility by emphasizing that the witness received compensation in exchange for an agreement to "assist" the party in the litigation.

The expert consultant is not necessarily a partisan, however. An attorney appreciates candid advice about the weaknesses as well as the strengths of a client's case, and the attorney may rely upon the expert consultant to provide an objective evaluation as an antidote to the attorney's inevitably partisan perspective as the client's advocate in our adversarial system of litigation.

Physicians who testify as expert witnesses, regardless of whether or not they also serve as consultants, must testify honestly and should not distort their testimony for partisan advantage. According to the American Medical Association (AMA):

> The medical witness must not become an advocate or a partisan in the legal proceeding. The medical witness should be adequately prepared and should testify honestly and truthfully.[9]

Physicians who have been accused of malpractice can play all three roles in the litigation. Malpractice defendants are occurrence witnesses regarding the events that gave rise to the claim, and they are expert witnesses insofar as they can express opinions about the diagnosis of the patient's presenting condition, the applicable standard of care, and possible noniatrogenic causes of the patient's unsatisfactory outcome. Physicians who are defendants in malpractice actions also can act as expert consultants in rendering advice to their attorneys. Much of this chapter's discussion of the role of expert consultants is thus fully applicable to physicians who want to take an active role in defending themselves against claims of medical malpractice.

IS THERE AN OBLIGATION TO PARTICIPATE IN LEGAL PROCEEDINGS?

In both criminal and civil actions, all parties have the right to compel attendance at trial of witnesses who have knowledge of relevant facts, and this right also applies in certain pretrial proceedings (grand jury proceedings, preliminary hearings, and depositions). Thus, a physician who has acquired direct knowledge of relevant facts in a professional or nonprofessional context can, like any other occurrence witness, be served with a subpoena which is a court order that compels a person to attend a trial or pretrial proceeding, to bring specified documents or other items, and to answer questions under oath.[38,43,52(§2451)] To disobey a subpoena is contempt of court, and violators can be fined or jailed.

For experts who are occurrence witnesses, such as treating physicians, it is not entirely clear whether the parties can compel them to give expert testimony.[14,21,24] In some jurisdictions, the parties can compel experts to testify about their observations and actions but not about their opinions. In other jurisdictions, the parties can compel experts to testify about opinions they previously formed but cannot compel experts to develop new opinions for purposes of litigation. Thus, in some jurisdictions treating physicians can be forced to answer only factual questions about the patient's history and symptoms and any tests or treatments that were administered, while in other jurisdictions physicians also can be required to testify about any opinions they had reached regarding the patient's condition, including the diagnosis, cause, and prognosis. A few cases even allow the parties to compel treating physicians to answer questions calling for expert opinion testimony on issues about which they had not previously formed opinions, although not if this would require the physician to undertake any additional research or preparation. An unwilling expert does not provide convincing testimony, however. Thus, even in jurisdictions that allow parties to use the subpoena power to compel opinion testimony from treating physicians, attorneys ordinarily seek voluntary cooperation, with appropriate compensation for the physician's time.

Regardless of the possibility of legal compulsion, a physician whose patient becomes involved in a legal dispute has an ethical obligation to assist the patient by participating in the ensuing legal proceedings. According to the AMA:

> If a patient who has a legal claim requests his physician's assistance, the physician should furnish medical evidence, with the patient's consent, in order to secure the patient's legal rights.[9]

It is therefore entirely appropriate for a treating physician to assist the patient's attorney in understanding the nature of a patient's current condition, its cause, and the patient's prognosis, in order for the attorney to make an appropriate claim on the patient's behalf in workers' compensation or Social Security disability claims or in personal injury litigation.

While treating physicians can be compelled to testify at trial and pretrial proceedings, participation as a retained expert witness or consultant is entirely voluntary. Nevertheless, a physician who is neither an occurrence witness nor a retained expert may, under extraordinary circumstances, be compelled to testify at a deposition or trial or make documents available for inspection and copying.[13,14,32,38,52(§2463)] As one leading authority explains:

> A growing problem has been the use of subpoenas to compel the giving of evidence and information by unretained experts. Experts are not exempt from the duty to give evidence, even if they cannot be compelled to prepare themselves to give effective testimony, but compulsion to give evidence may threaten the economic interests of experts who are denied the opportunity to bargain for the value of their services.[52(§2463)]

The courts have compelled participation of unretained experts who are not occurrence witnesses only in extraordinary circumstances,

when they have unique information not readily obtainable by other experts. For example, when the defendants in asbestos litigation sought to obtain records from Dr. Irving Selikoff of his studies relating to the carcinogenicity of tobacco, the New York courts quashed the subpoenas because the requests were unduly burdensome, while the federal courts upheld a narrower subpoena that ordered him to supply a computer tape containing some of this information.[26,32] One court upheld the subpoena for records of the Registry for Hormonal Transplacental Carcinogenesis in litigation concerning diethylstilbestrol (DES),[12,32] whereas another court recently denied a request to take the deposition of AIDS researchers on the grounds that cumulative requests might interfere with their research.[35] In recognition of the intellectual property rights of unretained experts and their freedom to withhold their expertise, the Federal Rules of Civil Procedure were amended in 1991 to add Rule 45(c)(3)(B).[3] This rule allows parties to obtain discovery "of an unretained expert's opinion or information not describing specific events or occurrences in dispute and resulting from the expert's study made not at the request of any party" only under extraordinary circumstances if the party seeking this information "shows a substantial need for the testimony or material that cannot be otherwise met without undue hardship and assures that the person to whom the subpoena is addressed will be reasonably compensated" (Fed.R.Civ.P. Rule 45(c)(3)(B)). In deciding whether to quash (cancel) or modify subpoenas directed to unretained experts, the courts will consider such factors as:[3,28,38,52(§2463)]

1. the degree to which the expert is called because of knowledge of relevant facts rather than to give opinion testimony;
2. the difference between testifying to a previously expressed opinion and forming a new one;
3. the possibility that the witness has unique expertise;
4. the likelihood that any comparable witness will willingly testify; and
5. the degree to which the witness may be oppressed by having continually to testify.

Thus, while the courts have the power in

extraordinary circumstances to compel physicians possessing unique expertise to share relevant background information and even divulge their previously formed opinions, it generally remains true that physicians who are not occurrence witnesses cannot be compelled to provide expert opinion evidence in civil proceedings.

BECOMING AN EXPERT WITNESS OR CONSULTANT

No legal or ethical duty obligates a physician to serve as a retained expert witness or consultant. On the other hand, providing expert services is consistent with the obligation to "assist in the administration of justice."[9] The quality of justice is greatly affected by the competence and integrity of expert witnesses. While members of the public and of the medical and legal professions justifiably decry the participation of "professional experts,"[20,21] the refusal of many leading physicians to become involved as expert witnesses leaves a vacuum that of necessity is filled by less scrupulous members of the profession. Insofar as honorable members of the medical profession refuse to serve as expert witnesses, the assumption by both lawyers and physicians that most medical experts are "hired guns" (or worse) is a self-fulfilling prophecy.[23]

Participation as an expert witness or consultant enables one to share one's knowledge and experience with attorneys and lay jurors. For many, this activity is stimulating and is intellectually and emotionally satisfying,[30] as well as financially rewarding.

Physicians seeking employment as expert witnesses or consultants sometimes advertise their services in legal publications or data bases.[21] They also can offer their services through agencies that act as liaisons between attorneys and potential experts.[21] These agencies generally collect a percentage of the experts' fees as compensation.

One excellent way to become acquainted with the activities of expert witnesses in an academic setting is to volunteer to participate in mock trial exercises at a local law school. Most law schools have courses in trial advocacy in which law students conduct direct and cross-examinations of witnesses, both in discrete exercises and in complete mock trials. By participating as expert witnesses in these exercises, physicians enhance the educational experience for the students while at the same time acquiring hands-on experience as expert witnesses and receiving feedback from the instructor about effective expert testimony.

FEES FOR EXPERT SERVICES AND RELATED ETHICAL CONCERNS

Ordinary occurrence witnesses cannot receive compensation from the parties apart from the standard witness fee (usually a small per diem fee plus an amount for travel expenses based on mileage to the courthouse), which must be paid when a subpoena to testify is served. As an occurrence witness, testifying only to facts, the physician is entitled to the normal witness fee but cannot receive additional compensation. Insofar as the physician will provide expert testimony, however, the physician can be compensated for time spent in preparation, and in most states the physician can also be compensated for the time spent in court beyond the normal witness fee.[21,24,31,33,43]

If invited to serve as an expert witness or consultant, it is important for the physician to reach a clear understanding regarding the fee. From a legal perspective, it is unethical to be paid for "testimony," but it is perfectly appropriate to be paid for "services" as an expert, which would include the time spent in preparation and in court, as well as travel time and out-of-pocket expenses.

Both the legal and medical professions consider it unethical for the compensation of an expert witness to be contingent upon the outcome of the lawsuit.[37] Lawyers in every jurisdiction are bound by state ethical codes based on either the American Bar Association's *Model Code of Professional Responsibility*,[5] adopted in 1970, or the *Model Rules of Professional Conduct*,[7] adopted in 1983. The *Code* expressly prohibits payment of contingent compensation to a witness: "A lawyer shall not pay, offer to pay, or acquiesce in the payment of compensation to a witness contingent upon the content of his testimony or the outcome of the case."[5] The *Model Rules* are less explicit, but they also indicate that payment of contingent compensation to an expert witness is improper. The *Model Rules* broadly prohibit the offer of "an inducement to a witness that is prohibited by law."[7] The comment to this rule explains that:

> [I]t is not improper to pay a witness's expenses or to compensate an expert witness on terms permitted by law. The common law in most jurisdictions is that it is improper to pay an occurrence witness any fee for testifying and that it is improper to pay an expert witness a contingent fee.[6]

The AMA declares bluntly: "It is unethical for a physician to accept compensation that is contingent upon the outcome of litigation."[9] Whereas the legal restrictions on contingent fees apply only to expert witnesses, the AMA's ethical standard would appear to apply to expert consultants as well.

Although the fees for services of an expert witness can be a fixed amount for an entire case, the fees usually are based on an hourly or daily rate of compensation.[13] For an expert witness, the hourly rate for time spent in preparation or in court should be commensurate with the physician's fees for other services. Because of the inconvenience of being away from one's office, fees for time in depositions or in court (including time in transit) may be higher than for time spent in preparation.[24,33,43] Also, because of uncertainty about the precise time when testimony will begin, a court appearance may preclude the physician from scheduling any other matters on a given day, which would justify compensation on a per diem basis for testimony at trial.[13] To avoid any question of whether payment is contingent on the outcome, the physician should be paid in full *before* appearing in court to testify.

For both expert witnesses and consultants, an agreement about fees should be set forth in a contract or a letter signed by the attorney that describes the nature and extent of the services and the basis of compensation, including any special rates applicable to time spent away from the office or in court. The agreement should obligate the client (and possibly the attorney as well) to pay all fees by the time of trial, and it should establish a schedule for interim payments (e.g., monthly, quarterly, or whenever fees exceed a specified threshold).[13] Attorneys understand the need for written evidence of the agreement on terms of employment and should readily comply with a request for such a document.

Before agreeing to serve as an expert witness or consultant, the physician should ascertain the identities of all parties and their attorneys to make sure there are no associates, relatives, or close friends connected with the case that would create a conflict of interest.[24,33,43] Although the attorney can be expected to initiate inquiry into possible conflicts of interest,[13] the physician should do so if the attorney does not.

Once a physician has agreed to serve as an expert on behalf of one party, it is inappropriate to engage in *ex parte* (private) communications with attorneys for the opposing party.[37] If the matter is pending in litigation, the rules of discovery provide the exclusive procedures for obtaining information from expert witnesses and consultants, and an attorney's attempt to circumvent these formal procedures would violate applicable disciplinary rules.[37] If no litigation is pending, an attorney's attempt to contact the opponent's expert might not be improper, but the retained expert should refuse to engage in *ex parte* communications out of loyalty to the client.

PRETRIAL ACTIVITIES OF EXPERT WITNESSES IN CIVIL CASES

Physicians who testify as expert witnesses in civil cases, either as treating physicians or as retained experts, generally engage in five categories of pretrial activities, which will be discussed separately below: 1) production of patient medical records; 2) medical examination of a party on behalf of the opposing party; 3) reports; 4) depositions; and 5) affidavits. For ease of exposition, the "friendly attorney" will refer to the attorney representing the patient of a treating physician or the attorney representing the party who retained an expert witness or consultant.

The activities of a physician in pretrial procedures will vary according to the physician's role in the litigation and the jurisdiction's rules of civil procedure. For purposes of pretrial discovery, the Federal Rules of Civil Procedure impose different obligations on four categories of experts: 1) occurrence witness experts whose information was not acquired in preparation for trial; 2) expert witnesses who were "retained or specially employed to provide expert testimony in the case" (Fed.R.Civ.P. Rule 26(a)(2) (B)); 3) nontestifying experts who were "retained or specially employed in anticipation of litigation or preparation for trial" but not expected to be called as witnesses at trial (Fed. R.Civ.P. Rule 26(b)(4)(B)); and 4) experts who were informally consulted but not retained.[13,38, 39,53(§2029)] (Actually, a fifth category consists of nonretained experts who were not occurrence witnesses and did not acquire their information in preparation for trial but may be subpoenaed in extraordinary circumstances based on their unique expertise.) Recent amendments to the Federal Rules of Civil Procedure have dramatically changed the discovery rules in federal courts,[13,38,53] and many states are likely to adopt similar procedures.

Production of Patient Medical Records

When patients file claims for benefits or lawsuits seeking compensation for damages based on allegations of injury, disease, or disability, they waive the confidentiality that ordinarily would protect the privacy of their medical records against disclosure to third parties. Thus, whenever the physical or mental condition of the plaintiff is at issue in litigation, the defendant will have the right to inspect and copy the plaintiff's medical records.

The procedures for production of these records vary according to the applicable law, local customs, and the preferences of the parties. The opponent can obtain copies of a party's medical records by submitting a request for production of documents to the party's attorney (Fed.R.Civ.P. Rule 34). In a few jurisdictions, the plaintiff is expected to provide the defendant with copies of the records without a prior request from the defendant, while in others the usual practice is for the defendant to obtain a signed release from the plaintiff and then procure the records directly from the physician or health care institution.

The latter procedure entails a risk of inappropriate disclosure and violation of patient confidentiality in two respects. First, the patient's release may have been forged or procured by fraud. Second, and more significantly, the physician or hospital inadvertently may release information about unrelated medical or emotional conditions that are not relevant to the current claim and as to which confidentiality was not waived. While physicians and health care institutions routinely honor signed releases for disclosure of patient medical records to other health care providers or insurers, they should take special care whenever the release directs that records be sent to an attorney. To minimize the risk of unauthorized or inappropriate disclosures, the safest procedure would be to release records only to the patient's attorney. Upon receipt of a release from an attorney, the physician should contact the patient to verify the signature and ascertain whether the attorney represents the patient or an opposing party.[24]

Medical Examination of a Party

Whenever the physical or mental condition of a party is at issue in litigation, the opponent is entitled to have the party examined by a physician or other suitably licensed or certified professional (Fed.R.Civ.P. Rule 35). Only in Mississippi is the physician-patient privilege deemed to bar court-ordered physical or mental examinations.[54(§2231)] In personal injury cases, for example, the defendant routinely retains a physician to conduct an examination of the plaintiff in order to evaluate the nature of the plaintiff's condition, its cause, and the extent and duration of any functional limitations. Although Federal Rule of Civil Procedure 35(a) and equivalent rules in many states allow the defendant to obtain a court order for such an examination "on motion for good cause," the practice in many jurisdictions is for the plaintiff's medical examination to be scheduled by agreement among counsel without need for a court order.

The examining physician is expected to prepare a report, copies of which will be furnished to attorneys for both parties. In federal practice, the defendant is required, upon request, to give the plaintiff "a copy of the detailed written report of the examiner setting out the examiner's findings, including results of all tests made, diagnoses and conclusions" (Fed.R.Civ.P. Rule 35(b)).

One potential source of dispute is whether the plaintiff's attorney is entitled to accompany the plaintiff to the examination.[19,54(§2236)] Attorneys who represent plaintiffs sometimes insist on being present to prevent the examining physician from eliciting statements by the plaintiff that would be admissible in court because they constitute "admissions of a party" and are not considered to be hearsay (Federal Rules of Evidence 801(d)(2)).[17] Attorneys who represent defendants object to the presence of the plaintiff's attorney as interfering with a proper examination, especially with tests designed to disclose feigned pain or limitations of motion or examinations of mental or emotional conditions. They also object that it converts the examination into an adversarial proceeding. The federal courts generally do not permit the party's attorney to attend, but they sometimes permit the party's physician or another observer to be present.[38,44,47,54(§2236)] State practices vary but more often permit attorneys or third parties to attend.[19,42,54(§2236)] In some states, including California, Illinois, and Michigan, the party has a statutory right to the presence of counsel.[54(§2236)] One court compromised by allowing the party's attorney to be present when the history was taken but not during the physical examination.[34] Some courts protect against inappropriate questions or conduct by the examining physician by allowing the party to tape record the session.[19,42] In Florida, court reporters sometimes record the medical examinations of workers' compensation claimants.[50] Unless the matter has been clarified by a prior agreement or by court order, the examining physician probably should insist on conducting a private examination. If the party objects, the physician should contact the attorney who requested the examination for guidance about whether to proceed with the examination.

Reports

Physicians routinely prepare reports on their patients for use in various contexts. Claims for insurance, Social Security disability or workers' compensation benefits frequently are decided based upon written medical reports without live testimony. In civil litigation, the role of medical reports from treating and examining physicians varies according to the jurisdiction.

Until recently, the Federal Rules of Civil Procedure placed little reliance on reports from physicians. Prior to 1993, the federal rules entitled a party to use written interrogatories to obtain four limited categories of information about the opponent's expert witnesses:[2,13]

1. the expert's identity;
2. the subject matter of the expert's expected testimony;
3. the substance of the facts and opinions to which the expert is expected to testify; and
4. a summary of the grounds for each opinion.

The answers to these interrogatories were prepared by attorneys based on information supplied by the physicians and usually were written in vague and conclusory language in order to minimize the extent of disclosure and avoid pinning the witnesses down.[2,13,38,53(§2031)] If this information were insufficient, a party did not have an automatic right to take the deposition of the opponent's expert witness but had to obtain permission from the court. With the increasing importance of expert witnesses, such permission was routinely granted, but the procedures were cumbersome and offered numerous opportunities for disputation and delay.[2,13,38]

Under the 1993 amendments to the Federal Rules of Civil Procedure, parties are now required to make certain mandatory disclosures without the necessity of requests from the opponent. (The district courts can opt out of these mandatory disclosure provisions, however, and many districts have not implemented them.[37,38]) With respect to expert witnesses, the rules require disclosure of the identity of each expert witness (Fed.R.Civ.P. Rule 26(a)(2)(A)), and this disclosure must "be accompanied by a *written report prepared and signed by the witness*" (Fed.R.Civ.P. Rule 26(a)(2)(B), emphasis supplied). The rule then specifies the content of the expert's report:

> The report shall contain a complete statement of all *opinions to be expressed and the basis and reasons therefor*; the *data* or other information considered by the witness in forming the opinions; any *exhibits* to be used as a summary of or support for the opinions; the *qualifications* of the witness, including a list of all *publications* authored by the witness within the preceding ten years; the *compensation* to be paid for the study and testimony; and a listing of *any other cases in which the witness has testified* as an expert at trial or by deposition within the preceding four years. (Fed.R.Civ.P. Rule 26(a)(2)(B), emphasis supplied)

To the extent that the report fails to disclose this information, a party may be precluded from using it as evidence at trial (Fed.R.Civ.P. Rule 37(c)). Thus, the physician's report must be sufficiently broad to encompass the anticipated trial testimony.

Under the Federal Rules of Civil Procedure, mandatory disclosure of expert reports applies only to experts specially retained for purposes of litigation and not to treating physicians whose information was acquired without regard to possible litigation.[2,38] The Federal Rules of Civil Procedure contemplate that depositions of treating physicians can be taken without the necessity of an expert report, just like any other occurrence witness.[2,38] Nevertheless, at least one federal court has indicated that a report should be provided if the physician's testimony would extend beyond recounting the facts observed during treatment and would include expression of expert opinions.[51] Also, local rules may mandate reports from treating physicians.

While the reliance on expert reports in federal litigation is a recent development, in some states, notably Pennsylvania,[1] the discovery rules have long required that opponents be provided with reports from each expert witness who was expected to testify. Pennsylvania enforces its discovery rules by forbidding experts from testifying at trial to matters outside the "fair scope" of the opinions and reasons stated in their expert reports. In one case, a physician whose report addressed only the absence of *negligence* during surgery was not permitted to express an opinion at trial about the *necessity* of that surgery.[46] In another case, a court ruled that a physician whose report contained only a "conclusory" opinion that the damage to a patient's hepatic duct occurred without negligence on the part of the defendant surgeon should not have been permitted to testify at trial about "an in-depth theory" that the tissues tore under tension from retraction and were not cut by the defendant.[27] Insofar as state practice requires reports from all experts, not just those specially retained for purposes of litigation, treating physicians must prepare reports if they are to testify about opinions or conclusions beyond their factual observations.

Even in jurisdictions in which the discovery rules do not mandate use of expert reports, attorneys frequently request written reports from their expert witnesses and consultants. These reports may be used to evaluate the case or to protect the attorney against charges that a claim or defense was asserted without a good faith basis. The reports of experts witnesses also may be shown to the opponents for leverage in settlement negotiations.

In all of these contexts, the expert report is an important document and requires careful preparation. Clarity and precision are essential. Although the report must be prepared by the physician, it is entirely appropriate and indeed necessary for the physician to confer with the friendly attorney in preparing the report.[13] In particular, the physician should ascertain from the attorney whether the applicable legal rules mandate any particular verbal formulas or "magic words" and make sure that the medical terminology with which the physician expresses the findings or conclusions will be properly interpreted in a legal context. (See Chapter 4 on trial testimony for further discussion of the importance of phrasing medical testimony to comport with applicable legal standards.) The opponents may be entitled to discovery of the draft reports and notes of testifying experts, so the preparation, retention, or destruction of these materials raises important strategic and ethical concerns.[10,13,31,33] Accordingly, the physician should confer with counsel before preparing any written report.

Depositions

A deposition is the out-of-court testimony of a witness that is taken under oath and recorded for use in trial preparation and possibly for introduction into evidence at trial. The deposition of a treating physician or retained expert usually is initiated by the attorney for the opposing party for purposes of discovery, but it also can be initiated by the friendly attorney for possible introduction at trial in lieu of live testimony from the expert witness. Because it is an out-of-court statement, a deposition is hearsay, but it can be used at trial if the witness is dead or otherwise unavailable. A witness is unavailable if he or she is beyond the reach of the trial court's subpoena power, which may be limited to a particular county or state and for federal courts extends beyond the state line up to 100 miles from the place of the deposition or trial (Fed.R.Civ.P. Rule 45).[52(§2461)] Even when the physician-witness is available to testify, the parties may agree to use of a deposition in lieu of live testimony in order to avoid the cost and inconvenience of calling a physician to the courthouse.[43]

The 1993 amendments to the Federal Rules of Civil Procedure now allow parties to take the deposition of an opponent's expert witnesses without obtaining a court order[37,38] (Fed.R.Civ.P. Rule 26(b)). Although the Rules previously required parties to obtain permission from the court before taking the deposition of an opponent's expert witnesses, in most jurisdictions it had become customary to do so by agreement of counsel without a court order, so in this respect the 1993 amendments served to confirm existing practice.[37,38]

The deposition of an expert is a critical event, and the witness should consult with the friendly attorney in preparation for any deposition. The witness may also wish to read texts and articles about expert depositions.[18,24,31,33] In addition, much of the discussion in the chapter about trial testimony is relevant to deposition testimony.

While most occurrence witnesses receive only the standard witness fee and mileage for appearing at a deposition, physicians (both occurrence witnesses and retained experts) customarily receive compensation at a professional rate from whichever side requests the deposition. Federal Rule of Civil Procedure 26(b)(4)(C) now requires that the party requesting the deposition of an opponent's specially retained expert witness must "pay the expert a reasonable fee for time spent in responding to discovery under this subdivision." The federal requirement of compensation for "for time spent in responding to discovery" arguably should include time spent preparing an expert report and a reasonable amount of time spent in preparation for the deposition. Some federal courts have allowed compensation for preparation, while others have not or have allowed it only as to preparation for depositions in complex cases.[38,53(§2034)] To the extent that the opponent does not compensate for deposition preparation by a retained expert, this cost remains the responsibility of the client and/or the friendly attorney. The federal provision mandates compensation from the opponent only for experts who are specially retained, whereas the practice in most states also requires the opponent to pay professional fees for taking the deposition of treating physicians. Insofar as treating physicians are not entitled to compensation from the opponents for time spent in discovery, they may be entitled to compensation from the patient or the patient's attorney under state rules or local customs.

The witness can be required to bring certain materials to a deposition and can be asked about these materials or any writings reviewed in preparation. The physician should not disclose any confidential documents without first verifying the patient's waiver or authorization. The witness should consult with the friendly attorney about materials that must be brought and about other materials that may be helpful, such as medical texts or published or hand-drawn illustrations and exhibits.

Depositions usually are taken in the office of one of the attorneys, but for the physician's convenience and to minimize cost, it can be taken at the physician's office. If so, it should be scheduled to avoid distractions, and care should be taken to prevent inappropriate access to medical records.[43] In general, the location and timing of the deposition should be at the convenience of the witness, and the physician can seek to reschedule any deposition scheduled without prior consultation.

The persons present at a deposition include the witness (often called the "deponent"), the attorneys for the parties, and the court reporter who records the testimony. In some cases the deposition is videotaped so that the judge and jury can see and hear the witness if the deposition is used at the trial. The plaintiff and the defendant also have a right to attend depositions. The court reporter usually is seated at one end of the table, with the witness and the interrogating attorney across from each other at that end. The friendly attorney usually sits next to the witness except when asking questions. The witness is entitled to decorum and quiet. The witness may request a recess when needed, during which private consultation with the friendly attorney is appropriate.[18,43]

The witness is placed under oath and asked questions, first by one attorney and then by the other. If the deposition is being taken for use at trial, the procedure is the same as for trial testimony, with the friendly attorney conducting a direct examination, the opposing attorney then conducting a cross examination, and the attorneys conducting further re-direct and re-cross-examination to follow up on particular points. If the deposition is being taken at the request of the opponent for purposes of discovery, the opponent's attorney asks most of the questions, and there may be little or no responsive questioning by the friendly attorney except to clarify any significant ambiguities or correct misleading impressions or mistakes.

The scope of inquiry is broader in a discovery deposition than in a deposition taken for use at trial. At trial, interrogation is restricted to questions seeking to elicit admissible testimony, whereas at a discovery deposition the witness can be asked questions that are "reasonably calculated to lead to the discovery of admissible evidence" (Fed.R.Civ.P. Rule 26(b)(1)).

The attorneys may object to certain questions. After stating an objection, the attorney often will allow the witness to answer, leaving it to the judge to decide later whether that portion of the deposition can be used in court. The witness should not answer until instructed to do so by the friendly attorney. The witness should listen carefully to objections, especially to those by the friendly attorney, which may be important cues. The witness has no right to object except to assert matters of confidentiality and privilege (e.g., physician-patient privilege or the privilege against self-incrimination), but the witness can cue the attorney to object by asking whether it is

necessary to answer a particular question.[43]

In a discovery deposition, the opposing attorney usually does not try to attack the witness but rather attempts to determine the extent of the witness's knowledge and subtly probes for weaknesses. In order to evaluate the potential strength of a physician's trial testimony, avoid surprises at trial, and prepare for cross-examination, the opposing attorney can be expected to fully explore all aspects of the anticipated direct examination, including the physician's qualifications, the physician's opinions, and the factual and scientific basis for those opinions. The most effective questioners attempt to put deposition witnesses at ease so that they will concede weaknesses or uncertainties, make overstatements, or create inconsistencies that can be used at trial to discredit the testimony. If the trial testimony is inconsistent with statements at the deposition, the deposition can be read aloud in court to "impeach" or contradict the witness.

The witness has a right to review the deposition transcript and ordinarily will be sent a copy of the deposition for a signature verifying its accuracy. Any errors by the witness in answering or by the court reporter in transcription should be noted in writing and sent to the attorney for transmittal to the court reporter. The court reporter must correct errors in transcription on the document itself; errors by the witness should be noted separately. At the conclusion of the deposition, the witness may be asked whether he wishes to "waive reading and signing" and rely on the accuracy of the court reporter. The pros and cons of doing so should be discussed with the friendly attorney, preferably prior to the deposition.[43]

Affidavits

The process of investigation and discovery sometimes reveals the existence of a core of undisputed facts that makes it possible for particular issues or even the entire case to be resolved without a trial because the law entitles one of the parties to prevail in whole or in part based on those undisputed facts. If so, one or both parties may file a motion for "summary judgment" which asks the court to enter judgment based on the undisputed facts (Fed.R.Civ.P. Rule 56). For example, the defendant may be entitled to summary judgment as a matter of law if the plaintiff failed to file suit within the time specified by the applicable statute of limitations, if the plaintiff has no evidence to support allegations of negligence by the defendant, or if the plaintiff has no evidence to support a causal connection between a defendant's negligence and the plaintiff's injuries. On the other hand, when there is undisputed evidence that the plaintiff was injured as a result of the defendant's negligence, the trial court can grant partial summary judgment on the issue of liability and limit the issues at trial to determining the extent of the plaintiff's damages.

Expert witnesses often play an important role in providing evidence to support or resist motions for summary judgment. The party seeking summary judgment usually needs supporting documentation in the form of one or more "affidavits," which are written statements under oath in which potential trial witnesses recite the undisputed facts on which the motion is based. The party opposing summary judgment usually provides counter-affidavits from potential witnesses to dispute the facts recited in the affidavits supporting the motion for summary judgment or to recite additional facts that demonstrate the existence of a factual dispute necessitating a trial of the issue.[39]

It is entirely appropriate for a physician's affidavit to be drafted by the friendly attorney to assure that it uses the precise language necessary to contradict particular statements in opposing affidavits or to meet standards established by applicable legal rules. Nevertheless, an affidavit is the sworn statement of the witness, so it must be honest and accurate. The attorney should consult with the physician in preparing the affidavit, and the physician must review the affidavit carefully and insist on any appropriate revisions before signing it. The physician can be questioned about the affidavit at any subsequent deposition or at trial.

ACTIVITIES OF THE PHYSICIAN AS EXPERT CONSULTANT

An expert consultant can assist the attorney at all stages in a dispute, from initially evaluating whether a claim should be asserted to assist-

ing at the trial itself. While an expert consultant is paid to assist one party to a dispute, the consultant best promotes that party's interests by retaining an objective perspective and communicating to the attorney the weaknesses as well as the strengths of the party's case.

Role of the Physician-Consultant Prior to Litigation

A conscientious attorney often will seek the services of an expert consultant at the earliest stages of a dispute.[13] A physician may be asked to educate the attorney concerning technical aspects of the case, explaining such matters as the notations and jargon in medical records. The physician-consultant can help the attorney evaluate the merits of the case. For example, in a malpractice case, the physician-consultant can identify possible factors that in theory could have contributed to an unfavorable outcome and help the attorney conduct an investigation to rule these factors in or out. In a personal injury case, the physician-consultant can evaluate the patient's prognosis and the extent to which the patient's condition is attributable to a recent accident as opposed to prior accidents or underlying disease processes. In toxic tort litigation, the physician-consultant can review medical literature for evidence supporting a causal link between a toxic exposure and a patient's current condition or a risk of future disease. A physician-consultant may be asked to design experiments or tests that could generate factual data to support a particular claim. If the tests generated useful data, the persons who conducted the tests would be potential expert witnesses to testify about the results at trial.

Role of the Physician-Consultant in Pretrial Proceedings

Once a decision has been made to initiate legal proceedings, the physician-consultant can assist the attorney in drafting the formal documents or "pleadings" by which a claim is asserted or defended. The physician working with the plaintiff's attorney can assist in drafting the "complaint," the document which sets forth the factual and legal basis on which recovery is sought. Likewise, the physician advising the defendant can assist in drafting the "answer," a document which may dispute the facts asserted in the complaint or assert additional facts that may be relevant and explain why recovery would not be warranted under the defendant's version of the facts.

The physician-consultant can also assist in the formal discovery proceedings by which the attorney obtains information about the case from the opposing party and other witnesses.[13,23,31,33] Each party is permitted to request the opposing party to make documents available for inspection and copying (Fed.R.Civ.P. Rule 34), to answer written questions ("interrogatories") under oath (Fed.R.Civ.P. Rule 33), and to appear in person to answer questions at a deposition (Fed.R.Civ.P. Rule 30). Witnesses who are not parties can be compelled to attend depositions and to bring with them relevant documents (Fed.R.Civ.P. Rule 45). The physician serving as a consultant can help the attorney in conducting this formal discovery by suggesting questions to ask in interrogatories or at depositions and by helping identify the relevant documents that might be in the possession of the opposing party or other witnesses.[13,23,31,33]

The consultant also can assist the attorney in responding to discovery initiated by the opponent. For example, the consultant can assist in drafting answers to interrogatories and can help prepare testifying expert witnesses for their depositions.[13,23,31,33]

Beyond assisting in development of the theoretical and factual foundation for the case, the expert consultant can work with the attorney in trial preparation. The consultant can identify other professionals who might serve as expert witnesses at trial, serve as liaison to these experts, and can evaluate the credentials of the opponent's experts.[13]

Role of the Physician-Consultant at Trial

The physician who serves as an expert consultant can continue to assist the attorney in last-minute preparation for trial and even in the courtroom.[13,23,31,33] A good consultant can help develop the paradigms and metaphors for translating technical information to a jury. The physician-consultant can help prepare expert witnesses for their trial testimony, especially by anticipating topics and questions that are likely to be explored on cross examination. Finally, the consultant can attend the trial itself, assisting in evaluation of jurors, suggesting additional questions to ask opposing expert witnesses, or focusing on the key points for closing argument.

Discovery from a Physician-Consultant

Unlike expert witnesses, whose reports are furnished to opponents and whose testimony frequently is taken at pretrial depositions, physicians who serve entirely in a consulting role usually remain behind-the-scenes and cannot be compelled to give testimony at depositions. In general, opposing parties are not even entitled to discover the identity of nontestifying experts who are specially retained to give advice concerning litigation.[13,38,53(§2032)]

The policy underlying the general rule against discovery from expert consultants is that a party should not be able to use an opponent's experts to prepare its own case. Also, because expert consultants work closely with the party's attorney, they frequently become acquainted with the thoughts, mental impressions, opinions, or conclusions of the attorney which constitute the attorney's "work product," and this work product generally is privileged against disclosure during litigation.[53(§2032)] Finally, depending on state law, the physician-consultant who works with an attorney may be able to receive confidential information that the client furnished to the attorney without loss of the attorney-client privilege. Thus, the consultation services of an expert are confidential, and the consulting expert is not generally subject to discovery.

Only under "extraordinary circumstances" will the court allow a party to obtain discovery about facts known or opinions held by an opponent's nontestifying expert consultants or even to ascertain their identity.[13,23,38,53(§2032)] The federal courts allow discovery of nontestifying consultants only "upon a showing of exceptional circumstances under which it is impracticable for the party seeking discovery to obtain facts or opinions on the same subject by other means" (Fed.R.Civ.P. Rule 26(b)(4)(B)). Such cases generally involve disputes about things that were altered or destroyed after an examination by the consultant but prior to any examination by the opponent, such as a tissue sample or a transient condition of a patient.[23,53(§2032)] Even if these exceptional circumstances exist, the scope of any inquiry would be limited to the essential facts or opinions that justified the discovery, such as providing copies of existing reports.

A special rule affords even greater protection against discovery with respect to experts who were contacted by an attorney but were not retained to assist in the litigation. No discovery whatsoever is allowed concerning experts who have no first-hand knowledge of relevant facts and who were informally consulted but not retained.[13,38] To the extent that nonretained experts are subject to discovery, it would not be based on the informal consultation itself but rather on "extraordinary circumstances" that independently justified discovery from these experts based on their unique expertise (see above).[53(§2033)]

PRETRIAL ACTIVITIES OF PHYSICIANS IN CRIMINAL CASES

The involvement of physicians in criminal cases differs greatly from that in civil litigation in two respects. First, criminal cases frequently involve expert testimony by physicians with special forensic training. Second, the pretrial procedures for ordinary physicians who are occurrence witnesses in criminal cases differ substantially from those in civil cases.

Physicians Who Are Forensic Experts

Forensic medicine is a specialized area of medicine concerned with presentation of evidence in judicial proceedings.[49] Although forensic medicine deals with testimony in civil as well as criminal cases, the two most well-developed areas of forensic medicine—forensic pathology

and forensic psychiatry—play special roles in criminal cases.

The physicians who most frequently become involved in criminal cases are those employed in the office of a coroner or medical examiner, whose regular duties include forensic investigation and who frequently specialize in forensic pathology. The coroner or medical examiner must evaluate all unexpected deaths or those that occur under suspicious circumstances in order to determine the cause of death and ascertain whether the manner of death was natural or unnatural (i.e., accident, suicide, or homicide).[29,31,48,49] In addition to completing a death certificate, the physicians who work with the coroner or medical examiner usually are called as witnesses in criminal trials to establish the cause and manner of death and testify about other details learned during the autopsy of the victim. The activities of physicians employed by a coroner or medical examiner are beyond the scope of this chapter and are considered in detail elsewhere.[48,49]

Forensic psychiatric opinion testimony is needed whenever the facts and circumstances raise substantial questions about the sanity of a criminal defendant at the time of the crime or the defendant's current competence to understand and participate in the criminal proceedings. Upon an appropriate factual showing, the defendant is entitled to have the court pay for a psychiatric evaluation of the defendant's competence or sanity. Psychiatrists who conduct such examinations, whether appointed by the court or retained by the defendant or the prosecution, must prepare reports. The standards employed in these evaluations are discussed in the chapter on mental incompetence (see Chapter 7).

Physicians Who Are Occurrence Witnesses

The physicians who are most likely to become occurrence witnesses in criminal cases are those who work in hospital emergency rooms and treat patients who are victims of criminal violence. These patients include not only victims of intentional criminal attacks—assault and battery (including child abuse, geriatric abuse, and sexual assault), stabbing and shooting—but also those injured in vehicular accidents caused by reckless or substance-impaired drivers. Although patients who are crime victims most frequently enter the hospital via the emergency room, other physicians who treat these patients can also become witnesses in criminal proceedings.

Physicians who treat the victims or alleged perpetrators of crimes may have a statutory duty to report certain information to public authorities (see Chapter 2).[29] These reporting requirements vary according to state law. With regard to patients who die, physicians are obligated to report death under suspicious, unusual or unnatural circumstances, such as: from violence or by apparent suicide; within 24 hours of hospital admission or surgery; when an inmate of a public institution; suddenly when in apparently good health; from an infectious disease that might constitute a threat to public health; or when there is no attending physician to certify the cause of death. The forensic investigation of these deaths by a coroner or medical examiner may lead to criminal prosecutions for intentional or negligent homicide. With regard to living patients, physicians are obligated to report infectious diseases, traumatic injuries from violent acts (e.g., gunshots and certain stabbings), and injuries that suggest abuse of members of vulnerable groups (e.g., children, impaired adults, the institutionalized elderly, and domestic abuse). Investigation of these injuries may lead to criminal prosecutions in which the reporting physician will be an important witness.

In addition to reporting pertinent information to public authorities, physicians should make reasonable efforts to preserve evidence of possible criminal or civil wrongdoing. The duty to preserve relevant information can be inferred from the AMA's opinion relating to medical testimony, which broadly declares: "As a citizen and as a professional with special training and experience, the physician has an ethical obligation to assist in the administration of justice."[9] The chapter on observation and description of trauma discusses the important evidence that physicians may encounter in treating various types of wounds, explaining how to preserve physical evidence (bullets, clothing, tissue samples) and how to document these observations through photographs, drawings, and notations

in medical records. Chapters 11 and 12 on abused patients provide details about the particular observations and evidence that may be relevant to proof of sexual assault or abuse, child abuse, spouse abuse, and geriatric abuse.

Pretrial activities of witnesses in criminal proceedings differ greatly from those in civil litigation. Whereas much of the pretrial investigation in civil cases consists of discovery undertaken after the filing of a complaint, most of the investigation in criminal cases occurs prior to the issuance of an indictment. In cases investigated by a grand jury, a physician may be subpoenaed to give testimony, but the proceedings are secret and the targets of the investigation are not entitled to attend. When a preliminary hearing is held to determine whether the evidence is sufficient to justify holding the defendant for trial, the hearing occurs before a judge in open court; the procedures resemble those in a trial. Whereas all parties in civil litigation can obtain subpoenas ordering occurrence witnesses to bring relevant documents and testify at a deposition, no such right exists under rules of criminal procedure. Criminal investigations thus depend quite heavily on the voluntary cooperation of persons having relevant information.

Once a physician has complied with any mandatory reporting requirements, there is no *legal* obligation to meet with either the prosecution or the defense prior to trial. Nevertheless, the *ethical* duty to "assist in the administration of justice" imposes an obligation on the physician to make reasonable efforts to cooperate with investigators or attorneys representing both the prosecution and the defendants in criminal proceedings. Absent special circumstances, such as a statute or court order mandating secrecy, a witness is permitted to meet with the defendant's counsel, and it is improper for the prosecutor to suggest otherwise.[11] Providing information to the prosecution assists in the administration of justice by facilitating conviction of the guilty and dismissal of charges against the innocent. Cooperation with the defense may assist in the administration of justice by encouraging appropriate pleas of guilty and by preventing unfair surprise to defendants at trial.[11] Also, physicians who have little or no relevant evidence about an alleged crime can benefit themselves by letting this be known to the defense in order to avoid being called to testify at trial by conscientious defense attorneys who might otherwise hope that the physician's testimony could be helpful in raising a reasonable doubt about the defendant's guilt.

Because these pretrial interviews are conducted without judicial supervision, the physician can meet separately with the prosecution and the defense without giving the other side notice or an opportunity to attend. On the other hand, the physician can insist on meeting only in the presence of investigators or attorneys for both sides, which might be desirable to avoid the inconvenience of multiple interviews, to protect against undue pressure from one side, or to eliminate suspicion that the physician was selectively favoring the other side.

New Mandatory Disclosures in Federal Criminal Prosecutions

Recent amendments to the Federal Rules of Criminal Procedure have substantially diminished the need for informal interviews with expert witnesses in federal prosecutions by providing for certain mandatory disclosures. The 1993 amendments added the following provision to Federal Rule of Criminal Procedure Rule 16:

> At the defendant's request, the government shall disclose to the defendant a written summary of testimony the government intends to use under Rules 702, 703, or 705 of the Federal Rules of Evidence [i.e., testimony from expert witnesses] during its case in chief at trial. This summary must describe the witnesses' opinions, the bases and the reasons therefore, and the witnesses' qualifications. (Fed.R.Crim.P. Rule 16(a)(1)(E))

If the defendant requests disclosure under this provision, the defendant must make a similar disclosure upon the government's request (Fed.R.Crim.P. Rule 16(b)(1)(C)).

This disclosure requirement applies to all expert witnesses, including employees of the government, treating physicians who are occurrence witnesses, or any specially retained expert witnesses. Thus, any physician who expects to testify in a federal criminal trial can also expect to be asked to help prepare a report summarizing the anticipated testimony.

The information that must be provided under these new criminal procedures is somewhat less detailed than that required under the new mandatory disclosure rules in civil litigation (see above), and the parties have no right to obtain additional information through depositions. Nevertheless, so long as these summaries are prepared in good faith, they should fulfill their intended purpose: "to minimize surprise that often results from unexpected expert testimony, reduce the need for continuances, and to provide the opponent with a fair opportunity to test the merit of the expert's testimony through focused cross-examination."[37] These mandatory disclosures should also reduce the pressure on physicians to provide this information informally to attorneys who represent defendants in criminal prosecutions. If the states were to adopt similar disclosure requirements, physicians would be relieved of the burden of informal interviews with defense counsel in criminal cases.

IMPROVING THE QUALITY OF EXPERT WITNESSES

Concerns about the ability and integrity of experts witnesses have been expressed by members of the medical and legal professions for over a century.[20,21,25,48] Reformers regularly advocate increased use of court-appointed experts in lieu of the current practice of partisan selection and preparation of expert witnesses.[21] Courts have been given the authority to appoint expert witnesses, yet they rarely avail themselves of this power.[21] Parties to civil litigation almost never ask the courts to appoint expert witnesses, apparently because the attorneys in our adversary system of justice are reluctant to relinquish their control over expert testimony.[21] An intermediate reform proposal would allow the parties to retain their role in designating experts but have the court appoint the witnesses and restrict pretrial contact with attorneys in order to minimize partisan witness preparation.[21]

State legislatures have begun to address the problem by enacting standards for expert witnesses, such as requirements that they be actively engaged in practice within the field or spend less than 20% of their time in court.[25] It is difficult to employ perjury as a sanction for expert testimony in which the witness expresses opinions rather than facts.[21,48] Nevertheless, perjury prosecutions have been initiated against experts who lied about their credentials,[48] and they could be brought against experts who give inconsistent scientific testimony in successive lawsuits.

Professional organizations have attempted to improve the quality of expert testimony by establishing guidelines or standards. Examples include the 1987 guidelines of the American Association of Neurological Surgeons (AANS)[4] and a 1989 statement of the American College of Surgeons.[8] Attempts at discipline by professional organizations are limited by the rights of free speech and prohibition on intimidation of witnesses (obstruction of justice), but these organizations can assist in the discrediting of experts who testify inappropriately.[41] The AANS now maintains a file of transcripts of expert testimony and depositions, cross-indexed by case name, name of the expert, and several key words, which serves as a neutral source of information.[40] The Defense Research Institute has established a computerized nationwide registry of approximately 18,000 experts from various medical and technical fields who have testified in civil litigation.[36] Sources such as these can be used to discredit or impeach a witness who has given inconsistent testimony in prior cases or has repeatedly worked with a particular lawyer.[41]

The success of efforts to improve the quality of expert testimony largely depends on the attorneys' ability to obtain information in pretrial discovery proceedings. Thus, despite the inconvenience and occasional unpleasantness of pretrial discovery, physicians should recognize that this process contributes to the quality of expert testimony as well as being essential to the adversary process of dispute resolution.

REFERENCES

1. 42 Pa CSA, Rules of Civ Proc Rule 40035
2. Advisory Committee Notes to Federal Rules Civil Procedure Rule 26 (reprinted at 146 FRD 627 (1993))
3. Advisory Committee Notes to Federal Rules Criminal Procedure Rule 45 (reprinted at 134 FRD 668 (1991))
4. American Association of Neurological Surgeons: The dos and don'ts of testimony. **AANS Newsletter** 1990(8):19, 1990
5. American Bar Association: **Model Code of Professional Responsibility**, in effect as of August 1983, DR-7-109(c) (reprinted in Gillers S, Simon RD Jr (eds): **Regulation of Lawyers: Statutes and Standards.** Boston, Mass: Little, Brown, & Co, 1992, 782 pp)
6. American Bar Association: **Model Rules of Professional Conduct**, as amended through August 1991, comment to Rule 34 (reprinted in Gillers S, Simon RD Jr (eds): **Regulation of Lawyers: Statutes and Standards.** Boston, Mass: Little, Brown, & Co, 1992, 782 pp)
7. American Bar Association: **Model Rules of Professional Conduct**, as amended through August 1991, Rule 34 (reprinted in Gillers S, Simon RD Jr (eds): **Regulation of Lawyers: Statutes and Standards.** Boston, Mass: Little, Brown, & Co, 1992, 782 pp)
8. American College of Surgeons: Statement on the physician expert witness. **Am Coll Surg Bull 74(8):** 6-7, 1989
9. American Medical Association, Council of Ethical and Judicial Affairs: **Current Opinions.** Chicago, Ill: American Medical Association, 1989, p 38, No. 907
10. Chu MC: Discovery of experts, in Rossi FF (ed): **Expert Witnesses.** Chicago, Ill: American Bar Association, 1991, pp 171-191
11. Cohen J: Should a witness allow an interview by criminal defense counsel? **NY Law J 215:**1(col 1), Feb 8, 1996
12. *Deitchman v ER Squibb & Sons, Inc,* 740 F2d 556 (7th Cir 1984)
13. Dombroff: **Expert Witnesses in Civil Trials: Effective Preparation and Presentation.** Rochester, NY: The Lawyers Co-Operative Publishing, 1987, 390 pp
14. Fairchild J: Right of independent expert to refuse to testify to expert opinion. **ALR 4th 50:**680, 1986
15. Federal Rules of Civil Procedure, 28 USC
16. Federal Rules of Criminal Procedure, 18 USC
17. Federal Rules of Evidence, Rule 801(d)(2), 28 USC
18. Fish RM, Ehrhardt ME: **Malpractice Depositions.** Oradell, NJ: Medical Economics, 1987, 152 pp
19. Fleming TM: Right of party to have attorney or physician present during physical or mental examination at instance of opposing party. **ALR 4th 84:** 558, 1991
20. Graham MH: Expert witness testimony and the Federal Rules of Evidence: insuring adequate assurance of trustworthiness. **U Ill Law Rev 1986:**43-90, 1986
21. Gross SR: Expert evidence. **Wisc Law Rev 1991:** 1113-1232, 1991
22. Hanley RF: Preparing the expert witness, in Rossi FF (ed): **Expert Witnesses.** Chicago, Ill: American Bar Association, 1991, pp 155-170
23. Hayes JL, Ryder PT Jr: Rule 26(b)(4) of the Federal Rules of Civil Procedure: discovery of expert information. **U Miami Law Rev 42:**1101-1186, 1988
24. Horsley JE, Carlova J: **Testifying in Court.** Oradell, NJ: Medical Economics, 1988, 150 pp
25. Huber PW: **Galileo's Revenge: Junk Science in the Courtroom.** New York, NY: Basic Books, 1991, 274 pp
26. *In re American Tobacco Co,* 880 F2d 1520 (2d Cir 1989)
27. *Jones v Constantino,* 631 A2d 1289 (Pa Super 1993), *appeal den,* 649 A2d 673 (Pa 1994)

28. *Kaufman v Adelstein*, 539 F2d 811 (2nd Cir 1976)
29. Kaufman HH, Lewin J, Munzner R, et al: Ethical and legal responsibilities of the neurosurgeon: selected topics. **Neurosurgery 28:**918-923, 1991
30. Klawans HL: **Trials of an Expert Witness.** Boston, Mass: Little, Brown, & Co, 1991, 277 pp
31. Leestma JE, Magee DJ: Pathology and neuropathology in the forensic setting, in Leestma JE (ed): **Forensic Neuropathology.** New York, NY: Raven Press, 1988, pp 1-23
32. Marcus RL: Evidence: discovery along the litigation/science interface. **Brooklyn Law Rev 57:**381, 1991
33. Matson JV: **Effective Expert Witnessing: A Handbook for Technical Professionals.** Chelsea, Mich: Lewis, 1990, 145 pp
34. *Mohr v District Court of Fourth Judicial District*, 660 P2d 88 (Mont 1983)
35. *Moore v Armour Pharmaceutical Co*, 927 F2d 1194 (11th Cir 1991)
36. Nora PF: National registry collects data on expert witnesses. **Am Coll Surg Bull 75(8):**16-17, 1990
37. Piorkowski JD Jr: Medical testimony and the expert witness, in American College of Legal Medicine (ed): **Legal Medicine: Legal Dynamics of Medical Encounters.** 3rd ed. St Louis, Mo: Mosby-Year Book, 1995, pp 141-155
38. Raeder MS: **Federal Pretrial Practice.** 2nd ed. Charlottesville, Va: Michie Butterworth, 1995, 1003 pp
39. Rossi FF: Pretrial consequences of liberal admissibility, in Rossi FF (ed): **Expert Witnesses.** Chicago, Ill: American Bar Association, 1991, pp 119-133
40. Rovit LR, Hauber C: The expert witness: some observations and a response from neurosurgeons. **Am Coll Surg Bull 74(7):**10-16, 1989
41. Spencer FC: The expert witness: one surgeon's opinion. **Am Coll Surg Bull 73(5):**11-14, 43, 1988
42. *Stoughton v BPOE #2151 (Brick Twsp Elks)*, 658 A2d 1335 (NJ Super 1995)
43. Taraska JM: The physician as a witness, in Taraska JM: **Legal Guide for Physicians.** White Plains, NY: AHAB Press, 1997, pp 9.1-9.56
44. *Tirado v Erosa*, 158 FRD 294 (SDNY 1994)
45. Underwood RH: "X-spurt" witnesses. **Am J Trial Advoc 19:**343, 1995
46. *Walsh v Kubiak*, 661 A2d 416 (Pa Super 1995), *appeal den*, 672 A2d 309 (Pa 1996)
47. *Warrick v Brode*, 46 FRD 427 (D Del 1969)
48. Wecht CH: Forensic pathology, in American College of Legal Medicine (ed): **Legal Medicine: Legal Dynamics of Medical Encounters.** 3rd ed. St Louis, Mo: Mosby-Year Book, 1995, pp 567-584
49. Wecht CH: Forensic use of medical information, in American College of Legal Medicine (ed): **Legal Medicine: Legal Dynamics of Medical Encounters.** 3rd ed. St Louis, Mo: Mosby-Year Book, 1995, pp 558-566
50. *Wilkins v Palumbo*, 617 So2d 850 (Fla App 1993)
51. *Wreath v United States*, 161 FRD 448 (D Kan 1995)
52. Wright CA, Miller AR: **Federal Practice and Procedure: Civil, Vol 9A.** 2nd ed. St Paul, Minn: West Publishing, 1994, 709 pp (and 1996 Suppl, 55 pp), §§2451-2466 (Rule 45)
53. Wright CA, Miller AR, Marcus RL: **Federal Practice and Procedure: Civil, Vol 8.** 2nd ed. St Paul, Minn: West Publishing, 1994, 688 pp (and 1996 Suppl, 64 pp), §§2001-2054 (Rule 26)
54. Wright CA, Miller AR, Marcus RL: **Federal Practice and Procedure: Civil, Vol 8A.** 2nd ed. St Paul, Minn: West Publishing, 1994, 740 pp (and 1996 Suppl, 24 pp), §§2231-2250 (Rule 35)

CHAPTER 4

TESTIMONY AT TRIAL

JEFF L. LEWIN, JD

The use of medical and other expert witnesses in civil and criminal litigation has increased dramatically in recent years.[21,43,45] Among the topics addressed in this chapter are the following:

1. how expert testimony differs from testimony of ordinary lay occurrence witnesses;
2. circumstances under which expert testimony is permitted or required;
3. qualifications of an expert witness;
4. the structure of expert testimony;
5. the content of expert testimony;
6. preparation for expert testimony;
7. the characteristics of effective expert testimony; and
8. cross-examination.

Trials are conducted in accordance with rules of criminal and civil procedure, and the testimony of trial witnesses in all such proceedings is governed by rules of evidence (see Chapter 1). The rules of evidence initially were created by judges, and they evolved within the common law system through appellate decisions in England and in the United States. In 1975, Congress adopted the Federal Rules of Evidence (hereinafter sometimes "Federal Rules" or "Rules"),[12]

a comprehensive code of evidentiary rules for the federal courts. In the ensuing two decades, roughly three-quarters of the states adopted evidence codes modeled in whole or in part on the Federal Rules of Evidence.[29] Accordingly, this chapter discusses physician testimony in relation to the Federal Rules of Evidence, making parenthetical reference to particular rules. Practices in individual states may vary, however.

TESTIMONY OF LAY AND EXPERT WITNESSES

As discussed in Chapter 1, the rules of evidence distinguish between two types of witnesses: occurrence witnesses and expert witnesses. When physicians testify, they frequently serve as both occurrence witnesses and expert witnesses. A physician who was a treating or consulting physician may testify as an ordinary occurrence witness with respect to any direct observations. The physician is an expert witness, however, whenever the testimony consists of inferences or conclusions, including professional opinions about the diagnosis of a condition, its cause, or its prognosis.

The rules governing expert testimony are quite complex and have been the subject of substantial controversy for well over a century.[20,21] Under the Federal Rules of Evidence, testimony of expert witnesses is governed by Rules 701-706.

Whereas lay occurrence witnesses generally are limited to testimony about direct first-hand observations "based on personal knowledge" (Rule 602), physicians and other expert witnesses are permitted to testify about inferences, conclusions, or opinions (Rule 702). Moreover, in forming an expert opinion, a physician is not confined to relying on direct observation but may base an opinion on information learned from third parties, such as treatises, journal articles, or notations in medical records. Even though the underlying information constitutes inadmissible hearsay (Rules 801, 802), it can provide the foundation for an expert's opinion as long as the facts or data are "of a type reasonably relied upon by experts in the particular field in forming opinions or inferences upon the subject" (Rule 703). Physicians are even permitted to testify to the content of certain statements made by their patients under a special exception to the hearsay rule which recognizes the inherent reliability of statements "made for purposes of medical diagnosis or treatment and describing medical history, or past or present symptoms, pain, or sensations, or the inception or general character of the cause or external source thereof insofar as reasonably pertinent to diagnosis or treatment" (Rule 803(4)).

On direct examination, lay witnesses may not be asked leading questions, which suggest a particular answer (Rule 611(c)), nor may they be permitted to give an unfocused narrative (Rule 611(a)), which risks introduction of irrelevant and inadmissible evidence.[38] Both of these rules are relaxed, however, for expert witnesses.

When testifying within their fields of expertise, expert witnesses are assumed to be less susceptible to leading questions, so courts frequently permit the friendly attorney to use leading questions during direct examination of an expert witness. Indeed, the use of leading questions may be essential to assist the jury in focusing on the issue which is the subject of the expert's opinion.

In order to fulfill the function of helping the jury to understand the evidence, an expert witness often must educate the jury about the underlying scientific principles, which may require an extended explanation that would be impeded by the usual question-and-answer format of direct examination.[9] To facilitate clarity of exposition, judges frequently allow expert witnesses to explain a scientific or technical principal to the jury in the form of a lecture that would be considered impermissible narrative testimony if a lay witness were testifying.

WHEN IS EXPERT TESTIMONY REQUIRED OR PERMITTED?

Traditional common law rules restricted the use of expert testimony insofar as courts allowed experts to testify only when "necessary." In particular, the common law did not permit use of expert testimony with respect to matters of common knowledge, but only to assist the jury in evaluating evidence that was "beyond the ken of the average layperson."[43,45]

The Federal Rules of Evidence are more receptive to the use of expert testimony.[45] Under Rule 702, expert testimony is not limited to situations where it is "necessary," but can be used whenever it would be "helpful" to the jury:

> If scientific, technical, or other specialized knowledge *will assist the trier of fact to understand the evidence or to determine a fact in issue*, a witness qualified as an expert by knowledge, skill, experience, training, or education, may testify thereto in the form of an opinion or otherwise.

Even under Rule 702, however, some courts continue to adhere to the view that expert testimony is inadmissible when the subject matter is within the knowledge or experience of laypersons.[43] An example of the more receptive approach was the decision of a federal appellate court upholding the admission of testimony by an experimental psychologist about the attractiveness of brightly colored elevator buttons and the accessibility of uncovered buttons.[4] Taking a more restrictive approach, another federal appellate court upheld the exclusion of testimony by an accident reconstruction expert, reasoning that where "the subject matter is within the knowledge or experience of laypersons, expert testimony is superfluous" and thus not helpful.[10]

Even the more restrictive approach is unlikely to present an obstacle to expert testimony by a physician, however, since courts generally respect the substantial education and training necessary to obtain a medical degree and recognize that the specialized knowledge possessed by physicians is far "beyond the ken of the average layperson." The testimony of a physician is likely to be "helpful" to the jury whenever it addresses an issue that is relevant to the dispute and represents a professional opinion based on recognized scientific principles and reliable data.

Expert testimony is frequently required as a matter of law to establish particular facts in civil or criminal cases. For example, in personal injury cases, expert testimony often is needed to establish that an accident, product or toxic exposure was a "substantial contributing factor" or cause of the plaintiff's injuries and also to establish the present and future consequences of those injuries. In a claim for professional malpractice, a jury ordinarily will not be permitted to find for the plaintiff unless a member of the profession testifies that the defendant's conduct failed to measure up to the profession's standard of care. In criminal cases, expert testimony often is essential to establish that the victim's traumatic injury or death was caused by a criminal act as opposed to accidental or natural causes. For example, only a physician may be able to determine whether a criminal assault was the cause of a child's cerebral hemorrhage or an elderly victim's heart attack.

Even where expert testimony is not required as a matter of law, it may help the jury understand the evidence and often supplies essential circumstantial evidence. For example, a physician who examined a victim's wound may be able to give an opinion about the instrument that caused the injury and the amount of force employed, which may help the jury decide whether the wound was inflicted intentionally or accidentally. In a personal injury case, a physician can help the jury understand the nature and severity of a patient's injuries by describing the pain and limitations of function ordinarily associated with those injuries. In a criminal case, expert testimony can link the defendant with the crime through ballistics tests, fingerprint identification, or tissue matching.

QUALIFICATION AS AN EXPERT

Unlike ordinary occurrence witnesses, whose testimony is limited to what they observed, expert witnesses are called upon to give opinions in their field of expertise, so their training and experience within their profession is crucial to the validity of their testimony. Testimony about the credentials of an expert witness is important for two reasons.[9]

First, as a matter of law, the trial judge must find that the witness is "qualified as an expert by knowledge, skill, experience, training, or education" within a particular field (Rule 702). The field itself may be broadly or narrowly defined. Any physician may be qualified to give testimony about general principles of medical diagnosis and treatment, but only a member of the particular school (allopathic, osteopathic, chiropractic), profession (physician, nurse) or subspecialty (e.g., general surgeon or neurosurgeon) may be competent to give testimony about the "standard of care" in a malpractice action, and special training in forensics may be a prerequisite to testimony on particular topics.[25,37,45,50] The trial judge has broad discretion in ruling on whether a witness is qualified as an expert in a particular field.[45]

Several cases involving neurosurgeons may help illustrate the variability in the extent of expertise that may be required. In one criminal case, where the issue was whether a patient's head injury was caused by a fall down a flight of stairs or by a baseball bat wielded by the defendant, a second-year resident in neurosurgery was deemed competent to provide expert testimony.[42] By contrast, in another criminal case an experienced neurosurgeon who had examined the defendant to determine whether he suffered organic brain damage was *not* qualified to give an opinion about the sanity of the defendant because the physician was not familiar with the legal definition of insanity.[40] In a personal injury case, a court ruled that two non-neurosurgeons—an orthopedic surgeon who operated on the plaintiff and a neurologist who examined the plaintiff on behalf of the defendant—were qualified by virtue of their training and experience to give expert opinions in the field of neurosurgery.[49] Thus, the primary purpose of testimony about the qualifications of an expert witness is to satisfy the judge that the witness is competent to provide expert opinion testimony within the particular field or fields that are to be the subject of inquiry.

Second, as a matter of persuasion, the witness must convince the factfinder (either judge or jury) that he or she is a competent and credible expert (i.e., an authoritative member of the profession, whose opinion is entitled to belief). Juries are impressed by training and experience, position as a teacher of others, and publications by the witness on the particular subject. As illustrated in the examples above, residents or specialists in other fields may be competent to render expert opinions, but their testimony may not be persuasive in the face of contrary testimony from a more authoritative expert. Depending upon the nature of the case and the details of each individual's background, an experienced, board-certified, and well-published specialist may be more or less persuasive than a senior resident who has worked extensively with a particular technique or condition.

Upon the completion of background questions addressing the expert's credentials and experience, the friendly attorney may "offer" the witness as an expert in a particular field or fields, thereby asking the court to rule that the witness is permitted to give opinion testimony in these areas.[47] At this time, the opposing attorney usually is permitted to interrupt the direct examination for "voir dire" cross-examination on the subject of the expert's credentials. The opponent may take the position that the witness is not an expert or does not possess expertise in the field in which the opinion testimony will be offered. Although the opponent rarely succeeds in excluding the expert's opinion testimony, the real purpose of this interrogation is to undermine the expert's credibility before the jury gets an opportunity to hear the substance of the expert's opinion testimony.[37]

The opposing attorney may offer to stipulate that the witness is an expert so as to curtail extensive testimony on the expert's qualifications. The friendly attorney usually declines to accept the stipulation, however, because it is important for the jury to hear these qualifications in order to evaluate the credibility of the expert's testimony.[7,9,38,47]

THE STRUCTURE AND CONTENT OF EXPERT TESTIMONY

Expert opinion testimony essentially has a syllogistic structure. The major premise is a general scientific principle or theory ("if A and B are true, then X is true"); the minor premise is a particular set of facts ("A and B are true"); the opinion is the logical conclusion ("therefore X is true").[27]

Expert testimony need not culminate in an opinion. An expert could give a dissertation on scientific or medical principles and leave it to the jury to apply those principles to the facts.[18] On the other hand, it is usually more persuasive for the expert to provide an opinion, and an expert opinion frequently is legally required for proof of particular matters.

In determining the admissibility of expert testimony, the trial court is limited to consideration of the relevance of the opinion and the reliability of the expert's major and minor premise. If the scientific and factual bases for the opinion are sound, the court cannot exclude the expert's opinion on the grounds that it disagrees with the expert's conclusion. The *Daubert*[8] opinion firmly established the distinction between the trial court's duty to evaluate the expert's "methodology" and its lack of authority to second-guess the expert's "conclusion."[6,19] Thus, in determining the admissibility of an expert's opinion, the trial court must answer the following questions:

1. Would the opinion be relevant to an issue in the case?
2. Does the expert's major premise or methodology have a reliable scientific basis?
3. To the extent that the expert's minor premise included facts or data that were not introduced into evidence, were these facts or data of the type reasonably relied upon by experts in the witness's field?

THE SCIENTIFIC BASIS FOR EXPERT TESTIMONY

With regard to the major premise underlying expert testimony, the proponent of scientific, technical, or medical evidence has the burden of demonstrating its reliability. The traditional common law standard of reliability is known as the "*Frye*" rule, based on a 1923 decision that upheld the exclusion of testimony relating to an early version of a polygraph test.[15] Under the *Frye* rule, the proponent of scientific evidence must establish that the principle or technique has "gained general acceptance in the particular field."[15]

The rationale for the *Frye* rule is that it promotes uniformity of decision and avoids the necessity of repeated trials in which reliability is the subject of conflicting expert testimony. The *Frye* standard has been criticized on a number of grounds: it tends to deprive the courts of novel but reliable evidence; it promotes excessive judicial deference to scientific opinion; and its application is inconsistent and uncertain because of vagueness about what constitutes "novel scientific evidence," about the scope of the "particular field" and about the degree of support necessary to constitute "general acceptance."[2,16,18,31,39,41,45]

The Federal Rules of Evidence, adopted in 1975, promoted a more liberal approach to admissibility. The Rules made no reference to *Frye*, and commentators were divided over whether it remained a valid test under the Rules.[2,16-18,31,39,45] A growing number of state and federal courts rejected the *Frye* test. Some of these courts employed a "relevancy" test under which the trial court determined whether the proffered evidence would be "helpful" to the jury, while others applied a "reliability" test in which the reliability and probative value of the testimony were weighed against its potential to mislead the jury.[2,16-18,31,39,45]

Critics complained that the demise of *Frye* had opened the courts to a flood of "junk science."[26] Upon closer examination, it appeared that the leading critic had himself engaged in junk litigation science, funded by partisan institutions, and had based his conclusions on anecdotal evidence, some of which was unsubstantiated and much of which was exaggerated and distorted.[5,33]

The extensive debate over the continued vitality of the *Frye* rule in federal courts eventually was resolved in 1993 by the United States Supreme Court's decision in *Daubert v. Merrell*

Dow Pharmaceuticals,[8] which declared that "*Frye* has been superseded" by the Federal Rules of Evidence and that its "general acceptance" test "should not be applied in federal trials." The Court said that trial courts retained an important "gatekeeping responsibility" under the Federal Rules of Evidence, and the "primary locus of this obligation" is the reference to "scientific" knowledge in Rule 702:

> The subject of an expert's testimony must be "scientific . . . knowledge." The adjective "scientific" implies a grounding in the methods and procedures of science. Similarly, the word "knowledge" connotes more than subjective belief or unsupported speculation. . . . [I]n order to qualify as "scientific knowledge," an inference or assertion must be derived by the scientific method. Proposed testimony must be supported by appropriate validation—i.e., "good grounds," based on what is known. In short, the requirement than an expert's testimony pertain to "scientific knowledge" establishes a standard of evidentiary reliability.[8]

The Court further explained that when "[f]aced with a proffer of expert scientific testimony," the trial court must make "a preliminary assessment of whether the reasoning or methodology underlying the testimony is scientifically valid." Rejecting *Frye*'s "austere" general acceptance standard, the Supreme Court envisioned a flexible inquiry into various factors bearing on scientific validity. The Court took special note of four of these factors:[8]

1. testability or falsifiability ("whether it can be (or has been) tested");
2. "whether the theory or technique has been subjected to peer review and publication";
3. "the known or potential rate of error"; and
4. "general acceptance" within a relevant scientific community ("A 'reliability assessment does not require, although it does permit, explicit identification of a relevant scientific community and an express determination of a particular degree of acceptance within that community.'").

By including "general acceptance" in this list, the Supreme Court retained the *Frye* standard as one of several relevant factors for assessing evidentiary reliability.

It is not yet clear to what extent the state courts will follow *Daubert* in abandoning *Frye*'s exclusive reliance on "general acceptance."[29,34] While several state courts have abandoned *Frye* in light of *Daubert*, others—including Arizona, California, Colorado, Florida, Illinois, Missouri, Nebraska, New Jersey, and New York—have persisted in their adherence to *Frye*.[34,35,43]

Also, it is not clear to what extent *Daubert* applies to traditional medical testimony. While some authorities have interpreted *Daubert*, like *Frye*, as applying only to novel scientific evidence, others have suggested it applies more broadly.[11,13,29,34] Regardless of the precise scope of *Daubert*, the decision is certain to influence judicial evaluation of medical testimony.

In an important and carefully reasoned decision, *In re Paoli RR Yard PCB Litigation*,[30] the U.S. Court of Appeals for the Third Circuit recently applied *Daubert* to determine the admissibility of medical testimony based on differential diagnoses which purported to link the plaintiffs' cancers with exposure to polychlorinated biphenyl (PCB). The court noted that the four factors identified in *Daubert* were "of only limited help" in assessing the reliability of the doctors' methodologies in performing differential diagnosis, because unlike traditional science, which is "designed to produce general theories," differential diagnosis "involves assessing causation with respect to a particular individual."[30(p758)] The court recognized that "although differential diagnosis is a generally accepted technique, no particular combination of techniques chosen by a doctor to assess an individual patient is likely to have been generally accepted."[30(p758)] The court concluded "that performance of physical examinations, taking of medical histories, and employment of reliable laboratory tests all provide significant evidence of a reliable differential diagnosis, and that their absence makes it much less likely that a differential diagnosis is reliable."[30(p758)] Nevertheless, the court ruled that "a doctor does not always have to employ all of these techniques in order for the doctor's differential diagnosis to be reliable,"[30(p759)] and it concluded that the trial court had erred in its wholesale exclusion of the opinion testimony of the plaintiffs' two physicians. The court said that "the opinion of a doctor who had engaged in few standard diagnostic techniques should be excluded unless the doctor ofers a good justification for his or her con-

clusion."[30(p761)] Accordingly, the court established a tripartite standard for evaluating the reliability of the physicians' differential diagnosis: 1) when the physician relied solely on patients' written self-reports of symptoms or illness without conducting an examination or reviewing medical records, the opinion was inherently unreliable and was properly excluded; 2) when the physician relied on a review of patient medical records without a personal examination, the opinion was presumptively unreliable unless plaintiffs could demonstrate its reliability; and 3) when the physician relied on a personal medical examination as well as review of medical records, the opinion was presumptively reliable unless defendants could demonstrate its unreliability. When the plaintiff's physician employed standard techniques of differential diagnosis, the defendants nevertheless might be able to demonstrate the unreliability of the opinion if they identified some other likely cause of the plaintiff's illness and the plaintiff's physician had no reasonable explanation for persisting in the belief that the defendants' actions were a substantial factor in bringing about that illness.[30(pp760,762)]

THE FACTUAL BASIS FOR EXPERT TESTIMONY

Traditionally, the law prescribed an artificial format for questioning an expert witness who had incomplete knowledge of the underlying facts: the hypothetical question. The attorney would ask the expert to provide an opinion based on an assumed set of facts, which the attorney would be obligated to prove through other witnesses. Essentially, the attorney provided the factual minor premise, the expert provided the conclusion, and the expert might or might not be asked to explain the theoretical major premise from which the conclusion was derived.[32,43,48]

The exclusive reliance on hypothetical questions has been criticized for two diametrically opposite reasons.[21,32,43,47,48] On one hand, hypothetical questions are ineffective because their length and complexity confuses juries, they frequently are interrupted by objections, and their artificiality renders them unpersuasive. On the other hand, hypothetical questions are too effective because they enable attorneys to summarize all of their key facts to the jury and essentially conduct closing arguments in the middle of the case.

Another alternative was for expert witnesses to attend the trial and base their opinions on the actual trial evidence. Having an expert witness attend an entire trial is generally impractical, however, both in terms of inconvenience to the expert and cost to the client.[47] Hence, attorneys rarely ask physicians to attend the trial and base their opinions on trial testimony.

The Federal Rules of Evidence expanded the permissible bases for expert testimony;[45] therefore, expert witnesses no longer are limited to answering questions based on hypothetical facts. Under the Rules, an expert's opinion can be based upon the actual trial evidence or upon information conveyed to the expert prior to trial (Rule 703). Moreover, the facts or data upon which the expert relies need not be introduced into evidence, nor must they even be potentially admissible in evidence, so long as they are "of a type reasonably relied upon by experts in the particular field" (Rule 703).

When an opinion is based in part on information that was not itself admissible into evidence, the court must determine whether it was "reasonably relied upon." In so doing, the court generally should defer to the profession, but not necessarily to the testifying expert.[3,18,21,30,32,45] For example, a federal appeals court in 1989 reversed a verdict for the plaintiff because the trial court had erred in allowing a neurologist to base his opinion that the plaintiff suffered from post-concussive syndrome on a "topographical brain map" (a computerized enhancement of the electroencephalogram) without determining its trustworthiness or its acceptance in the relevant scientific community.[24] When the proponent establishes that the profession regularly or customarily relies on a particular type of information, the court must apply an objective standard to decide whether that practice is reasonable.[45]

Thus, to the extent a physician's opinion is not based on a hypothetical question or on actual trial testimony, it can be based on any of the following information:

- the physician's direct observations, including those obtained through examination of the patient;
- statements by the patient (admissible hearsay under an exception for statements for purposes of medical diagnosis or treatment, Rule 803(4));
- review of medical records (admissible hearsay under an exception for records of regularly conducted activity, Rule 803(6)); and
- reports or verbal statements by other medical experts or other data that would not otherwise be admissible into evidence, so long as physicians reasonably rely on such information (Rule 703).

The expert is allowed to give an opinion without disclosing the underlying facts or data (Rule 705), but the testimony usually is more persuasive if the jury knows what facts were relied upon and can evaluate their accuracy. Whenever testimony is based on observations or opinions of others, the witness should explain to the fact finder that physicians regularly rely on such information. This is especially important if the testifying physician has not examined the patient.

Insofar as the expert has based an opinion on facts that would not be admissible into evidence, substantial controversy exists about whether the expert is permitted to inform the jury of these facts in the course of presenting the opinion.[3,21,28,44,45] To avoid an error that would necessitate a new trial, it is essential that the expert consult with the attorney to determine the extent to which underlying information should be disclosed during the testimony. Even if the witness is not permitted to disclose the inadmissible facts during direct examination, the opposing counsel may "open the door" to introduction of this evidence by inquiring into the basis of the expert's opinion on cross-examination.

In testifying about the facts, witnesses are supposed to rely primarily on their memories and may not bring notes to the stand. A witness may refer to documents that have been admitted into evidence, such as a patient's medical records. Other notes and files may be brought to court in case they are needed to refresh the witness' memory in the event of a memory lapse while testifying (Rule 612), but they should not be brought to the witness stand unless they will be introduced into evidence. Some judges are lax about this procedure, however, and allow experts to testify from their notes or records without requiring that these documents be formally entered into evidence.

THE EXPERT OPINION

Expert testimony need not be in the form of an opinion. As mentioned above, an expert may give a dissertation on scientific or medical principles and leave it to the jury to apply these principles to the facts.[18] On the other hand, it is usually more persuasive for the expert to provide an opinion, and in many instances an expert opinion is legally required in order to satisfy the burden of proof.

In the past, many courts restricted the scope of expert opinion testimony by forbidding experts to express opinions on the "ultimate issue" in a case, such as whether the defendant in a malpractice case was "negligent" or whether an accident was the "cause" of a plaintiff's injuries.[34,43,45] The "ultimate issue" rule received harsh criticism from legal scholars, and by the 1960s it had been rejected in most jurisdictions.[34,45] The Federal Rules of Evidence expressly declare that an opinion otherwise admissible "is not objectionable because it embraces an ultimate issue to be decided by the trier of fact" (Rule 704(a)). While experts are now free to express *factual* conclusions, they may not state *legal* conclusions.[43,45] Where an opinion involves mixed issues of law and fact, courts may allow the witness to express the opinion if it would be "helpful" to the jury but not if it is phrased in terms of "inadequately explored legal criteria."[45] Also, Rule 704(b) restricts expressions of opinion about the mental state of a criminal defendant when the mental state is an element of the crime (e.g., "intentional" or "premeditated") or a defense (e.g., insanity or diminished capacity).[45]

In presenting the opinion itself, the expert may be required to include certain "magic words" or verbal formulations to meet the applicable legal standards. Some of these verbal formulas relate to the applicable standard of proof, some relate to proof of particular categories of facts, and some relate generally to the expression of expert opinions.

First, the phrasing of an expert's opinion must be consistent with the applicable legal standard of proof, which differs in criminal and civil cases. In criminal cases, proof of guilt must be "beyond a reasonable doubt," so the expert generally must be able to opine that the particular proposition is "certain" or "reasonably certain" to be true. (The expert is not expected to say that a fact is true "beyond a reasonable doubt" and may be forbidden from doing so, for this phrase refers to the legal standard that the jury must apply in evaluating the evidence rather than the expert's degree of certitude.) In a civil case, proof must be by a "preponderance of the evidence," which means that the proposition must be "more probably true than not true." Thus, on such questions as whether an injury was caused by an accident or whether the defendant violated a standard of care, the expert usually need only state that the proposition is "probably" true. Some courts allow juries to base a finding on expert testimony that a proposition might "possibly" be true, but many have held that such testimony was legally insufficient, and some courts do not allow any testimony in terms of possibilities.[18,34,43]

Second, expert opinions often must contain precise verbal formulas in order to satisfy legal rules describing the burden of proof for particular elements of a claim or defense. For example, to establish that an agent or event was the legal cause of a person's injuries, in some jurisdictions the physician must state that it was a "substantial contributing factor" in causing the injuries, while in others the physician must state that it was a "competent producing cause" of the injuries. With respect to claims for the permanence of existing injuries or for the future development of new diseases, conditions, or complications, some jurisdictions allow recovery only if medical testimony establishes that such injuries are "reasonably certain" to occur, while others require testimony that such injuries are "reasonably probable."

Third, in some jurisdictions, courts require that all expert testimony be expressed with "a reasonable degree of professional certainty."[2,7,20, 34,43,47,50] For physicians, some jurisdictions require that testimony be expressed with "a reasonable degree of medical certainty" or "reasonable medical certainty," while other jurisdictions require testimony in terms of "reasonable (degree of) medical probability."[34,45] The magic words "reasonable medical certainty" have achieved talismanic status in the interrogation of medical witnesses, so one would expect the phrase to have a definite and ascertainable meaning. Unfortunately, the phrase seems to have various meanings in different jurisdictions, generating substantial confusion among lawyers and judges as well as among physicians who are called upon to provide expert testimony.[34,43]

The phrase "reasonable medical certainty" was first used in Illinois, and attorneys in the rest of the nation adopted this usage through imitation of models provided in an influencial work on trial technique written by a prominent Chicago trial lawyer.[34] Because the phrase was adopted by attorneys without prior guidance from the courts, its meaning has been influenced by idiosyncratic local doctrines relating to admissibility and sufficiency of proof,[34] including the rules described in the preceding paragraphs, which explains the diversity of interpretations.

In the vast majority of jurisdictions, the phrase "reasonable medical certainty" is interpreted as a substantive comment on the underlying probabilities. In most states, the courts interpret "reasonable medical certainty" as meaning that the proposition is "more likely than not" to be true, and in many of these jurisdictions the phrase is used interchangeably with "reasonable medical probability."[34,43] Ignoring the existence of alternative interpretations, one leading medicolegal authority misleadingly advises: "'Reasonable medical certainty' is a catch phrase meaning 'more likely than not' in a medical sense."[50(p560)] In a few jurisdictions, most notably in Pennsylvania, the courts interpret the phrase as requiring a higher degree of certainty, sometimes approaching scientific certainty. Under this stringent interpretation, a physician's opinion that there was a 75% likelihood of recovery with proper treatment would not suffice to establish with "reasonable medical certainty" that the malpractice was the cause of the patient's death.[22,34] Finally, in a handful of jurisdictions, most notably in Illinois, the phrase "reasonable medical certainty" is not interpreted as a substantive comment on the existing probabilities, but rather as a shorthand way of indicating that the testimony represents a considered professional opinion, based on accepted scientific principles and methodologies.[34] Indeed, one leading academic scholar accepts this as the definitive interpretation of the phrase, ignoring the fact that it represents a distinct minority viewpoint.[20]

In criticizing the cases that generated the phrase "reasonable medical certainty," the nation's leading evidentiary scholar, John Henry Wigmore, wrote in 1923:

> This is a good example of that legal quibbling which creates for the law of trials a disrespect in the minds of competent physicians. . . . This is only one of the many instances in which the subtle mental twistings produced by the Opinion rule have reduced this part of the law to a congeries of nonsense which is comparable to the incantations of medieval sorcerers and sullies the name of Reason.[51(§1976)]

While the liberalization of evidence law under the Federal Rules of Evidence has diminished the importance of this phrase in many jurisdictions, existing confusion about the meaning and purpose of the phrase remains a potential semantic trap for physician witnesses.

In sum, the requisite terminology for expert opinion testimony and the meaning of the various phrases vary dramatically depending on the jurisdiction and the context. It is therefore imperative for the physician to consult with the friendly attorney prior to trial in order to ascertain the legal standard of proof for the proposition in question, the precise terminology which must accompany the expression of the opinion in court, and the local interpretation of any mandatory verbal formulas.[2,18]

PREPARATION FOR EXPERT TESTIMONY

Witness preparation is fundamental to the adversary process of dispute resolution. The author of a comprehensive analysis of the doctrinal and ethical problems of witness preparation in civil litigation provided the following introduction to the topic:

> Witness preparation is any communication

between a lawyer and a prospective witness . . . that is intended to improve the substance or presentation of testimony to be offered at a trial or other hearing. Witness preparation enables lawyers to present witnesses who are thoroughly familiar with the subject matter of their testimony and who are prepared to say what they know in a clear, coherent manner. American litigators regularly use witness preparation, and virtually all would, upon reflection, consider it a fundamental duty of representation and a basic element of effective advocacy.

At the same time, for many other lawyers and most nonlawyers, witness preparation represents the worst qualities of the legal system. Because witness preparation is ordinarily conducted in private, it is difficult for the lawyer and witness to avoid the appearance that they have invented a convenient story for the jury. . . . Moreover, the line between preparing and prompting (or "coaching," the usual term of opprobrium) is rarely clear even for the most scrupulous.

* * *

The doctrinal uncertainties in witness preparation often result in misunderstandings in the application of legal rules to particular witness-preparation practices. . . .

* * *

Witness preparation is also permeated by ethical uncertainty. It presents one of the most difficult ethical dilemmas regularly encountered by lawyers. . . . Any attempt to eliminate the doctrinal uncertainty that dominates the area of witness preparation must fully consider the competing goals of partisan representation and truth seeking that are present in the adversarial system of justice.[1]

The need for witness preparation is especially acute for expert witnesses,[7,23] on whom the law places far greater demands than it does ordinary lay witnesses. In contrast to ordinary lay witnesses, who primarily are expected to answer discrete factual questions about their direct observations with respect to a limited set of relevant events, expert witnesses are expected to express well-considered professional opinions, to base those opinions on all of their prior training and experience and on a variety of sources of information, to express those opinions using precise verbal formulas, but at the same time to make their testimony comprehensible to lay jurors by translating arcane technical jargon into everyday language, conveying complex concepts through commonplace analogies,

and using a variety of demonstrative exhibits.

While preparation is especially important for expert witnesses, it is also especially fraught with ethical dilemmas. Insofar as expert testimony is less rooted in discrete factual observations, it provides far more opportunity for distortion through omissions and half-truths. In response to this problem, one leading commentator proposed that the preparation of expert witnesses be transformed "from a confidential and partisan process into an open proceeding" in which all communications with an expert witness would be shared with the opponent and any meetings with the expert would be open to all parties.[21] In the absence of such reforms, physicians must understand that witness preparation remains an essential part of U.S. litigation, and they must be ready to confront the ethical dilemmas inherent in this process.

EFFECTIVE MEDICAL EXPERT TESTIMONY

This chapter cannot provide comprehensive guidance on how to be an effective expert witness. Before appearing to testify at a deposition or at trial, physicians may want to read one or more books or articles on the topic,[14,25,32,36,37,48] as well as consulting with the friendly attorney. A few key points are noted here.

Courtroom Etiquette and Demeanor

Courtroom decorum and etiquette are important. The witness should be aware that his or her actions will be observed by the jury from the time the witness enters the room, and every activity—the walk to the witness box, the swearing in, and the exit—must be done with appropriate decorum. The witness should arrive promptly when scheduled to testify, take a seat in the public seating area, and wait for a break in the proceedings to contact the attorney by sending a note via the bailiff.

The judge is the authority in the court and must be treated with deference and respect. Ordinarily, only the attorneys are permitted to address the court, and witnesses are limited to answering questions posed by the attorneys. The witness can address the judge only if the judge asks the witness a question, if the witness believes a question inquires about privileged information, or if the witness is asked a leading ("yes or no") question which cannot fairly be answered without an explanation.

The witness should focus on conveying the evidence to the fact finder, usually a jury. Although engaged in a question-and-answer dialogue with the attorney, answers should be directed to the jury. The witness may not volunteer information to the jury except in response to questions. Except when testifying, the witness may not speak with jurors at all until the trial has concluded.

Trials are open to the public and often are reported by the media. It is inappropriate for expert witnesses to discuss the case with the media or observers until after they have testified, and it is better not to make any comments until the trial has ended.

General Suggestions for Effective Expert Testimony

An effective expert witness is one who succeeds in conveying new and often complex information to the jury with clarity and focus. In general, the attributes of an effective witness are those of an effective teacher: dignity, strength, and confidence without arrogance; thoughtfulness, thoroughness, and accuracy; honesty and objectivity; clarity of organization; focus on the essential points; a conversational tone; use of simple language without condescension; use of examples and analogies from everyday life; use of exhibits and illustrations; and use of interesting rhetoric, gestures, and emotion, without being overly dramatic or exaggerated.[9]

Effective expert testimony frequently relies heavily on "demonstrative evidence" in the form of diagrams, drawings, models, charts, chronologies, photographs, x-rays, videotapes, or more elaborate computer-generated graphics that make the testimony more vivid and comprehensible to the jury.[46] To work effectively with demonstrative evidence, the expert witness and the attorney must collaborate in the preparation of the exhibits and the planning for their

incorporation into the testimony.

It is appropriate for the witness to pause before each answer to make sure both the witness and the jury understand the question. Leaving a short pause is especially important on cross-examination in order to avoid being rushed into an inaccurate answer and to allow the friendly attorney an opportunity to object to improper questions.

If either attorney objects to a question, the witness should not answer but should wait for a ruling from the judge. The judge may rule immediately or summon the attorneys for a "sidebar conference" at the bench; in rare cases, there may be a recess to consider the objection.[32,37]

Establishing Expertise

The initial portion of an expert's testimony addresses the expert's qualifications. It is awkward to proclaim one's own expertise, but it is essential for the jury to understand the expert's qualifications in order to assess the quality of the testimony, especially if there will be conflicting testimony from an opposing expert. To avoid either false modesty or boastfulness, the expert should work with the friendly attorney to portray the witness's expertise in its best light.[47] Some of this information may be presented most effectively by introducing the expert's *curriculum vitae* into evidence as an exhibit.[7,38,47]

The preliminary questions about a physician's field of expertise can provide an occasion to humanize the witness in the eyes of the jury, conveying warmth and compassion for patients, a sense of humor, or other qualities that may favorably influence juror perceptions. The background questions also provide an opportunity to educate the jury, defining technical terms in lay language and explaining the fundamental scientific concepts in a neutral context, prior to the expression of an expert opinion.

Presentation of Expert Opinion Testimony

Responsibility for organizing the presentation of the expert's opinion testimony primarily rests with the attorney who will conduct the direct examination. The following discussion is meant to explain the alternative ways in which attorneys may decide to present an expert's testimony and may enable physicians to provide useful input into the preparation of their testimony.

The traditional form of examination asks whether the witness has formed an opinion (with the requisite degree of certainty) about a particular subject, to which the answer should be "yes" (or "no"); the attorney then asks the witness to state that opinion.[38,47] On the other hand, rather than immediately eliciting the substance of the opinion, the attorney may first inquire about its scientific and factual basis.

The expert is permitted to express an opinion without explaining either the scientific theory or the facts on which it rests (Rule 705). Nevertheless, the bare expression of an opinion without any supporting foundation is not very convincing, so the expert should be prepared to explain both the scientific and the factual basis for the opinion. The witness and the attorney should reach a clear understanding as to whether this explanation will come before or after the expression of the substance of the opinion.

In most lawsuits, the scientific basis of the expert's testimony is not controversial, in which case the expert is not legally required to testify about the underlying theories or techniques. (When the scientific basis of the expert's testimony is controversial, the judge usually will hold a pretrial hearing to determine the admissibility of the expert's opinion.[8]) Nevertheless, to be persuasive, the expert ought to provide some explanation, in lay terminology, of the basic methodology or theoretical underpinnings of the testimony.

In explaining the scientific basis for the opinion, it may be helpful to read to the jury from a leading treatise or periodical on the subject. Although the written statement of an outside authority is "hearsay," in a majority of jurisdictions it may be received into evidence under the "learned treatise" exception to the hearsay rule if the witness can establish that the work represents "a reliable authority" in the field (Rule 803(18)).[9,38,45]

With regard to the factual basis for the opinion, attorneys usually ask physicians about their examination and treatment of the patient immediately following the testimony about qualifications, so that the jury already understands the basis for the opinion before the witness is asked to express it.[7,47] A treating physician should emphasize the time and care taken in obtaining the patient's history and in conducting the physical examination. To the extent that the testimony is based on notations in medical records, the witness should emphasize the extent to which physicians rely upon the accuracy of these records. An expert witness who has not examined the patient should establish that treating physicians regularly rely upon advice from specialists who base their professional opinions on oral or written information about the patient's medical history.

If the attorney decides to use one or more hypothetical questions, the witness should work quite closely with the attorney in phrasing the questions. Each hypothetical question must incorporate every relevant fact on which the opinion is based, and it must be entirely accurate.

CROSS-EXAMINATION

Dramatic fictional presentations have generated an unwarranted fear of cross-examination, which rarely is as intense or confrontational as it is usually portrayed. In one respect, physicians should have less reason to fear cross-examination than lay witnesses, for they are being questioned about matters on which they have special expertise. On the other hand, experts are subject to particular types of cross-examination which make them more vulnerable than lay witnesses. The discussion here identifies the general types of cross-examination that a physician can expect to encounter and suggests how to respond appropriately to both the substance of the question and the demeanor of the cross-examining attorney. (Preparation of the expert for cross-examination is the responsibility of the friendly attorney.)

The Substance of Cross-Examination

Beyond attacking the credibility of the witness, the topics of cross-examination generally follow the structure of expert witness testimony, focusing on the qualifications of the expert, the scientific basis for the opinion, the factual basis for the opinion, and the expression of the opinion.

All witnesses can be cross-examined with respect to possible bias or prejudice. Most lay occurrence witnesses who are not parties should be relatively immune to this sort of questioning, whereas experts, because they are being paid for their services, are particularly vulnerable. The physician should be prepared to answer questions about the amount of the fee without any hesitation or embarrassment. The treating physician may be asked about loyalty to the patient. The nontreating physician may be portrayed as a hired gun, especially if the witness obtains a substantial percentage of income from appearing as an expert or testifies in most cases for the same side.

Physicians often are cross-examined about limitations on their expertise. The opponent will emphasize any differences between the subject of the testimony and the physician's precise areas of specialization.

Physicians can be cross-examined about the scientific basis for their opinions. The opponent can be expected to cast doubt upon the testimony by asking whether medicine is always an exact science and whether physicians ever disagree about matters of theory, about particular diagnoses, or about the most appropriate treatments for various conditions. A witness should be prepared to concede that nothing is certain or that other interpretations or conclusions are "possible." The cross-examiner may go further and ask the witness to admit that a previously expressed opinion is "speculative" or "conjectural" in an attempt to have the court exclude the testimony of the witness, for testimony that is "speculative" or "conjectural" is not legally admissible. A witness should refuse to accept this characterization so long as the opinion is based on "probabilities" as opposed to "possibilities" and on known facts or valid inferences as opposed to mere assumptions.

Just as the expert can rely upon a "learned treatise" in testifying, the cross-examiner can use such treatises to impeach the expert. A passage from an authoritative text or periodical that supports the cross-examiner's position is read to the expert, who is then asked whether he or she agrees with the proposition. If the witness agrees with the authority, the point has been established; if the witness disagrees, the testimony is inconsistent with the authority. Impeachment with a learned treatise is especially powerful if the expert has relied upon the treatise in testifying or admits that it is a reliable authority. If the witness denies that the work is authoritative, then the opponent must establish its reliability through the testimony of another expert witness unless it is so well known that the judge can take "judicial notice" of its reliability. A common technique for partially defusing impeachment with a treatise is to deny from the outset that any treatise is absolutely reliable, emphasizing that the various chapters or sections of a work may not be equally authoritative and that there is substantial disagreement within the profession with regard to certain statements in even the most highly regarded works.[48] In preparation for trial or deposition testimony, the witness should review any treatises, periodicals or pamphlets which may be deemed reliable authorities for possible inconsistency with anticipated testimony and call them to the attention of the friendly attorney.

Physicians can be cross-examined about the factual basis for their opinions, especially if there is a disagreement among occurrence witnesses about the underlying facts. If the physician's opinion was based on particular facts, either actual or hypothetical, the physician can be asked whether the opinion might differ if one or more of those facts were different. The cross-examiner can go even farther and construct a comprehensive hypothetical question based on a set of facts most favorable to that side. The physician must answer the hypothetical question unless it does not include sufficient information to enable the physician to form an opinion.[14,37,48]

Finally, as is true of all witnesses, an expert witness can be confronted with prior statements in a deposition or elsewhere that are inconsistent with the testimony at trial. In preparation for trial, the physician should review any expert reports or depositions in the case, as well as any of the physician's own published works on the subject, to make sure that the trial testimony is consistent with these prior statements or that any inconsistencies can be explained.[32,37,48]

Demeanor on Cross-Examination

On cross-examination, the witness is presumed to be uncooperative and resistant to suggestive questioning, so the opposing attorney is permitted to use leading questions, which call for a "yes" or "no" answer. Indeed, attorneys are taught to rely almost exclusively on leading questions on cross-examination. On cross-examination, the attorney is not so much interrogating as using the witness to establish a few points that the witness can be expected to concede.

If a simple "yes" or "no" answer is appropriate, it is best to comply, for a witness who refuses to do so may sound evasive. On the other hand, if a definitive answer is not possible, or if it would be misleading unless accompanied by an explanation, the witness should so state.[32] If pressed further by the attorney, the witness can ask the judge whether a "yes" or "no" answer is required or whether the witness will be permitted to explain the answer. Even if no explanation is permitted at that time, the friendly attorney will have been alerted to ask for an explanation on the "re-direct" examination which is permitted as a follow-up to cross-examination.[14,23]

For questions that can be answered accurately with a simple "yes" or "no," attorneys differ about whether it is advisable to attempt to elaborate or explain the answer during the cross-examination or to wait for re-direct examination. Much depends on the relative competence and experience of the attorney and the witness, their personalities, the predilections of the judge, the nature of the case, and various other situation-specific factors. This issue should be discussed with the friendly attorney in preparation for testifying, along with the related matter of how any anticipated problem areas on cross-examination will be clarified or corrected on re-direct examination.

It is important to listen carefully to the question. The witness should limit the answer to the particular question without volunteering additional information and without presuming to anticipate the next logical question. If a question is vague, unclear, or ambiguous, the witness should so state and request that it be rephrased. The witness should be on guard for questions out of context, should avoid speculation, and

should not answer a question calling for an opinion outside the expert's area of competence.

Demeanor on cross-examination should be firm, patient, and polite. The friendly attorney should object to repetitive or argumentative questions, but it may be appropriate for the witness to respond: "I believe I've already answered that question." or "That's not a fair question." The witness should resist temptation to argue with the attorney and avoid sarcastic remarks.

References

1. Applegate JS: Witness preparation. **Texas Law Rev** 68:277-352, 1989
2. Black B: A unified theory of scientific evidence. **Fordham Law Rev** 56:595-695, 1988
3. Carlson RL: Policing the bases of modern expert testimony. **Vand Law Rev** 39:577-593, 1986
4. *Carroll v Otis Elevator Co*, 896 F2d 210 (7th Cir 1990)
5. Chesebro KJ: Galileo's retort: Peter Huber's junk scholarship. **Am U Law Rev** 42:1637-1726, 1993
6. Chesebro KJ: Taking *Daubert*'s "focus" seriously: the methodology/conclusion distinction. **Cardozo Law Rev** 15:1745-1753, 1994
7. Corboy PH, Smith TA: The medical expert, in Rossi FF (ed): **Expert Witnesses.** Chicago, Ill: American Bar Association, 1991, pp 287-333
8. *Daubert v Merrell Dow Pharmaceuticals,* 509 US 579 (1993)
9. Dombroff MA: **Expert Witnesses in Civil Trials: Effective Preparation and Presentation.** Rochester, NY: The Lawyers Co-operative Publishing, 1987, 390 pp (and 1995 Suppl, 317 pp)
10. *Ellis v Miller Oil Purchasing Co,* 738 F2d 269 (8th Cir 1984)
11. Faigman DL, Porter E, Saks MJ: Check your crystal ball at the courthouse door, please: exploring the past, understanding the present, and worrying about the future of scientific evidence. **Cardozo Law Rev** 15:1799-1835, 1994
12. Federal Rules of Evidence, 28 USC
13. Fenner GM: The *Daubert* handbook: the case, its essential dilemma, and its progeny. **Creighton Law Rev** 15:939, 1996
14. Fish RM, Ehrhardt ME. **Malpractice Depositions: Avoiding the Traps.** Oradell, NJ: Medical Economics Books, 1987, 152 pp
15. *Frye v United States*, 293 F 1013 (DC Cir 1923)
16. Giannelli PC: The admissibility of novel scientific evidence: *Frye v United States* a half-century later. **Columbia Law Rev** 80:1197, 1980
17. Giannelli PC: *Daubert*: interpreting the Federal Rules of Evidence. **Cardozo Law Rev** 15:1999-2026, 1994
18. Giannelli PC, Imwinkelried EJ: **Scientific Evidence.** 2nd ed. Charlottesville, Va: The Michie Company, Vol 1, 1993 (and 1996 suppl)
19. Gottesman MH: Admissibility of expert testimony after *Daubert*: the "prestige" factor. **Emory Law J** 43: 867, 1994

20. Graham MH: Expert witness testimony and the Federal Rules of Evidence: insuring adequate assuarance of trustworthiness. **U Ill Law Rev 1986:**43, 1986
21. Gross SR: Expert evidence. **Wisc Law Rev 1991:** 1113-1232, 1991
22. *Hamil v Bashline*, 392 A2d 1280 (Pa 1978)
23. Hanley RF: Preparing the expert witness, in Rossi FF (ed): **Expert Witnesses.** Chicago, Ill: American Bar Association, 1991, pp 155-170
24. *Head v Lithonia Corp*, 881 F2d 941 (10th Cir 1989)
25. Horsley JE, Carlova J: **Testifying in Court.** Oradell, NJ: Medical Economics Books, 1988, 150 pp
26. Huber PW: **Galileo's Revenge: Junk Science in the Courtroom.** New York, NY: Basic Books, 1991, 274 pp
27. Imwinkelried EJ: The "bases" of expert testimony: the syllogistic structure of scientific testimony. **North Carol Law Rev 67:**1-27, 1988
28. Imwinkelried EJ: A comparativist critique of the interface between hearsay and expert opinion in American evidence law. **Bost Coll Law Rev 33:**1-35, 1991
29. Imkinkelried EJ: The next step after *Daubert*: developing a similarly epistemological approach to ensuring the reliability of nonscientific expert testimony. **Cardozo Law Rev 15:**2271-2294, 1994
30. *In re Paoli RR Yard PCB Litigation,* 35 F3d 717 (3rd Cir 1994)
31. Jasanoff S: Science on the witness stand. **Issues Sci Techn 6:**80, 1989
32. Leestma JE, Magee DJ: Pathology and neuropathology in the forensic setting, in Leestma JE (ed): **Forensic Neuropathology.** New York, NY: Raven Press, 1988, pp 1-23
33. Lewin JL: Calabresi's revenge? Junk science in the work of Peter Huber. **Hofstra Law Rev 21:**183-204, 1993
34. Lewin JL: The origins of legal uncertainty about "reasonable medical certainty." **Md Law Rev** (In press, 1997)
35. Lyons T: Frye, Daubert and where do we go from here? **RI Bar J.** Vol 45, Jan 5, 1997 (WESTLAW)
36. MacHovec FJ: **The Expert Witness Survival Manual.** Springfield, Ill: Charles C Thomas, 1987, 171 pp
37. Matson JV: **Effective Expert Witnessing: A Handbook for Technical Professionals.** Chelsea, Mich: Lewis, 1990, 145 pp
38. Mauet TA: **Fundamentals of Trial Techniques.** 3rd ed. Boston, Mass: Little, Brown, and Co, 1992, 451 pp
39. McCormick M: Scientific evidence: defining a new approach to admissibility. **Iowa Law Rev 67:**879-916, 1982
40. *Nowitzke v State*, 572 So2d 1346 (Fla 1990)
41. Osborne JW: Judicial/technical assessment of novel scientific evidence. **U Ill Law Rev 1990:**497, 1990
42. *People v Rogers*, 557 NYS2d 375 (NY App Div 1990)
43. Piorkowski JD: Medical testimony and the expert witness, in American College of Legal Medicine (ed): **Legal Medicine: Legal Dynamics of Medical Encounters.** 3rd ed. St Louis, Mo: Mosby-Year Book, 1995, pp 141-155
44. Rice PR: Inadmissible evidence as a basis for expert opinion testimony: a response to Professor Carlson. **Vand Law Rev 40:**583-596, 1987
45. Rossi FF (ed): **Expert Witnesses.** Chicago, Ill: American Bar Association, 1991, 549 pp
46. Siemer DC: Demonstrative evidence and expert witnesses, in Rossi FF (ed): **Expert Witnesses.** Chicago, Ill: American Bar Association, 1991, pp 251-283
47. Stein ER: The direct examination of the expert witness, in Rossi FF (ed): **Expert Witnesses.** Chicago, Ill: American Bar Association, 1991, pp 193-222
48. Taraska JM: The physician as a witness, in Taraska JM: **Legal Guide for Physicians.** White Plains, NY: AHAB Press, 1997, pp 9.1-9.56
49. *Thorne v U-Haul of Metro DC, Inc*, 580 A2d 672 (DC App 1990)
50. Wecht CH: Forensic use of medical information, in American College of Legal Medicine (ed): **Legal Medicine: Legal Dynamics of Medical Encounters.** 3rd ed. St Louis, Mo: Mosby-Year Book, 1995, pp 558-566
51. Wigmore JH: **A Treatise on the System of Evidence in Trial at Common Law.** 2nd ed. Boston, Mass: Little, Brown, and Co, 1923, Vol IV, 972 pp

CHAPTER 5

RELATIONS BETWEEN PATIENTS AND PHYSICIANS IN MEDICAL DECISION-MAKING

HOWARD H. KAUFMAN, MD

The process of medical decision-making is founded on the relationship between patients and physicians. The nature of this relationship is one of the basic issues in medical ethics. This relationship has its underpinnings in morality as well as the practical effects of decisions, and determines how the physician should act.[26] However, the standards for the relationship have been imposed by physicians, are therefore somewhat insulated from outside influences, and may not be very responsive to societal changes. In the past several years, previous standards have been modified by a shift from a paternalistic model to a participatory model, with a greater emphasis on physician accountability.[9,59]

On the other hand, all societies impose rules to control the conduct of their citizens and their actions. In the United States, the liberal political philosophy of the founders protected personal freedom and privacy and led to a particular way to resolve conflicts. Dworkin discusses the liberal viewpoint:

> Does a state protect a contestable value best by encouraging people to accept it as contestable, understanding that they are responsible for deciding for themselves what it means?

Or does the state protect a contestable value best by itself deciding, through the political process, which interpretation is the right one, and then forcing everyone to conform? The goal of responsibility justifies the first choice, the goal of conformity the second. A state cannot pursue both goals at the same time.[22]

Dworkin concludes that the former goal is the proper one. For a pluralistic society to function, it is necessary to recognize individuals' rights to make decisions for and about themselves above all other principles, and this tolerance is the price required for our "adventure in liberty." Under today's legal standards, patients or their surrogates have a right to determine what will happen to them based on their own values, while physicians have the responsibility to educate them and act as their advocates.[14]

Indeed, physicians are expected to know and abide by laws and regulations in addition to the precedents established by court cases, with significant penalties, including time loss and costs, attached to violating them or being perceived to violate them. On the other hand, if a situation arises in which the law conflicts with ethics, there is a moral obligation to pursue an ethical course.[9,18]

This chapter outlines issues concerning the relationship between physician and patient in a legal context. There are several other monographs on medical law which examine these issues from different perspectives and highlight various aspects (see Appendix immediately following this chapter).

THE PATIENT-PHYSICIAN RELATIONSHIP

The patient-physician relationship is governed by constellations of legal doctrines—contract law and tort law. In a relationship governed by contract law, both parties freely agree to enter a relationship based on the fulfillment of promises. The concept of the patient-physician relationship as an arms-length contract has been limited because the physician has greater bargaining power and information and because the relationship is intimate. Tort law intervenes by establishing a relationship in which a physician is required to act reasonably with regard to the standard of care while honoring the patient's risk/benefit preferences through informed consent. The fiduciary relationship between doctor and patient involves a duty of loyalty to protect the patient from the physician's advantage of power, requiring the physician to act in the patient's best interest first and promoting patient trust.[49]

According to the law, a physician has no duty to agree to treat a patient, even if the patient is in danger of harm. This is somewhat different from ethical considerations. However, a few states do have statutes which require citizens to provide aid in emergency situations.[4] In such circumstances, in which pay is not expected, the physician is not liable unless the care provided is characterized by gross negligence. An extension of this concept involves legislation in a number of states which grants immunity from ordinary liability for physicians providing pro bono care.[46] The physician who is an employee of a hospital which is required to accept emergencies and who has agreed to do this as part of the employment must care for all such patients.[70] Another interesting issue involves laws and cases that prevent physicians from refusing to treat certain classes of patients. These derive from the Rehabilitation Act (1973) and the Americans With Disabilities Act (1990), which prevent exclusion of handicapped persons from programs supported by federal funds.[61,66]

A related issue involves the duty to treat patients who may pose a risk to the physician. Patients may be dangerous because they are violent or may have a communicable disease. This risk varies with specialty. For instance, 40% of psychiatrists report having been attacked by patients.[24] Another type of dangerous patient is one with acquired immune deficiency syndrome (AIDS), a subject that will be discussed in the chapter dealing with infectious diseases (Chapter 16). Traditionally, no citizen is required to accept risk to benefit another, but the obligations of a physician are different. The argument that the physician has an obligation to assume risk relates to the voluntary commitment to service and the collegial responsibility to share risks so that they are not concentrated in a few physicians.[58] On the other hand, there must be circumstances so dangerous that it is not reasonable to mandate someone to assume such risks. The issue has not been fully resolved.

Once the physician does agree to accept the patient,[4] there is a contractual relationship which is consensual. The agreement may be explicit, though oral, between a patient and a physician or it may be based on an agreement with a third party, such as a health maintenance organization, for the physician to care for the patient. The agreement may be implied, such as when the physician gives advice on the telephone, writes a prescription, or even makes an appointment to see a patient for a particular problem. The contract may be expanded, such as when a physician guarantees an outcome (a poor idea), or restricted, such as when a specialist limits the scope of care to a particular problem. Here the specialist is responsible if he/she directs the care of a patient or gives advice which is used in that care. A relation may or may not persist for a physician caring for a chronic condition, depending on how active and how severe the disease is and how frequently the patient is seen. There is no relationship between a patient and a physician who sees the patient for a third party, such as for an insurance examination, unless the physician gives the patient advice.[36,70]

Once a relationship has been established, the

physician has a duty to the patient, which is to provide a proper "standard of care" while keeping the patient informed and educated and while respecting autonomy and confidentiality. Care must be timely and adequate. At one time, the standard was based on that of the locality. However, with increased communications and mobility, in most areas of practice physicians must meet a national standard. Specialists are expected to meet a higher standard, and standards are now being established by specialty societies which are being used for legal guidance.[9,68]

Failure to meet a standard is termed "negligence," which includes doing what an ordinarily prudent person would not do or not doing what an ordinarily prudent person would do. If this is related to an act of the physician, it is "active" liability. If related to the act of someone who is in his/her employ or for whom he/she is responsible, it is "passive" liability. (In such circumstances the physician is responsible to choose, train, supervise, and ensure the other's performance.) In a hospital context, there may also be a responsibility for a "borrowed servant," an employee of a hospital whom the physician directs. Likewise, liability may be imposed on a hospital or group if they fail to assure physician performance.[36,68]

There are times when a physician is not available to care for a patient due to illness of the physician, caring for another patient, being off call, being on vacation, having rotated off service, or other reasons. Many of these situations are so accepted that nothing must be done other than to assure adequate substitute care. Under circumstances where the substitution will be for long periods or for important events (e.g., childbirth), the patient should be notified and permitted to make alternative plans if desired.[36,68,70]

A relationship is terminated when the patient is cured of the condition for which help was sought or is transferred to another physician's care, perhaps because of a complex problem, or is transferred back to the primary physician after a particular problem is solved. The relationship is also terminated when the physician and patient agree to terminate it or when the patient terminates it.

In addition, there are instances when a physician wishes to or it is advisable to terminate a relationship (e.g., the patient may not pay bills, may not follow advice, or may miss follow-up appointments). The patient may also threaten suit. Under such circumstances, the physician must assure follow-up care if possible, failure to do so being termed abandonment. Under these circumstances, the physician must evaluate the patient's condition, inform the patient of the medical problem and of his/her intent to withdraw from the case, and must carefully document this. The patient should be helped to find a new physician and must be given adequate time to do so.[36,68]

A major problem arises when the patient requires treatment and the insurer refuses to pay for it, placing the physician in an untenable position. The physician must provide adequate care, and this problem is discussed in detail in the chapter on managed care organizations (Chapter 23). If society decided to change the traditional obligation for the purpose of rationing, it could modify the physician's fiduciary relationship with the patient through legislative action, placing the locus for decision-making in the political arena, although this could be extremely problematic.[49]

INFORMED CONSENT

Once a relationship is established, health care requires diagnosis and treatment. These are a joint effort of the physician and patient based on a process called "informed consent." Consent is required for one person to touch another. Touching someone without consent is a crime called "battery" and a tort called "assault," even if no harm results. When a physician does something to a patient, not only must permission be obtained in order to avoid battery, but informed consent must be obtained, which requires information, competency, and voluntariness.[8,10,11,67]

The legal requirement for informed consent, based on the right of privacy, was enunciated in 1914 by Judge (later Supreme Court Justice) Benjamin Cardozo in a case in which surgery was performed without the patient's consent:

> Every human being of adult years and sound mind has a right to determine what shall be done with his own body; and a surgeon who performs an operation without his patient's

consent commits an assault, for which he is liable in damages.[63]

This statement is the embodiment of the common-law right of self-determination. It indicates a general requirement of consent and a more specific requirement of informed consent as well as the right of privacy, which includes the right to refuse treatment.[8,50,51] A decision must be voluntary and in no way coerced.

The term "informed consent" first appeared in the case of *Salgo v. Leland Stanford Jr. Univ. Bd. of Trustees*,[62] involving a patient who was paralyzed following transaortic arteriography. Based on a professional practice standard, the court stated that the physician had a duty to disclose "any facts which are necessary to form the basis of an intelligent consent by the patient to the proposed treatment."[31]

Since the 1970s, the courts have used a "patient-centered" standard in deciding issues of informed consent.[44] In 1972, in *Canterbury v. Spence*,[15] a standard was established of what information was material for a reasonable person to make a decision. This involves the nature of the risk and likelihood of this adverse event as well as the significance a reasonable person would attach to the risk given the circumstances.[5] However, in acute disabling conditions, such as a spinal cord injury, it has been suggested that patients may initially lack a full perspective on the problem, and decision-making should be deferred for some time.[56] If the physician does not obtain informed consent, and if harm results, then he/she is guilty of negligence.[8,10,67] There are times when a hospital also has liability, such as if it tolerates an incompetent physician or if its employee is responsible for obtaining permission.[10,67]

Different states have various statutes and court rulings that specify the indications and specifics for documented informed consent. The types of diagnostic and therapeutic procedures for which documentation is required include most invasive procedures, and these may be listed in detail in hospital policies. Proof of informed consent can be documented on a form or even on a videotape.

The physician must give information about: 1) the nature of the illness; 2) the proposed therapy in terms of its nature, its risks, what sort of success is to be expected, and what may be the results of forgoing it; and 3) the alternative therapies including their possible risks and benefits.[10,67]

One question is how much to discuss. There should be specific, substantial discussion about all aspects of the issues, especially common risks, even those of minor consequence, and any risks of major harm and death. The patient has the right to know and should be given any information which might sway the decision. The physician should also consider what is in the literature about the problem, what any prudent physician would say, and what the community standard might be. In at least one state, Texas, the state medical society developed a list of appropriate facts which should be given when obtaining informed consent for each of a number of operations. If such a list is not established, it is probably wisest to discuss even uncommon risks with the patient. Any question the patient asks, including how experienced the physician is in dealing with the problem, must be answered.[67]

It is the treating physician who has the responsibility to educate the patient and obtain the permission (although the authority to do so may be delegated). The presence of a third party, particularly someone who is a health care provider and may assist in answering questions, may be helpful.

The physician must comply with the patient's decision if it meets the criteria for informed consent. In any situation where the physician cannot honor a decision because of personal philosophy, help should be sought from sources such as an ethics committee, minister, or social worker. If agreement is not reached, withdrawal from the case and transfer of the patient is appropriate. If this is not possible, the physician may elect to apply to a court for a decision on the issues.[67]

There are times when a physician may obtain consent even if he/she will not be treating, such as if the physician were recommending a course of treatment or giving information or if he/she remains the primary care physician even during the care of another (such as a surgeon).

In order to have decision-making capacity to give informed consent, the patient must have competency (i.e., the ability to understand the consequences of one's decision, which requires the capacity to understand the relevant facts and to make a rational judgment based on those facts and one's value system).[33] It is the responsibility of the physician to judge mental competence,[8,9] which is discussed in Chapter 7. Whenever a decision seems inappropriate, it is the physician's responsibility to seek the help of the court on behalf of the patient.[8]

There are two groups who cannot give consent: minors and persons who are incompetent.[10,11,67]

Informed Consent for Minors

Minors (from birth to between 16 and 21 years, depending upon the state) cannot give informed consent because they are considered to lack knowledge, experience, and judgment, and so are not expected to be able to make adequate decisions. Parents, because of their bonds of affection and their legal and financial responsibility, are given the power to act on the behalf of their minor children. Generally, one parent is sufficient to give permission. If parents are divorced, the parent with custody or both parents may be needed to give permission. If parents are unavailable, a legal guardian or another relative may give consent.[8,9,27]

Parents can decide that treatment should be stopped, and their decision must be respected even if it leads to their child's death, as was established by the Indiana Supreme Court's 1982 Baby Doe decision (see *Bowen v. American Hospital Association*[12]). However, in certain circumstances in which prognosis is favorable, abandoning treatment may constitute child abuse, which may lead to problematic situations. The Baby Doe regulations,[3] which followed the Child Abuse Amendments of 1984, amending Child Abuse Prevention and Treatment Act of 1974 (Pub. L. No. 98-457 (1984)), amending Child Abuse Prevention and Treatment Act of 1974 (codified at 42 USC §§5101-5115, amended, 110 Stat. 3063 (October 3, 1996)), were an attempt to establish reasonable protection for children. Although they generally mandated care, they also provided exceptions in certain circumstances (i.e., if the patient is comatose, if care would prolong dying, or if care would be futile and inhumane).[8,72] This subject is also discussed in Chapter 6 on decisions at the end of life.

There are exceptions to the requirement of parental consent because of the sensitivity of the situation or the need to assure confidence so that the minor will come for help or will provide information or because of the status of the minor. Depending on the jurisdiction, exceptions include pregnancy, abortion, venereal disease, drug abuse, child abuse, or psychiatric problems. In addition, minors may be considered mature (after at least 14-15 years old) or to be emancipated. They could be emancipated if they live apart from their parents, support themselves, are married or have a child, or are in the military. If the parents' decisions appear inappropriate, the physician may need to try to protect a child by going to the court for clarification (since the state under the power of parens patriae acts as the protector of children). A classic problem is a child who is a member of the Jehovah's Witnesses and who needs a blood transfusion; this requires individualized consideration.[8,48,67]

Informed Consent for Incompetent Persons

Patients who are incompetent are another special class. Patients may be temporarily incapacitated (e.g., from medications), and the decision of whether to delay procedures needs to be individualized. Permanent incapacity may be total or partial, depending on the circumstances. Emotional or intellectual competence may require determination by an expert, as discussed in the chapter on competence, and/or a court order. Patients who are in a permanently vegetative state constitute a subset for which criteria are now available.[53,67] Anencephalic patients are another subset which has been well defined.[40] Brain-dead patients constitute another incompetent group, about which there is general agreement, and again this will be discussed later. Withholding and withdrawing care from such patients will be discussed in the chapter on the decisions at the end of life.

It should be noted that if a married person is competent, the right to give consent remains with the person, and there is no obligation to obtain the permission from the spouse. A person must be appointed as legal guardian to give consent for an incompetent spouse.[6,67]

Other Issues Regarding Informed Consent

One unusual problem that has been considered is the possibility of the consent by others for an incompetent person to become an organ donor of a paired organ or part of an organ (which would not usually be fatal). In this instance, there is the consideration of whether the potential donor could appreciate the help that this would give others and whether there would be personal benefit from improving another's health or preventing their death. There have been varying decisions on this point.[48,67,74] When the potential donor is a minor and a sibling, in at least two cases the courts have decided that giving an organ would create benefits justifying the small risk and have authorized donation.[23]

Another problem is what to do if, during surgery, an unexpected condition is discovered. It might be prudent to awaken the patient, discuss it, and obtain the appropriate informed consent. This would be true particularly if the new treatment concerned reproduction, loss of a limb or an organ, or other high risk.[10,67]

Another issue that might arise involves subsequent discovery of risks of prior treatment (e.g., silicone breast implant). The physician should attempt to notify the patient of the risk of bodily harm or death.[67]

There are situations in which informed consent is not required. There are emergencies in which there is immediate risk of death or serious bodily harm, and in these instances it is proper and even necessary for the physician to act. In addition, there are situations in which providing full information would make a patient too distraught to act or would exacerbate the illness, so discussion with the patient is limited under the rubric of "therapeutic privilege." In this setting, a full discussion should be held with the next of kin and the situation documented. At times, a patient may wish to waive the right to be informed, and here again a full discussion should be held with the family and the situation documented. The physician should also be sensitive to cultural and ethnic belief systems which have different norms and in which the patient defers to the physician, the family, or society for decision-making.[32] There are times when government rules dictate testing (e.g., blood alcohol concentration level) or treatment (e.g., vaccination). The physician who complies in good faith should be protected from liability. If there is a question, clarification can be requested from the court.[8,10,48,67]

TREATMENT WHEN CARE IS FUTILE

One issue that is being much debated is what to do in situations in which care is futile and yet such care is demanded. This subject is becoming critical because of the rising costs of health care, as well as the need to define what is appropriate or inappropriate. A few facts illustrate the problem. A large proportion of medical costs are expended in the last year of life. Only 10% of people treated in an intensive care unit (ICU) eventually leave the hospital.[8] Those over 65 years old constitute 11% of the population but consume 30% of health care expenditures. In addition, between 25% and 35% of medical care is said to be inappropriate or to carry risks equal to potential benefits.[65] However, only 10% to 12% of health care cost is spent on patients who die, and at most 27% of this (or 3% of total costs) might be saved by eliminating unwanted and futile care.[25]

The definition of what is futile is complex, but in general futile means of no ultimate value to the patient because the treatment is unable to achieve its physiological objective. Futility involves two aspects: 1) the chance that care will help, and 2) the quality of improvement that the care will provide. Both aspects can create difficulties. There is no agreement on how frequently a treatment should be successful for it to be used. Likewise, it is not clear what impact the treatment should have on a person's life to be considered useful. However, treatment may be considered inhumane "where it aimlessly prolongs an already pain-wracked existence, or where it inflicts new pain or discomfort without benefiting the patient."[39]

Based on a goal of benefiting the patient, a definition of treatment has been suggested. A treatment is futile if it had not helped the last 100 patients, if it would not be appreciated by a patient (i.e., if a patient were in a permanently vegetative state), or if it did not enable enjoyment of life (i.e., allow a patient to leave an ICU or the hospital). Physicians should not offer futile care because of professional responsibilities, including not deceiving a patient by offering a miracle.[65]

Judgment is to some degree subjective. Health care workers, even in critical care settings, have been shown not to agree on these issues.[57] The physician should provide information to help patients and families make individual decisions. On the other hand, many parties, including payors, hospital administrators, and lawyers, as well as governmental watchdogs, are intruding into patient-physician decision-making and influencing that decision-making based on considerations of costs as well as perceived benefits and risks. Physicians should carry out studies to better determine when care is futile and should educate and promote discussion with a view toward promoting societal decisions about futile care and legislation to solve the problem.[65] This subject will be discussed in several other chapters. A number of studies have begun to suggest that it will be possible to devise formulas to determine when care will be futile.[60]

To fully resolve the issues, patients, physicians, and society must come together, consider from all points of view pluralistic values and best information, agree on definitions of futility in general and in specific situations, and obtain more information about the effects of treatment. Organized medicine should drive consideration of this issue and develop guidelines, but legal standards will also be required.[27] An American Medical Association (AMA) task force has been constituted to try to define futile care. At the present time, there has been some agreement about limiting treatment in patients in a permanently vegetative state, where considerable law has developed, and in terminal cancer patients.

Basic questions are: "what are the rights of individuals and families to request care," and "what are the rights of the physician to refuse care when it is inappropriate." The problem of how the physician can restrain inappropriate treatment has been made more worrisome by several court cases.[20,65] In the Helga Wanglie[37] case in 1991, a court in Minneapolis mandated care for a vegetative patient because the husband requested it.[7,17] Care was also mandated in the cases of Baby K,[38] a neonate with anencephaly, and Baby L,[55] who was mentally retarded, blind, deaf, and quadriplegic. These cases indicate that there is lack of judicial support for withholding care. However, other recent cases may indicate some shift in this situation. A jury ruled that two physicians at Massachusetts General Hospital acted properly in withdrawing life support from a comatose woman despite the objections of her daughter, who was her surrogate decision-maker.[30,47] Unfortunately, this case did not clearly resolve all the issues involved, and at least an appellate court review would be required for it to have great legal import.[16] Laws were passed in Virginia (1992) and Maryland (1993) empowering physicians not to treat if ethically or medically inappropriate, but the interpretation of these laws has not been tested in courts.[20] Institutional policies may be developed to empower physicians,[20] as was done at the University of California, Los Angeles, in 1993, although this has not been tested.

Because of the lack of societal agreement about such circumstances, it is hard to recommend that physicians go against surrogates' wishes, even though physicians are not ethically obligated to provide care which is not helpful and indeed may have an obligation to patients and society not to do so.[9] This issue must be discussed and clarified by national consensus if physicians are to have the authority to stop futile treatment.[14] It has been suggested that guidelines be developed to assist such decisions, that physicians be empowered more, and that outside parties participate in decision-making.[45,52] Otherwise, there will be continued reliance on the courts when such cases arise, and outcomes may be inappropriate. There will always arise situations, particularly in borderline cases, which place the physician in ethical and legal quandaries and may require inappropriate care.[29,43]

ALLOCATION OF RESOURCES OR RATIONING

Allocation of resources or rationing requires consideration of how much money society wants to devote to medical care and, of this total amount, who is to get what portion, presumably on some just basis. This has only been done in a fragmented *ad hoc* fashion in the United States.

Based on the principle of "maximizing overall benefit to patients," the AMA Council on Ethical and Judicial Affairs has stated that acceptable criteria for allocation are likelihood of benefit, duration of benefit, change in the quality of life, urgency, and amount of resources required. When patients require similar resources and the chances of benefiting from treatment are equal, decisions should be made on a first-come, first-served basis. Inappropriate criteria are ability to pay, contribution of the patient to society, *perceived* obstacles to treatment, contribution of the patient to the medical condition, and past use of medical resources. The Council suggested developing allocation mechanisms which do not rely on physicians, but pointed out that centralized mechanisms and decentralized mechanisms are both problematic. The Council recommended patients be informed of the process. Guidelines for allocation of ICU beds and organs for transplantation were presented.[19]

In cases of absolute scarcity in individual situations, physicians can fulfill their tort obligations by acting reasonably.[49] However, this can cause conflicts of interest when the physician has obligations to two patients or to a patient and society. To avoid requiring physicians to make such decisions *ad hoc*, one author suggests that expert arbiters aid in decision-making when allocation of resources is an issue.[21]

Societal decision-making remains problematic, although efforts are being made to clarify the issues. Oregon created a pilot program for rationing based on ranking treatments in the order of usefulness, costing out the treatments, determining the funds available, and eliminating payment for treatments below the level at which funds would not be available. Implementation required a waiver from the federal government. This was denied in 1992 on the basis that the plan was inconsistent with Medicaid provisions since it used quality of well-being as a measure to prioritize care, which was said to illegally discriminate against the disabled.[31] The problems in the Oregon deliberations and the need for a democratic and just process with adequate sophistication have been pointed out.[28] In addition, it has been noted that the principle stating that "it is better to spend a sum for many inexpensive tests or treatments versus one expensive one" may not be just to the one person who could receive tremendous benefit.[73] Recent work on this subject involves how to determine the dollar worth of medical interventions in terms of years of functional life and satisfaction, how much different members of society are owed and should request, and what they are willing to pay for themselves and for others.[4,13] A national discussion about developing criteria for prioritization and mechanisms for doing this is necessary.

Confidentiality and Reporting

One of the most important considerations in the patient-physician relationship is the requirement of confidentiality. The right of a patient to expect protection of confidentiality has been recognized by professional codes from the time of the Hippocratic Oath, by the AMA from its earliest years, and by state medical societies. It is also obvious that without this expectation and protection, patients would be reluctant to discuss important but sensitive aspects of their medical problems with physicians. State licensure statutes also often mandate confidentiality. Because the law of England, from which U.S. law derives, did not encompass this right, all states, beginning with New York in 1928, enacted statutes allowing physicians to claim privilege from testifying about medical information in courts. Some statutes establish liability for disclosing confidential information in other circumstances. Court rulings, based on traditional medical ethics, the aforementioned statutes, licensure statutes, and public policy needs, have extended this privilege to other situations. The right to confidentiality extends even after death and is transferred to the legal representative or executor and to the next of kin.[34,35,69]

The definition of what is confidential information may be specified by state or federal law.

An example is information about alcohol and drug abuse. Because of the sensitive nature of information related to alcohol and drug abuse, including its prevention and treatment, federal law to guarantee confidentiality was enacted in the 1970s and amended in 1986 and again in 1992.[2] Regulations implementing these statutes were issued in 1975 and 1987.[1] If no statute applies, confidential information is defined as that which the patient would expect and want to be confidential, including information acquired in the context of the patient-physician relationship, information that is relevant and necessary for care, and information that is not absolutely required by society. To assure accuracy, the patient has the right to review, correct, and have copies of records and other relevant artifacts such as radiographs (unless there is an issue of therapeutic privilege).[34,35,69]

In most cases, confidentiality is not absolute. Confidentiality can be waived by the patient or can be overridden because of societal needs. A patient or legal guardian can authorize or request release of medical information in any circumstance, although consent must be voluntary, informed, and competent. There are also circumstances in which reporting of information about patients is mandatory or discretionary. Reporting of certain medical information may be compulsory by statute or regulation because of considerations of public welfare.[41] These include:

- vital statistics, including births and deaths
- abortions
- disease registries
- certain contagious diseases (this will be discussed in the chapter on infectious diseases)
- transplant requisites (i.e., brain death)
- occupational diseases and injuries
- child abuse and elder abuse
- wounds by particular means (e.g., guns and knives) or under particular circumstances (e.g., suspected homicide or suicide)
- excessive radiation exposure
- medical device failures
- environmental pollution
- prescriptions of certain drugs.

Requirements for Reporting to the CDC

When determining what diseases need to be reported one must consider two classes of patients, the living and the dead. As far as the living, there are several disease categories that the Centers for Disease Control (CDC) require be reported to them (state agencies may have their own requirements). These include:

- diseases or conditions to be reported immediately by telephone to the County Health Department (highly infectious diseases)
- diseases or conditions reported weekly to the County Health Department (certain infectious diseases)
- diseases to be reported weekly by numerical totals to the County Health Department (certain infectious diseases)
- illnesses of unusual prevalence or clusters of unexplained health occurrences to be reported to the State Health Department (includes AIDS, birth defects, cancer, hemophilia, lead poisoning, dengue, occupationally related illnesses, and unusual or ill-defined conditions).

Animal bites to humans must be reported to the CDC if the animal is rabid or could possibly be so. Communicable disease should be reported, and of note is the premarital requirement for testing for syphilis. The debate raging around AIDS reporting will be discussed in Chapter 16. Trauma must be reported, particularly where there is a question of a criminal act, negligence, defective products, or accidents. The issue of which victim of criminal acts should be reported revolves around who may or may not be vulnerable: children, the adult impaired, or victims of domestic abuse. Heinous acts such as gunshot wounds and some stabbings, along with other vicious woundings, are to be reported. Then there is the question of persons who pose a danger to themselves or others, which includes those with a seizure disorder, where laws vary from state to state, and those involved in accidents that may have resulted from alcohol or drug ingestion. Reporting considerations about patients who may have evidence of alcohol or drug abuse and who are involved in accidents are discussed in Chapter 14.

If there is a necessity to report a problem in a patient admitted to a hospital or nursing home, the institution should report the problem. In some instances, laboratories are also obligated to report positive findings on certain tests. In outpatient settings, reporting to the CDC is the responsibility of the individual physician.

Issues of Disclosure

In addition, medical information can be required by court order or by subpoena (requirement to appear) of a court or governmental administrative agency. In the case of a court order, the patient will have been notified about such an order, and failure to object indicates a waiver of confidentiality. However, the physician may still have concern and should verify the patient's permission to release information. If there is a question, the physician may ask the parties to bring the issue to the judge to resolve it, or a lawyer may be retained to bring this inquiry directly to the judge. In a courtroom, where the lawyers of the parties are present to represent them, a ruling may be requested from the judge.

Rules about disclosure vary from state to state. Several specific issues need to be considered.[34,35,69] In terms of transmission of information between physicians, since patients voluntarily undertake relationships with their various physicians, a conditional privilege between releasing and receiving physicians might be assumed. However, it is wise to obtain authorization, which initially may be oral but eventually should be confirmed in writing. Photographs can be particularly sensitive artifacts. Confidentiality requires specific permission to even photograph patients. If a patient who requires care for mental or physical disease is determined by reason of incompetence to be a danger to self, the physician has immunity to participate in commitment procedures. The assessment of competence will be discussed in Chapter 7, and the rights of the patient to refuse treatment are discussed in Chapter 6. If the patient is determined to be a danger to others, for instance because of a predisposition to violence (*Tarasoff v. Board of Regents*[71]) or because of a communicable disease, and if the patient refuses to adjust the behavior, the specific individual at risk should and must be notified. There may even be an obligation to warn the public (*Naidu v. Laird*[54]).[34,36] On the other hand, if a patient is competent and not a danger, even a spouse is not entitled to confidential information.

Law enforcement officers generally require appropriate court orders to obtain confidential information, except for situations with mandated reporting requirements. Of note, the U.S. Supreme Court (*Schmerber v. California*[64]) has authorized the warrantless seizure of a blood sample for assessment of alcohol level if this is in connection with an arrest, there is probable cause, and the collection method is acceptable. However, this does not permit the use of information obtained for the purpose of medical diagnosis and care. This subject will be discussed in Chapter 12E on forensic pathology.

There are circumstances in which there is media interest in a patient. In the case of a public official or a celebrity, the public has an interest in the person and the press has the privilege to inform. Information may be released, but this should be limited and circumspect and subject to the approval by the patient. In the case of a newsworthy event, a person may be involved who is not known to the public. There are no good rules about release of information in this situation, but the best thing would be to obtain consent for whatever will be communicated.

One very frequent question is what to tell private insurance companies or other insurers about a patient. One should have authorization to release information to the insurance company, and then should report only what is needed. This subject is also discussed in the chapter on payors (Chapter 24).

There are times when a physician is employed by a third party to assess a patient. Here the allegiance is to that third party and not the patient. An exception arises if the physician offers unsolicited advice or treatment, in which case a relationship is initiated and therefore a duty to the patient exists. Sometimes a physician is hired by a third party to treat. The physician should let the patient know of this relationship and request authorization from the patient for release of information.

In a clinic or hospital, numerous employees have access to medical records as a consequence of their positions, but such people are legally bound to protect confidentiality. Researchers and teachers may be given limited access. In addition, patient information is now used without permission by hospital physician committees and hospital review groups (for statistical studies, review for privileges, and quality assurance) as well as by regulatory and licensing agencies. This subject is also discussed in the chapter on medical records.

There are certain legal situations, the institution of which by nature overrides confidentiality. These include: 1) child custody disputes (because of the interest of the child); 2) litigation by the patient involving his or her medical problems ("patient litigation exception"); 3) contest of a patient's will; 4) legal actions by a physician, such as for non-payment of bills; and 5) legal actions by a patient, such as filing a malpractice claim or even retaining an attorney, with regard to a physician discussing the case with his/her own attorney.

In the case of a lawsuit by the patient, the physician may be contacted by an attorney for the opposing side. If there is authorization from the patient, a court order, or a subpoena requiring release of information, the physician should comply. Without authorization, the response should be governed by the local laws. In some jurisdictions, courts have held that instituting a suit obviates confidentiality and that it is efficient to allow "informal discovery" to promote access to information for the opposing lawyer. In other jurisdictions, courts have held that the patient has a right to protect self-interest and that information should not be made freely available. In any case, the physician is not compelled to cooperate with opposing counsel without the involvement of friendly counsel.

It is thus wise for the physician to: 1) become informed about the local law; 2) notify the patient prior to any disclosure (to give the patient an opportunity to object); and 3) request legal authorization (either consent from the patient, or, if the patient objects, a court order) prior to any disclosure.

Another question is whether medical information should be made available to individuals involved in an adoption. Because of the distress that could be caused to the natural parent, the adoptive parents, or the adoptee, such disclosures are strongly discouraged.

Failure to follow legal guidelines about confidentiality creates liability on several bases, including: 1) contract theory (breach of promise of confidentiality); and 2) tort theory (breach of duty of privacy or confidentiality, which has a shorter statute of limitations).

If false information is transmitted (called defamation and termed libel if written or slander if oral) and if the information is by nature defamatory (e.g., alleges criminal misconduct or infection with a venereal disease) or the information can be shown to cause damage to the person's reputation, the patient can sue. If the defendant had acted intentionally or recklessly or with malice, the plaintiff can request punitive damages.

If confidential information is released inappropriately in a legal case, this information might be excluded, and if a decision were based on this information, the decision might even be reversed.[34,35,69]

In every state the law requires that when a patient dies, the attending physician must declare death and fill out a death certificate, which includes the condition that resulted in death and the time it occurred. The medical examiner/coroner must be notified if there has not been a physician recently involved in the patient's care or under certain circumstances such as violent, accidental, or mysterious death including: 1) dead on arrival; 2) death from possible criminal actions; 3) death from industrial accidents; 4) death from vehicular accidents; 5) death from burns, chemicals, electricity or radiation; 6) death less than 24 hours after hospital admission, perioperative deaths, or deaths from therapeutic misadventures; and 7) death while in a public institution or in custody of the law.

The medical examiner/coroner will make a determination of whether an autopsy is required. If an autopsy is not required, then the next of kin, who has a property interest in the body, may request a total or limited autopsy. The decedent may have made wishes known before death, but the next of kin has the ultimate decision-making power.[8,42]

CONCLUSIONS

The relationship between patients and physicians is in a state of flux. A recent review has put the situation in perspective.[6] Historically, there has been an evolution from the tradition of the physician as a paternalistic and authoritarian expert in charge of medical care to a democratic, even libertarian, view of the right of the patient to request or refuse care to a system in which resources are believed to be limited and outside forces, including government and managed care entities, regulate services. It is clear that the patient should have autonomy but that this requires responsibility and must be limited to a certain degree. Physicians must continue to act as advocates and educators, but must develop guidelines for care (requiring new research to determine what is useful) and should be given the authority to use such guidelines. Third parties must develop institutional ethics to assure useful care is given and should be kept distant from the relationship between patients and physicians.

REFERENCES

1. 42 CFR §§21 et seq
2. 42 USC §290dd-2
3. 45 CFR §8455 (1985)
4. Annas GJ: **Standard of Care. The Law of American Bioethics.** New York, NY: Oxford University Press, 1993
5. Ausman JI: Informed consent. **Surg Neurol 44:** 495-497, 1995
6. Balint J, Shelton W: Regaining the initiative. Forging a new model of the patient-physician relationship. **JAMA 275:**887-891, 1996
7. Belois PL: The conservatorship of Helga M. Wanglie. **Issues Law Med 7:**369-377,1991
8. Berger AS: **Dying and Death in Law and Medicine. A Forensic Primer for Health and Legal Professionals.** Westport, Conn: Praeger, 1993
9. Bernat JL: **Ethical Issues in Neurology.** Boston, Mass: Butterworth-Heinemann, 1994
10. Bianco EA, Hirsh HL: Consent to and refusal of medical treatment, in American College of Legal Medicine (ed): **Legal Medicine. Legal Dynamics of Medical Encounters.** 3rd ed. St Louis, Mo: CV Mosby, 1995, pp 274-296
11. Bisbing SB, McMenamin JP, Granville RL: Competency, capacity, and immunity, in American College of Legal Medicine (ed): **Legal Medicine. Legal Dynamics of Medical Encounters.** 3rd ed. St Louis, Mo: CV Mosby, 1995, pp 27-45
12. *Bowen v American Hospital Association,* 476 US 610, 106 SCt 2101 (1986)
13. Brock DW: **Life and Death: Philosophical Essays in Biomedical Ethics.** Cambridge, Engl: Cambridge University Press, 1993
14. Brody H: The physician's role in determining futility. **J Am Geriatr Soc 42:**875-878, 1994
15. *Canterbury v Spence,* 464 F2d 772, 787 (DC Cir 1972)
16. Capron AM: Abandoning a waning life. **Hastings Cent Rep 25:**24-26, 1995
17. Capron AM: In re Helga Wanglie. **Hastings Cent Rep 21:**26-28, 1991
18. Council on Ethical and Judicial Affairs, American Medical Association: **Code of Medical Ethics: Current Opinions.** Chicago, Ill: American Medical Association, 1992
19. Council on Ethical and Judicial Affairs, American Medical Association: Ethical considerations in the allocation of organs and other scarce medical resources among patients. **Arch Intern Med 155:** 29-40, 1995
20. Daar JF: Medical futility and implications for physician autonomy. **Am J Law Med 21:**221-240, 1995
21. Dubler N, Nimmons D: **Ethics on Call. Taking Charge of Life-and-Death Choices in Today's Health Care System.** New York, NY: Vintage Books, 1993
22. Dworkin RM: **Life's Dominion. An Argument About Abortion, Euthanasia, and Individual Freedom.** New York, NY: Alfred A Knopf, 1993
23. Dwyer J, Vig E: Rethinking transplantation between siblings. **Hastings Cent Rep 25:**7-19, 1995
24. Eichelman BS, Hartwig AC: **Patient Violence and the Clinician.** Washington, DC: American Psychiatric Press, 1995
25. Emanuel EJ, Emanuel LL: The economics of dying. The illusion of cost savings at the end of life. **N Engl J Med 330:**540-544, 1994
26. Ficarra BJ: Ethics and bioethics, in American College of Legal Medicine (ed): **Legal Medicine. Legal Dynamics of Medical Encounters.** 3rd ed. St Louis, Mo: CV Mosby, 1995, pp 351-363
27. Fins JJ: Futility in clinical practice: report on a Congress of Clinical Societies. **J Am Geriatr Soc 42:** 861-865, 1994
28. Fleck LM: Just caring: Oregon, health care rationing, and informed democratic deliberation. **J Med Philos 19:**367-388, 1994
29. Fowler FJ Jr (ed): The Proceedings of the Conference on Measuring the Effects of Medical Treatment. **Med Care Suppl 33,** 1995
30. *Gilgum v Massachusetts General Hospital,* Super Ct Civ Action No. 92-4820, Suffolk Co, Mass, *verdict,* 21 April 1995
31. Goldworth A, Silverman W, Stevenson DK, et al (eds): **Ethics and Perinatology.** New York, NY: Oxford University Press, 1995
32. Gostin LO: Informed consent, cultural sensitivity, and respect for persons. **JAMA 274:**844-845, 1995
33. Gunn M: The meaning of incapacity. **Med Law Rev 2:**8-29, 1994
34. Hirsh HL: Disclosures about patients, in American College of Legal Medicine (ed): **Legal Medicine. Legal Dynamics of Medical Encounters.** 3rd ed. St Louis, Mo: CV Mosby, 1995, pp 312-342
35. Hirsh HL: Medical records, in American College of Legal Medicine (ed): **Legal Medicine. Legal Dynamics of Medical Encounters.** 3rd ed. St Louis, Mo: CV

Mosby, 1995, pp 297-311

36. Howard ML, Vogt LB: Physician-patient relationship, in American College of Legal Medicine (ed): **Legal Medicine. Legal Dynamics of Medical Encounters.** 3rd ed. St Louis, Mo: CV Mosby, 1995, pp 265-273

37. *In re Wanglie*, No. PX-91-283 (Hennepin Cty, Minn, Probate Ct, June 28, 1991)

38. *In the Matter of Baby K*, 832 F Supp 1022 (ED Va 1993) aff'd, 16 F3d 590 (4th Cir), *cert denied*, 115 SCt 91 (1994)

39. Jecker NS, Pagon RA: Medical futility: decision-making in the context of probability and uncertainty, in Goldworth A, Silverman W, Stevenson DK, et al (eds): **Ethics and Perinatology.** New York, NY: Oxford University Press, 1995

40. Kaufman HH, Bodensteiner J, Simmons GM, et al: Anencephaly, in McComb JG, Venes JL (eds): **Neural Tube Defects, Volume 1.** Park Ridge, Ill: American Association of Neurological Surgeons (In press)

41. Kaufman HH, Lewin J, Munzner R, et al: Ethical and legal responsibilities of the neurosurgeon: selected topics. **Neurosurgery 28:**918-923, 1991

42. Kaufman HH, Lynn J: Brain death. **Neurosurgery 19:** 850-856, 1986

43. Kopelman LM: Conceptual and moral disputes about futile and useful treatments. **J Med Philos 20:** 109-121, 1995

44. Laine C, Davidoff F: Patient-centered medicine. A professional evolution. **JAMA 275:**152-156, 1996

45. Law, Medicine & Health Care: Medical futility. **Law Med Health Care 20:**307-339, 1992

46. Manuel BM: No good deed goes unpunished. **Bull Am Coll Surg 80:**28, 29, 50, 1995

47. Mass jury: Doctors were right to withdraw life support. **Am Med News.** May 8, 1995

48. McMenamin JP, Bigley GL: Children as patients, in American College of Legal Medicine (ed): **Legal Medicine. Legal Dynamics of Medical Encounters.** 3rd ed. St Louis, Mo: CV Mosby, 1995, pp 456-487

49. Mehlman MJ, Massey SR: The patient-physician relationship and the allocation of scarce resources: a law and economics approach. **Kennedy Inst Ethics J 4:** 291-308, 1994

50. Meisel A: The legal consensus about forgoing life-sustaining treatment: its status and its prospects. **Kennedy Inst Ethics J 2:**309-345, 1993

51. Misbin R (ed): **Euthanasia. The Good of the Patient–The Good of Society.** Frederick, Md: University Publishing Group, 1992

52. Morreim EH: Profoundly diminished life. The casualties of coercion. **Hastings Cent Rep 24:**33-42, 1994

53. Multi-society Task Force on PVS: Medical aspects of the persistent vegetative state. Parts 1 and 2. **N Engl J Med 330:**1499-1508, 1572-1579, 1994

54. *Naidu v Laird*, 539 A2d 1064, 1073 (Del 1988)

55. Paris JJ, Crone RK, Reardon F: Physicians' refusal of requested treatment. The case of Baby L. **N Engl J Med 322:**1012-1015, 1990

56. Patterson DR, Miller-Perrin C, McCormick TR, et al: When life support is questioned early in the care of patients with cervical-level quadriplegia. **N Engl J Med 328:**506-509, 1993

57. Raffin TA: Withdrawing life support. How is the decision made? **JAMA 273:**738-739, 1995

58. Reamer FG (ed): **AIDS & Ethics.** New York, NY: Columbia University Press, 1991

59. Rodwin MA: Patient accountability and the quality of care: lessons from medical consumerism and the patients' rights, women's health and disability rights movements. **Am J Law Med 20:**147-167, 1994

60. Rowe JW: Health care myths at the end of life. **Bull Am Coll Surg 81:**11-18, 1996

61. Royal MA: Patients with human immunodeficiency virus (HIV) infection and acquired immunodeficiency syndrome (AIDS), in American College of Legal Medicine (ed): **Legal Medicine. Legal Dynamics of Medical Encounters.** 3rd ed. St Louis, Mo: CV Mosby, 1995, pp 516-530

62. *Salgo v Leland Stanford Jr Univ Bd of Trustees*, 317 P2d 170, 181 (Cal App 1957)

63. *Schloendorff v. Society of New York Hospitals*, New York Supreme Court, Vol 211, NY, pp 129-130

64. *Schmerber v California*, 384 US 757 (1966)

65. Schneiderman LJ, Jecker NS: **Wrong Medicine. Doctors, Patients, and Futile Treatment.** Baltimore, Md: Johns Hopkins University Press, 1995

66. Tarasaka JM: AIDS, infectious diseases and the health care practitioner, in Tarasaka JM: **Legal Guide for Physicians.** White Plains, NY: AHAB Press, 1995, pp 13.01-13.100[3]

67. Tarasaka JM: Consent and informed consent, in Tarasaka JM: **Legal Guide for Physicians.** White Plains, NY: AHAB Press, 1995, pp 6.01-6.100[18]

68. Tarasaka JM: The bases of civil liability for health care providers, in Tarasaka JM: **Legal Guide for Physicians.** White Plains, NY: AHAB Press, 1995, pp 4.01-4.08[4]

69. Tarasaka JM: The disclosure of patient information, in Tarasaka JM: **Legal Guide for Physicians.** White Plains, NY: AHAB Press, 1995, pp 3.01-3.100[6]

70. Tarasaka JM: The doctor/patient relationship, in Tarasaka JM: **Legal Guide for Physicians.** White Plains, NY: AHAB Press, 1995, pp 2.01-2.100[5]

71. *Tarasoff v Board of Regents*, 551 P2d 334, 340 (Cal 1976)

72. Urofsky MI: **Letting Go; Death, Dying & the Law.** New York, NY: Maxwell Macmillan International, 1993

73. Veatch R: Research on "big-ticket" items: ethical implications for equitable access. **J Law Med Ethics 22:** 148-151, 1994

74. Weedn VW, Kellerman E: Organ donation and transplantation, in American College of Legal Medicine (ed): **Legal Medicine. Legal Dynamics of Medical Encounters.** 3rd ed. St Louis, Mo: CV Mosby, 1995, pp 372-403

APPENDIX

SOURCES OF DETAILED LEGAL DISCUSSIONS OF THE STATUTES, RULES, AND
COURT CASES IN MEDICAL LAW RELATING TO PATIENT DECISION-MAKING

American College of Legal Medicine: **Legal Medicine. Legal Dynamics of Medical Encounters.** 3rd ed. St Louis, Mo: Mosby-Year Book, 1995, 670 pp. (An encyclopedic treatise which references laws, rules, and court cases. Many of its authors have both medical and law degrees. The college represents legal medicine in the House of Delegates of the AMA.)

Annas GJ, Law SA, Rosenblatt RE, et al: **American Health Law.** Boston, Mass: Little, Brown and Co, 1990, 1000 pp. (A standard, comprehensive, detailed text.)

Berger AS: **Dying and Death in Law and Medicine. A Forensic Primer for Health and Legal Professionals.** Westport, Conn: Praeger, 1993, 228 pp. (A review of medical and legal issues faced by patients at the end of life. The book discusses the most important statutes and court cases.)

Bernat JL: **Ethical Issues in Neurology.** Boston, Mass: Butterworth-Heinemann, 1994, 364 pp. (A comprehensive discussion of ethics, particularly as applied to patients with serious neurological disease. The author provides an excellent review of the statutes and judicial decisions that relate to these problems.)

Council on Ethical and Judicial Affairs, American Medical Association: **Code of Medical Ethics. Current Opinions with Annotations (1994 Edition).** Chicago, Ill: American Medical Association, 1994, 177 pp. (Although basically a discussion of the ethics which are a basis for the law, this edition for the first time cites many landmark court decisions, state attorney general opinions, and selected articles from the medical, legal, and ethics literature.)

Hoefler JM: **Deathright: Culture, Medicine, Politics, and the Right to Die.** Boulder, Colo: Westview Press, 1994, 291 pp. (A discussion of the forces that influence the development of law and a review of the development of right to die law in the courts and the legislatures.)

Meyers DW: **The Human Body and the Law.** Edinburgh: Edinburgh University Press, 1990, 367 pp. (An excellent, well-referenced treatise on health care law.)

Meyers DW: **Medico-Legal Implications of Death and Dying.** Rochester, NY: Lawyers Co-operative Publishing Co, 1981, 639 pp. + cumulative supplements. (An excellent, well-referenced treatise on health care law regarding situations at the end of life.)

Taraska JM: **Legal Guide for Physicians.** White Plains, NY: AHAB Press, 1995, 1281 pp. (A loose-leaf guide to the laws affecting health care. This is updated annually.)

CHAPTER 6

Decisions at the End of Life

Howard H. Kaufman, MD

Dying is the ultimate crisis, the extinction of the individual who has lost control of his/her fate and often is in physical and mental anguish. Although dying and death are an inevitable part of living and therefore must be accepted, they are also a defeat of life and so are dreaded and resisted.

In recent decades, evolving medical technologies have begun to permit the support of vegetative functions in circumstances that in the past would have led to a rapid demise. Such care may result in prolongation of a life which is excessively burdensome because of a permanently disabling condition or a painful terminal disease or may stabilize vital signs in a person for whom consciousness has been lost permanently. Concerns about the use of scarce resources and the excessive expense of treatment have become important considerations. Lastly, there has been a change in the model of the relationship between patients and physicians, from an approach in which the physician decides for the patients how they are to be treated to an approach in which patients are to be informed and educated and then have the right and responsibility to decide for themselves whether treatment is desired. These circumstances have forced our society to confront many new questions about how to deal with the dying process, including how long to pursue cardiorespiratory support and to administer nutrition and hydration.

When considering treatment during the dying process, it must be remembered that life is sacred and that personal growth occurs even with suffering. On the other hand, artificially prolonging dying may not always be humane. Traditional medical ethics teach that the role of the physician is to stop dying and restore health. But inevitable death should be "peaceful and dignified." In addition, the patient has the right to expect to be told the truth, to participate in the decision-making process, and to be given the opportunity to make personal, legal, and financial arrangements for death.[18,19,191] Current studies, including an extensive investigation, the Study to Understand Prognosis and Preferences for Outcomes and Risks of Treatment (SUPPORT), reveal that physicians often do not know patients' wishes, that many patients, even the elderly, do want aggressive treatment, and that such care can offer prolonged life. Problems arise when the patient demands futile care or when there are pressures on the physician to restrict care to minimize costs.[127] These issues require the physician to remain committed to advocacy for the patient and for society at large to agree upon shifts of priority, as will be discussed in this and other chapters.

The law is constituted to protect citizens from abuses and to promote their welfare. On the other hand, our political system emphasizes liberty, as specified in the privacy and due process clauses in the United States Bill of Rights, and the right of self-determination in the common law. These rights have been the basis of a series of state and federal legal opinions which specify that the individual can refuse medical care even if this means death. However, the next question is how to deal with patients who have lost competency. This has led to the development of advanced directives and refinement of surrogate decision-making. Then there is the problem of how to deal with people who were never competent, namely how to avoid inappropriate care while at the same time protecting their right to treatment when it will be beneficial.

There are a number of specific classes/situations which require so-called "end-of-life" decisions. These include three major classes and within each class are several specific situations:

1. The competent—including the right to refuse treatment, physical incapacity, terminal illness, aging, suicide, and physician-assisted death.
2. Those who have lost competency—including advance directives, dementia, brain death, the permanent vegetative state, and organ donation.
3. The never competent—the fetus, the anencephalic, the infant, the older child/adolescent, and the adult.

A substantial body of law dealing with these issues has been reviewed in detail in several outstanding treatises (see Appendix at the end of Chapter 5).

END-OF-LIFE DECISION FOR COMPETENT PERSONS

The Right to Refuse Care

The right to refuse care is illustrated by the right of a member of the Jehovah's Witnesses to refuse a blood transfusion, even if the refusal will result in death. There are many legal cases in which this right has been affirmed.[13,19,68,96,195]

This right can only be compromised for a competent person if it conflicts with certain interests of the state. These were discussed in *In re Conroy*[102] and include: 1) preserving life (which might then involve the determination of competence); 2) preventing suicide; 3) protecting innocent third parties (e.g., controlling communicable disease and mandating care for a mother of minor children); and 4) safeguarding the integrity of the medical profession (although if this compromised a patient's right to refuse care, the physician might be compelled by court order to transfer the care of the patient to another physician or to cease certain care). Two groups who cannot give consent and thus cannot refuse treatment are minors and people who are deemed incompetent.[23,25,190]

Physical Incapacity

Certain patients, although not terminally ill, are so severely incapacitated and/or suffering that they wish to stop support, including nutrition and hydration. Two landmark cases were: 1) Perlmutter, a victim of amyotrophic lateral sclerosis, who successfully petitioned a court to permit him to stop his respirator (*Satz v. Perlmutter*[174]); and 2) Bouvia, a severely disabled victim of cerebral palsy described as a woman so incapacitated by cerebral palsy that she "must lie physically helpless subject to ignominy, embarrassment, humiliation and dehumanizing aspects created by her helplessness" who petitioned the court successfully for the right to not be forced to have tube feedings (*Bouvia v. Superior Court*).[18,29,99] In such cases, the physician must bear in mind the patient's right to refuse care.

Terminal Illness

Some patients are terminally ill and expected to die in a short period no matter what treatment is given. It has been pointed out that the incidence of distressing symptoms in dying patients is not known. However, there are ways of dealing with the most distressing symptoms. Another problem is that the needs of dying patients are not fully understood, and service and funding for these needs are not generally available. In addition, patient preferences with regard to care have not been studied extensively. These subjects deserve more study, but it is clear that enlarged infrastructure and increased funding is necessary to meet these needs.[55]

Still, it is known that in some patients who are burdened with uncontrollable pain and suffering, treatment adds additional discomfort and is ultimately futile. It is appropriate under these circumstances to discontinue unwanted treatment.[18,19,191] It has been shown that patients can be comfortably maintained despite minimal, if any, intake of food or even water, and aggressively treated patients may actually have complications of treatment (and increased tumor growth).[133] Even the diagnosis of depression may not preclude honoring a request for forgoing treatment if competence remains, particularly since the depression may be appropriate.[188] When considering treatment, one must honor the patient's right to refuse care.

Aging

The demographics of the United States are changing with regard to the number and percentage of people over 65 years old. This group of citizens has been growing steadily because of increased life expectancy and now number 30 million people (12% of the population). This figure will increase because of the multitude of aging "baby boomers." Their number is expected to double in the next 40 years, especially the "old old," defined as those aged 85 years and more, who will increase from 3 million to over 20 million. More than one-half of the elderly are females, of whom one-half are widows. While in general the elderly are gaining in affluence, elderly women are less affluent.

Many of these elderly are healthy, and the enlarging knowledge about preserving wellness as well as the application of that knowledge to preserve wellness may mean that even more of the elderly will be robust. However, a significant number of the elderly suffer from chronic problems which impact on the quality of their lives. Data from the 1980s suggest at age 65 years, when men will live to 80 years and women to 84 years, 10%-20% of their remaining life will be dependent; at 75 years, when men will live to 84 years and women to 87 years, 25%; and at 85 years, when men will live to 90 years and women to 93 years, 50%.[170] Of those over 65 years,

two million are in nursing facilities and seven million will spend some time in a nursing facility. Eighty percent of nursing home inhabitants have mental impairment; half of them are ill with Alzheimer's disease. While in a nursing home all are constrained by the rules of the institution, and one-half by physical or chemical restraints.[65]

Most problematic is impairment of mental health. This problem was studied by the White House Mini-Conference on Emerging Issues in Mental Health and Aging, February 1995, whose resources, papers, and reservations form an important source for understanding and planning.[75] The following was noted: 18%-25% of people over 65 years old have mental health problems, including delirium, dementia, depression, mania, psychosis, and anxiety; many persons currently in their 40s and 50s are already afflicted with depression, anxiety, and substance abuse; much has been learned about prevention, diagnosis, and treatment in the last decade; much more research is needed; and there needs to be improvement in the funding and systems to deal with this problem.

In the U.S. today, one-third of the federal budget goes to aid older people, essentially creating a welfare state for the elderly. The older 12% of the population account for 50% of deaths and consume 30% of all health expenditures, particularly in the last year of life and especially in the last month of life.[55] If current trends continue, the cost for medical care of older people will continue to rise, although the change appears to be due to their increasing numbers since the lifetime medical care of individuals does not rise very much for older individuals and the cost of care at the end of life actually decreases as they age.[88,120,170,203] Nevertheless, more extensive use of hospices, rather than hospitals, and the implementation of advance directives, which would lead to desired and more appropriate care, could result in savings of several billion dollars a year.[70,131,170] Projections suggest that, given current trends, this will mean the Medicare Trust Fund will become bankrupt about the year 2001 and, thereafter, health care will lead to large federal deficits.[34]

The growing number of elderly individuals, both vigorous and impaired, in a time of contracting resources, will force those individuals to consider how much medical care they want and society to consider what is their due.[31] The needs of the elderly will have to be balanced against other societal needs, including food, housing, and education, as well as health care (including the needs of various generations, such as immunizations for children, maternal care and trauma care for young adults, and cancer care and geriatric care for older individuals). It has been suggested that there should be more research on the disabling diseases of the elderly.[203] It should be remembered that mental dysfunction is seen with various ailments and is often reversible.[65] Another issue is how to determine the effectiveness of such treatments as cardiopulmonary resuscitation (CPR), enteral feeding, and dialysis.[203]

Of course, the elderly have an interest in living as long as they are able to enjoy life, and indeed can continue to grow mentally and spiritually. Also, as members of the human community, they have a right to expect respect and humane treatment and repayment for their contributions in working and raising families. On the other hand, it is in their best interests to learn to meet death with equanimity. Indeed, many elderly do not wish aggressive care that provides little chance of success but which causes suffering.[203] Death as a result of aging and loss of will to live is a natural event.[134] In addition, some have suggested that since the elderly have had the opportunity for a full life, they should not make demands which will compromise the welfare of future generations and thus are obliged by an "ethics of responsibility" to place a limit on their expectations.

The suggestion has been made that in order to give each generation an equal share of the resources of society, there should be rationing of health care purely on the basis of age. However, since exceptions might have to be made for individuals who are extremely valuable to society or who remain very healthy and vigorous, rules would have to be complex and would still risk being subjective and arbitrary.[120,144,203]

Another suggestion is to develop a system for allocation of resources by category of treatment rather than rationing by age or other patient-specific criteria. This would require a cost/benefit analysis so that reasonable treatment, particularly primary care and long-term care, would

be given. On the other hand, very expensive care that offers only limited assistance or treatment that does not lead to improved quality of life would not be initiated.[120,144,203]

Discussion of such options must be done publicly in order to establish fair guidelines based on trust and solidarity so that all generations will buy into the system.[34,144] Considerations may include place in the queue, potential quality of life, and, to a lesser extent, value to society, and will have to include allocation decisions for all generations.[96] Perhaps it should be mandated that all Medicare recipients fill out advance directives.[34]

Suicide

Suicide has been described as a self-inflicted, self-intended cessation of life. Suicide is an act carried out to remove oneself from an unbearable situation and is characterized by helplessness and hopelessness. It is the result of the conjunction of three factors: the individual's personality, the general situation, and the specific problem leading to the act. Suicide may be made a criminal act by state law, and this is the case in a number of states, but the law is rarely, if ever, invoked in the U.S. to punish a person for attempting suicide.[195]

The physician may be concerned with suicide in several circumstances: 1) in a patient who may be suicidal, where preventive action is indicated, 2) in a patient who may request help in carrying out suicide, where a response must be made, and 3) in a victim of a suicide attempt, such as a self-inflicted gunshot wound to the head, where care is required.

Suicide is often the result of correctable circumstances, and therefore prevention and treatment generally are indicated. If a patient is suspected of being suicidal, the physician should facilitate treatment of depression and improvement in the patient's environment.[27] Much can also often be done to deal with the cause of stress, for example, aggressive pain control for a cancer victim, an area of interest to neurosurgeons.

When faced with a patient who has attempted suicide (e.g., a self-inflicted gunshot wound to the head), if the physician accepts that the underlying depression can be treated and that a patient will benefit by care, he/she obviously should do so. Therefore, the judgment to treat should be based on the prognosis of the injury itself as well as other mitigating circumstances, such as the presence of terminal disease. As a violent injury, suicide should be reported to the proper authorities, as discussed elsewhere.

However, there are instances of debilitating disease or terminal disease when suffering cannot be relieved, and then suicide may be considered "rational."[53] The circumstances in which assisted suicide or a request for euthanasia has been thought, at least by some, to be appropriate will be discussed below.

Physician-Assisted Death (Assisted Suicide and Euthanasia)

Physician-assisted death (PAD) includes a physician giving medication to relieve pain and suffering which might also hasten death (double effect), giving information about suicide, and helping at suicide (physician-assisted suicide—PAS). PAD also includes overtly ending the patient's life (voluntary active euthanasia) since there are terminally ill patients who because of physical or mental incapacity cannot end their own lives and would require help in dying. Generally discussed in relation to terminally ill patients, there is also the question of whether PAD should be permitted in patients who, while not terminally ill, are experiencing intolerable pain and incapacity because of incurable diseases or disabilities.

A logical extension of the right of self-determination is to honor the request of a terminally ill patient for the physician to hasten dying. The arguments include the following: needless suffering is not in the patient's best interest and therefore under certain circumstances death may be a lesser harm; the patient has the right to ask that this suffering be stopped; and the physician is the person who has the expertise and thus an obligation to carry out the patient's wishes.[110,140,141] Such reasoning involves the physician's obligation to care for a patient (rather than to treat) and interpretation of historical traditions and ethical considerations (including autonomy) which support PAD.[143]

Several authors have discussed the patient's constitutional right to die.[59,68,176] Dworkin concludes that the issue of controlling one's fate:

> . . . involves decisions not just about the rights and interests of particular people, but about the intrinsic, cosmic importance of human life itself. In each case, opinions divide not because some people have contempt for values that others cherish, but, on the contrary, because the values in question are at the center of everyone's lives, and no one can treat them as trivial enough to accept other people's orders about what they mean. Making someone die in a way that others approve, but he believes a horrifying contradiction of his life, is a devastating, odious form of tyranny.[68]

Strict safeguards could be created to prevent abuses.[185] Decisions as to whether PAD is appropriate need to be individualized based on the patient's situation.[152] This requires considering seven issues: eligibility (e.g., terminal disease); mental competence or capacity; consent; voluntariness; witnesses; a definition of what constitutes abuse; and a requirement to report, investigate, and punish abuse.[37] One suggestion includes the requirement for case-specific oversight by palliative-care consultants who would aid in decision-making as well as more general oversight and education by palliative-care committees.[141] In addition, if there are conditions under which suicide is legally acceptable, a second person should not be liable for helping someone exercise that right.[19] However, it has been argued that regulation is not possible and that abuses could not be prevented because of the privacy/confidentiality inherent in the patient-physician relationship and because of the impossibility of adequately defining the medical situation, the mental and emotional state of the patient, and the reactions of the physician.[37]

It has been suggested that assisting death is morally different from allowing death to occur by withholding or withdrawing care, that this practice would compromise the trust placed in physicians, and that the result would be the excessive application of euthanasia.[31,99,110,122,137,157] Even assuming acceptance of PAD in principle, the patient's prognosis may be wrong or a new treatment or cure may be developed and be of benefit. More importantly, it is possible to improve the care of many terminally ill patients by directing attention to the patient's level of depression and pain. It is thought that 90% of cancer victims could have their pain controlled, but that pain is still a problem in 50%.[44] Recently, guidelines for pain control have been published by such bodies as the American Pain Society and the Agency for Health Care Policy and Research.[98] More widespread hospice care would also be very helpful. One example of a correctable problem is suicide in patients with human immunodeficiency virus, where the distressing complications and secondary depression may have a number of treatable etiologies.[118] In addition, the elderly, debilitated, and/or impoverished individual may feel obligated to consider or may be persuaded to commit suicide, but health problems in such individuals are often correctable and should not be used as a reason for suicide.[201] In the case of a debilitating but nonterminal illness, the state has a special interest in limiting suicide since it would be inappropriate.[176] Thus, there are many arguments for prohibiting the various forms of euthanasia.[41,201]

Understanding the issues regarding PAD requires considering the concepts of deontology, consequentialism, and clinical pragmatism in terms of the effects on patient care and public policy on legalizing PAS and possibly voluntary active euthanasia.[73] A recent collection of writings of the major thinkers in the field presents various arguments about experiences with euthanasia.[201]

One comprehensive approach is that of Heifetz,[96] who suggested the following guidelines: 1) Competent patients who are physically able should be allowed to commit suicide (and not ask someone to assume any burden for them). 2) Competent patients unable physically to commit suicide should be able to request euthanasia. 3) Patients in a permanent vegetative state, since they would not suffer from lack of food or water, should have care withdrawn. 4) Retarded handicapped newborns should have euthanasia since withdrawing care would cause suffering. 5) Retarded children and adults who are unaware of relationships, have no interest in living, and are a burden on others could have euthanasia. 6) Retarded children and adults who are aware of relationships should have care.

A knowledgeable second party should evaluate any patient considering PAD. Physicians should not be required to perform euthanasia if they do not believe that they can.

A related issue is a mentally incompetent patient who, while still competent, expressed a wish not to live if dementia developed. This will be discussed later. A more difficult question concerns patients who do not have the mental capacity, because of youth, retardation, or dementia, to make such decisions. They may or may not be aware, and they may or may not be suffering. The criteria for euthanasia and the determination of who would make the decision will require extensive deliberation.[31,195]

Much can be learned from the Dutch experience with euthanasia.[60,97,142,163] The issue was addressed seriously after Dr. Schoonheim, who had been convicted for the euthanasia of Mrs. Barendregt, was exonerated by the Dutch Supreme Court in 1976. The Dutch Medical Association drew up guidelines in 1984, a report was published by the State Commission on Euthanasia in 1985, and a number of court decisions agreed that euthanasia was appropriate under specific circumstances. Initially, each case had to be reported and investigated. This led to underreporting, so in 1991 the rules were changed to allow prosecutors to review each case and elect not to investigate. However, there is no legislation legalizing euthanasia and the situation is still ambiguous. The most recent guidelines were issued by the Dutch government in 1994. These rules allowed euthanasia if the following criteria were met: an incurable disease with unbearable mental or physical suffering, no other solution, a voluntary and persistent request, and concurrence of a second physician. The patient need not be terminally ill. More recently, several court cases have indicated acceptance of euthanasia for those who cannot request it, such as deformed babies.[66] Surveys have suggested that in over one-half of all Dutch cases of euthanasia, the patient has not requested it.[146]

By 1991, 57% of the Dutch citizens believed that lethal injections should be given on request, about 32% said it depended on the situation, and 9% opposed the practice. A survey of 405 Dutch physicians in 1990-1991 revealed that 49% had performed euthanasia, another 38% would be willing to do so, and only 13% could not imagine doing so.[146,197] At the end of 1995, two cases were being considered by the Dutch Supreme Court in which physicians euthanized newborns with severe congenital anomalies at the request of the parents.[101] On the other hand, to decrease the emotional stress on physicians, the Royal Dutch Medical Association in 1995 revised its policy to encourage PAS as opposed to voluntary active euthanasia for patients capable of carrying out the act.[67]

Information concerning the Dutch euthanasia experience suggested that of 129,000 deaths in 1990, 2,300 (1.8%) involved voluntary active euthanasia and 400 (0.3%) were PAS. In 1,000 patients, life was terminated without request, but one-half of the patients had discussed this previously and in all but two cases another professional or the family was consulted. Seventy percent of euthanasia patients had been expected to die within 1 week, and only 10% in more than 3 months. The underlying disease was most often cancer (83%), severe neurological disease (e.g., multiple sclerosis or amyotrophic lateral sclerosis) (10%), or acquired immune deficiency syndrome. The most common reasons for the request were weakness and exhaustion, physical dependence, loss of dignity, and disfigurement. Severe pain was a less common factor, although it has also been suggested that sophistication in pain control and other aspects of terminal care was limited.[60] Eighty-eight percent of Dutch physicians reported a willingness to carry out euthanasia, although one-half had never done so. Morphine was the most common drug used for euthanasia, although barbiturates and curare were recommended. Interestingly, one-half of requests were not honored. Only 2% of deaths were assisted, and only in very circumscribed circumstances. It is worrisome that the Dutch physicians assist suicide for depression and use voluntary active euthanasia without consent, often have not utilized consultations, and have not been careful about documenting cases.[97]

On an institutional level, some Dutch hospitals, nursing homes, and institutions for the disabled have developed policies concerning euthanasia, but not as many have developed policies about other aspects of decision-making at the end of life. Many institutions inform their doctors and nurses of their policies, but few inform their patients. (The situation in the United States has not been surveyed.[95])

Of concern is that in the U.S. there is less of a feeling of mutual support among the population and physicians and there is a greater possibility that economic factors may influence physicians and patients to opt for assisted death.[108]

Another landmark was the passage in 1996 of a carefully crafted law in the Northern Territory of Australia making euthanasia legal, the first place where this has actually been done.[172] It will be instructive to track experiences in Australia.

In 1995, 75% of the American public favored voluntary active suicide and less so PAS, as did physicians, although a significant number of physicians opposed these practices and less than half would be willing to participate in them.[16,44, 45,50,60,88,124,157,163] The American Medical Association (AMA) has appointed a task force to oppose assisted suicide,[78,84] although the mission of this group has been altered to emphasize consideration of issues related to futility.[76]

The consideration of PAS has been accelerated by the actions and discussions of Dr. Jack Kevorkian and Timothy Quill (a well known advocate of PAS), although because of the differences in approach, the former has been particularly criticized on a number of issues.[99] On the other hand, juries have thrice (1994, 1996, and 1996) acquitted Dr. Kevorkian on charges of assisting suicide, deciding he was acting to relieve suffering rather than to kill the patient as a primary motivation.[8]

Many states have laws forbidding PAS, and voluntary active euthanasia is not accepted in any state. Attempts made in Washington (1991) and California (1992) to enact laws specifically allowing PAS were defeated by margins of 54% and 46%, respectively, due in part to campaigns by medical groups.[99] A law allowing PAS was passed in 1994 in Oregon,[151] but it left several issues unresolved.[11,43] The Oregon law was declared unconstitutional in 1995 by a federal district court because of conflict with the equal protection guarantees of the Fourteenth Amendment as applied to the disabled (*Lee v. State of Oregon*[123]) (declaring the Act unconstitutional as a denial of equal protection to terminally ill persons).[146] This decision is being considered on appeal by the Federal Court of Appeals for the Ninth Circuit, which, given the ruling striking down a Washington state ban on PAS (vide infra), will likely reverse the district court ruling and uphold the Oregon law.[79,85] On the other hand, as discussed below, the U.S. Supreme Court heard the arguments about the issue in January 1997, and it may make a decision later in the year which could decide the law within the United States. Laws allowing PAD have been and will be considered in several other states.

Two federal appellate court decisions may indicate a change in the legal acceptance of PAD. In March 1996, a Washington state ban on PAS was declared unconstitutional by the Federal Court of Appeals for the Ninth Circuit in *Compassion in Dying v. Washington*,[4] a case brought by four physicians and three patients. This decision was based on a liberty interest protected by the Fourteenth Amendment in "determining the time and manner of one's death" for competent, terminally ill adults who request the right to choose to die. The court ruled that the state's interest in protecting life was less weighty near death—especially "a protracted, undignified, an extremely painful death," and it noted "the compelling similarities between right-to-die cases and abortion cases." This decision seemed to establish a positive constitutional right to PAD. The court also emphasized the need to establish regulations.

In April 1996, the Federal Court of Appeals for the Second Circuit struck down a similar law in New York (*Quill v. Vacco*[164]), a case brought by three physicians and three patients. This decision was based on the equal protection clause of the Fourteenth Amendment, the court determining that there was no basis for prohibiting "persons in the final stages of terminal illness from having assistance in ending their lives when others are allowed to hasten their deaths by requesting stopping of life support." To counter the argument that there was a difference between allowing death to occur by stopping life support and administering a drug to *cause* death, the court stated that in the former case, death might occur because of dehydration and starvation, which was also "not natural." Therefore, both situations, where the intent was to cause death, were similar. In this case, too, the need for regulations was emphasized.[12,42]

Many groups, including the AMA, as well as the attorneys general from 15 states, have petitioned the U.S. Supreme Court to rule on these judgments. The Supreme Court agreed to hear appeals of these two cases, which it did in January 1997, and a ruling is expected in July. This will hopefully be a landmark decision, establishing or rejecting a federal constitutional right to PAD. In addition, the U.S. House Judiciary Constitution subcommittee held the first congressional hearings on assisted suicide in May 1996.[81] Depending on the Supreme Court's ruling, the U.S. Congress might adopt a federal policy encouraging or discouraging PAD insofar as it might be permitted under state law.

Actions at Death

The patient, at the time of dying, may wish to "settle his/her affairs." This may take the form of arranging for disposition of belongings or making known information about his/her own or others' activities.

If the patient dies without a will (intestate), the state will dispose of the property according to its statutes, which may not be in accordance with the patient's wishes or may result in greater taxes. Accordingly, the patient may give property directly (inter vivos) or make a will with the transfer made only after death (testamentary). In only a few states, the patient may make an oral ("noncupative") will, which is problematic because it may not be transmitted accurately and can be challenged. In some states, the patient may also record wishes in writing (a holographic will), although again such wills can also be subject to challenge. Physicians may serve as witnesses to such acts and also may need to certify that the patient was competent when the will was made.[18]

END-OF-LIFE DECISIONS FOR THOSE WHO HAVE LOST COMPETENCY

Advance Directives and Surrogate Decision-Making

The right to direct (and refuse) treatment either directly or through a surrogate extends into the future in case of incapacity. This was first established in the case of Karen Quinlan, a patient in a vegetative state.[104] In this case it was decided that, given what was known about her ideas, Karen Quinlan would not have wanted to be maintained in a vegetative state.

The right to direct (and refuse) treatment is embodied in the concept of advance directives, which include the living will and the right to appoint a surrogate.[68,99] The living will was first suggested by Louis Rutner in 1969 and first authorized by statute in California in 1976.[18] A model law for the living will was offered by the National Conference of Commissioners on Uniform State Laws (NCCUSL) in 1984. All states now have living will statutes or allow the appointment of surrogates, and most have both provisions.[18,38,65,88] The advantage of a living will is that it makes the patient's wishes explicit. Appointment of a surrogate through a durable power of attorney or advance directive has the advantage of allowing more flexibility, but may not always lead to the care the patient would have wanted. However, surrogate laws need not refer to specifics, are less politically controversial, and are therefore easier to enact.

There may be times when a patient has both a living will and a durable power of attorney and a conflict arises. In different states, either document may be given precedence, while in some, including South Dakota, the latest document controls.[99] However, if there is no legal requirement, one could defer to the surrogate, who may have the knowledge and understanding to modify directives appropriately in the face of an unanticipated situation.[148]

The patient should make family and friends aware of the presence of documents about advance directives and where they are kept, and hospitals should have a copy on record. Unfortunately, there are not adequate procedures to inform physicians about such wishes, as indicated by studies showing advance directives are not forwarded from nursing homes when patients are transferred to hospitals.[79]

In many instances, there are no advance directives because the patient neglected to prepare them. Patients may deny the severity of their medical problems or refuse to consider their mortality and so have not discussed this issue.[19] Since up to 75% of patients lack deci-

sion-making capacity when such choices are required and only about one in 10 patients has created advance directives, there is a great need for educational efforts to inform people about their rights and options in this regard.[88,171,202] It is clear that over 80% of patients are interested in such decisions.[165] It has been argued that the physician must become more active in encouraging patients to create advance directives during emergency and routine contacts, and that they should be reimbursed for their time in doing this![70]

The absence of advance directives may create great difficulties, as noted in the case of Quinlan. Even more problematic was the case of Cruzan (*Cruzan v. Harmon*[57]) in which the U.S. Supreme Court affirmed the refusal of the Missouri Supreme Court to allow stoppage of food and water for a patient in a permanent vegetative state based on the lack of "clear and convincing evidence" of the patient's intentions, establishing the need for formal advance directives. The Missouri Supreme Court subsequently permitted stoppage based on new information about the patient's prior wishes.[99] In a similar case, the Michigan Supreme Court prevented removal of an incompetent patient's gastrostomy tube (*In re Martin*[103]). In this case, the patient's wishes were not specific, he appeared to the court to be contented, the treatment did not cause discomfort, and the family disagreed on removing the tube. Unfortunately the discussion, as in many cases, did not address the quality of life issues which were the heart of the case.[64]

In 1991, a federal law, the Patient Self-Determination Act, was enacted to assure the right to direct future care by mandating policies for a variety of institutions to inform patients about advance directives, to educate staff, and to document patient receipt of information.[65,142] This law includes requirements for hospitals and other providers receiving federal funds to inform patients of their legal options for refusing or accepting medical treatment by these advance directives. While of laudable intent, this law has not been very successful in influencing patients to create advance directives.[179] It appears that giving information to patients before hospital admission (or even in a physician's office) can increase the rate significantly compared to giving the patient information after admission.[58]

Aggressive intervention can also increase advanced directives.[170]

An informative booklet, "Shape Your Health Care Future with Health Care Advance Directives," containing all needed forms was developed in 1995 by the AMA, the American Bar Association (ABA), and the American Association of Retired Persons, and is available from the AMA. The problems and complexities involved in creating and using advance directives and the strategies to investigate them have been discussed in detail.[193] If there are no advance directives, decisions need to be made by surrogates based on "substituted judgment" (i.e., an educated evaluation of what the patient would have wanted). Some jurisdictions require "clear and convincing evidence" of what the patient would have wanted, which is a very high standard, while others require only a "fair preponderance" of the evidence, as in the case of Karen Quinlan.[104] As mentioned before, it was decided that given what was known about her ideas, Quinlan would not have wanted to live in a vegetative state.

If the patient had never been known to express an opinion (or had never been competent), decisions should be made on "best interest," that is, what a reasonable person would want based on balancing benefits and burdens of the decision. Decision-making power may, by law, be given to someone with power of attorney, a guardian, spouse, adult children, parents, and other relatives (in order).[19]

It is now well established that in circumstances approved by the physician and society, the surrogate can elect to withhold or withdraw care, including administering nutrition and water.[18,154] The provision of nutrition and water to people who cannot eat or drink has been included as medical treatment since the California Court of Appeals ruled for the family of Clarence Herbert on the issue of having tube feedings discontinued (*Barber v. Superior Court*[17]).[99] Statements by the President's Commission in 1983 and the AMA Council on Ethical and Judicial Affairs in 1986 emphasize that withholding and withdrawing care are equally acceptable.[18,19,21,191] Since state laws about provision of water and nutrition vary, physicians should become aware of the details of the statutes and court decisions in their jurisdiction.

The problem is determining exactly what criteria should be used and who should make these decisions.[99] In general, private parties act as they see fit, and courts become involved only when a suit is filed. If a particular decision by a surrogate does not seem reasonable, the physician may seek a court order for clarification of what to do.

One situation which must be anticipated in advance is the desire for cardiopulmonary resuscitation (CPR) in case of cardiac arrest. A great deal of information has been accumulated about prognosis in such areas as cancer and heart disease and, therefore, when resuscitation may or may not reasonably be expected to be effective in terms of survival to hospital discharge.[142] An uncritical approach to this problem would result in forcing many people to prolong their dying in dismal circumstances. Patients and physicians should discuss the patient's prognosis, and patients should be allowed to elect not to be resuscitated. Reasonable reasons for "do not resuscitate" (DNR) orders include poor prognosis, poor quality of life before arrest, or a poor quality of life anticipated after resuscitation. This decision must be based on probability and is a matter of judgment. State laws on this subject first appeared in the 1980s. Since 1988, the Joint Commission on Accreditation of Healthcare Organizations (JCAHO) has required for hospital accreditation that a process be in place to inquire about the patient's wishes, although it is not mandatory for the patient to make a declaration. The Patient Self-Determination Act required that a mechanism for inquiry be in place for recipients of Medicare and Medicaid funds.[142] Where no declaration is available, it is wisest to proceed with CPR. If a declaration has been made, and of course this should be documented, the wishes of the patient or surrogate should be followed. The decision-maker may decide to permit only some measures, possibly less burdensome ones, and here too, these wishes should be followed.[191]

An interesting issue is whether DNR orders should be suspended when a patient goes to an operating room. As many as 15% of patients with DNR orders undergo surgery, and the fact of giving consent for surgery implies the desire for treatment. In addition, cardiac arrest in the operating room is usually due to correctable problems, and resuscitation is usually successful. If a patient has a DNR order, the issue should be discussed and agreement reached regarding circumstances in which resuscitation should or should not be attempted.[65,122,194] This "required reconsideration" should be documented on the operative consent form.[6]

There are a number of states with out-of-hospital DNR provisions, so that a person can have the wish not to be resuscitated honored in emergency situations. However, in some states (e.g., North Dakota), emergency medical personnel are exempted from liability for resuscitating, since they might not have access to DNR information. A variety of strategies, such as identification bracelets, are being developed to make such information available.[99]

If issues concerning care arise, it is best to try to resolve them privately whenever possible, since the judicial process is time consuming, confrontational, intimidating, and expensive.[21] If proper procedures are followed, the physician is less likely to encounter a problem.[21,191] Bioethics committees can be helpful in focusing the issues and educating the surrogates and physicians, but their role is advisory.[7] However, since criminal or civil liability can be attached to either using or withholding/withdrawing life support, there may be times when it is prudent or even required in some states to obtain clarification and authorization from a court to withhold or withdraw treatment.

There may be circumstances that involve specific legal issues. Examples include those in which there is a conflict with the state's interest, as well as cases involving disagreement within a family, disagreement between the family and a physician or other parties, abuse or other violence, malpractice, unreasonable decisions, or pregnant women, or cases in which it is not clear who has responsibility or there are other legal uncertainties.[7,191] In addition, there are circumstances in which other parties must be involved. For example, patients in nursing homes are considered vulnerable, and in certain jurisdictions provisions have been made to ensure their protection by requiring involvement of an ombudsman.[191]

The legal power of advance directives and the decisions of surrogates are demonstrated by a recent court decision awarding damages of $16.5 million against a hospital in Flint, Michigan, for not giving adequate information to a surrogate to enable an informed decision on whether to initiate life support; several other such cases have been brought.[129]

Dementia

A related problem involves patients with dementia. Dementia, particularly Alzheimer's disease, is an example of a major societal problem.[24] Although there are over 50 causes of dementia, Alzheimer's disease is responsible for the overwhelming number of cases, now estimated as high as four million, with one-third to one-half of patients requiring continuous or nursing home care and accounting for one-half to two-thirds of those in nursing homes. Aggregate costs to date for these patients have been estimated at over $80 billion.

Alzheimer's disease occurs with increased incidence with age, with estimates in the following ranges: aged <65 years, <1%; 65-74 years, 1%; 75-84 years, 7%-16%; and >85 years, 25%-48%. Since those over 85 years old constitute the fastest growing segment of our population, it has been further estimated that in less than 50 years, there will be possibly over 12 million Alzheimer's victims whose annual care costs will total about $150 billion.

Dementia involves deterioration of cognitive and behavioral function to the point where patients are unable to care for themselves and are unaware of their plight and even their surroundings. The disease is insidious in onset, and slow and variable in course. Depending on the patient and the realization of the problem, it may or may not cause great fear and suffering, but this is sometimes difficult to determine. In fact, for a long period, the patient may be able to experience considerable pleasure in many aspects of life and thus deserves aggressive medical treatment. During further decline, the patient continues to have rights and always has value. The patient must be treated with respect and dignity and always deserves to be relieved of suffering and to have routine nursing care. On the other hand, when there is no benefit from the medical treatment, either because the dementia has proceeded to the point where awareness is completely lost or there is a disease in which the burdens of treatment outweigh possible benefits, the patient has the right not to be treated. Indeed, justice mandates that resources not be wasted on such treatment.[24,31]

The questions are how to care for such patients as they deteriorate and when care should be stopped. To make such determinations requires consideration of the following: the prior personality and attitudes of the patient; the degree of dementia; the rights (and perhaps obligations) of its victims, their families, and our entire society; how to streamline appropriate care; and how to mobilize resources for that care.[24,35]

One interesting argument revolves around advance directives. Either before or after learning of the disease, the patient may set limits on care, and because of the right of autonomy, should be able to do so. However, it has been argued that since the patient could not truly understand dementia before experiencing it and since treatment in the early stages of dementia can be in the patient's best interest and lead to improved quality of life, there should be limits to this autonomy, and treatment plans should be reconsidered and renegotiated with the patient and/or family periodically. Care must be individualized based on the patient's previous wishes, quality of life, opinions of their families and other surrogates who knew the patient well, and the burdens and benefits of treatments required as different medical problems arise.[24,35]

Last is the issue of what to do at the point when the decision is made that no treatment is indicated. Withholding and withdrawing treatment, including food and water unless requested, is currently accepted as appropriate (vide supra). However, explicit discussions about how to do this are still required.[24,88]

The next step would be to consider the possibility of euthanasia for patients who are no longer sentient. Currently in the U.S., this is not considered ethically or legally acceptable. For euthanasia to be acceptable, criteria for a level of dementia and a process for determining that level would have to be evolved, as well as a method for euthanasia which is acceptable to society and particularly to those who would need to practice it.[24]

Brain Death

Two important and related conditions are brain death and the permanent vegetative state (vide infra). The question of what is life and when it is lost must be considered. In philosophical terms, there is perceived to be something unique about a human being separate from organic or somatic functioning. From ancient times, it was believed that the locus of this unique quality resided in the brain.[60,159] The mind is identified more specifically with the neocortex, where self-awareness and reasoning are thought to be located. Following this concept, it is not until neocortical functioning occurs that a true human being exists, and once this is lost, human life is over.

However, it is now possible to support vegetative functions in patients whose brains have irreversibly ceased all function, and even more easily in those who have lost only neocortical function.[22,72,150,155] This situation has resulted in a need "to define death by criteria that do not depend primarily on the cardiorespiratory function that life support systems artificially preserved."[60] When these criteria are met, care should not be continued.

There are several excellent recent reviews about the clinical determination of brain death.[26,63,115,153] A group of consultants to the President's Commission for the Study of Ethical Problems in Medicine and Biomedical Research and Behavioral Research refined previous criteria.[130,135,161] The consultants advocated that laws should define brain death as "irreversible cessation of all functions of the entire brain."[116,135,161] Their criteria involve clinical evidence of loss of brain function and a period of observation which can be shortened by confirmatory tests, particularly cerebral blood flow studies. These criteria provide the current standard and have proven to be reliable. Criteria for the declaration of brain death in children aged less than 5 years have been considered problematic. However, in the last few years, reliable guidelines have been developed.[113,119] Unfortunately, the most modern criteria are not necessarily being used in either adults[115] or children.[138]

A model brain death law, the Uniform Determination of Death Act (UDDA), was approved in 1980 by the President's Commission, the AMA, the ABA, and the National Conference of Commissioners on Uniform State Laws. The UDDA states that brain death is equivalent to death recognized by cardiopulmonary standards. However, it reserves actual criteria and determination to the medical profession.

Since Kansas passed such a law defining brain death in 1970, over 90% of the states have statutes specifying brain death as a way of defining death and leaving the criteria to the medical profession. In the remaining states, the concept is established by common law. These statutes vary and may have particular requirements, such as specifying two physicians' concurrence on the diagnosis, so the physician should be familiar with the state law. In a few cases, criminals and their lawyers have attempted to avoid responsibility for homicide by attributing death to physicians who have stopped support of brain-dead patients, but the courts have ruled against them (*State v. Fiero*[184] and *People v. Eulo*[158]).

There is an imperative to define death when it occurs. On the one hand, a living person should not be treated as dead. On the other hand, a dead person also should not be treated as being alive, for to do so would violate the trust of the family and society that the physician can recognize death, require health care workers to treat a dead body, expend resources without benefit, and might be perceived as an indignity to and abuse of the body. Exceptions can be made in rare circumstances, for example in an attempt to salvage a viable fetus from a brain-dead woman.

Consent of the family is not necessary to stop cardiopulmonary support of a brain dead patient. Indeed, asking the family for permission to stop support is inappropriate and puts an unnecessary burden on them. But the physician does have an ethical duty to explain the situation, including the fact that the patient's cardiac and respiratory function would have ceased without support. It is reasonable to delay the declaration long enough for the family to gather or to obtain a second opinion if requested. When brain death has been caused by criminal assault, the medical examiner/coroner should be notified. The declaring physician should not benefit by the patient's death and should have no other interest, such as being part of a transplant team.[7,18,21,191]

Permanent Vegetative State

A related class of patients is those who have permanently lost consciousness. Descartes stated the concept of consciousness with elegant simplicity, "Cogito ergo sum." Consciousness has been defined as "our immediate sense of the present and what amounts to memory (the source of the revisions of reality . . .)."[162] As to the exact location of consciousness in the brain, ". . . on the basis of modern evidence for the massive parallel processing of information within the brain, . . . consciousness is not a unitary phenomenon but rather a continually changing, updated and edited version of the world that derives from many neurological sources."[162]

A task force including representatives from the American Academy of Neurology, the American Academy of Pediatrics, the American Neurological Association, the American Association of Neurological Surgeons, and the Child Neurology Society have considered this subject in depth.[145] Their report begins with the definition:

> The vegetative state is a condition of complete unawareness of the self and the environment accompanied by sleep-wake cycles with either complete or partial preservation of brain stem and hypothalamic autonomic functions.[145]

The report includes an extensive literature review of the various causes and epidemiology of the persistent vegetative state and the duration after which it can be known to be permanent. It notes there are currently estimated to be 10,000 to 25,000 adults and 4,000 to 10,000 children in a persistent vegetative state and that their care costs between $1 and $7 billion/year.

The question therefore arises as to how to treat such patients, with the options being: care at some level, no treatment (including withholding food and water), considering them dead (and as organ donors), or terminating their vegetative functions through euthanasia. In most cases, considering their prior feelings through substituted judgment, or, if these are not known, through best interests, would not seem to warrant treatment. Since care would be futile (and costly), families and friends and society would be best served by withholding or withdrawing treatment. However, to treat them as dead would require a definition as reliable as brain death and a societal consensus, both of which are problematic, and utilizing euthanasia would require a consensus on euthanasia and specifically its use in impaired but not terminal patients.[175]

A pronouncement by the Executive Board of the American Academy of Neurology on the persistent vegetative state clearly indicates nutrition and hydration need not be given and can be discontinued.[5] This concept has been accepted in a number of legal decisions. The seminal court case was Quinlan,[104] in which the New Jersey Supreme Court granted Quinlan's father the right to stop unwanted ventilatory support on her behalf based on the right of privacy. In Cruzan,[57] the U.S. Supreme Court upheld the Missouri Supreme Court's refusal to approve cessation of nutrition and hydration because there was not "clear and convincing evidence" of the patient's intentions sufficient to overcome the state's interest in preserving life, although this was eventually permitted by a probate court based on the right of due process after new evidence revealed the presumed wishes of the patient. (Missouri soon thereafter enacted a medical power of attorney law.[99]) All other subsequent state decisions have concurred that the surrogate could make such decisions for such patients.[7,13,18,19,88,191,195] Many state legislatures have now passed laws specifically allowing withdrawal of life support in instances of persistent vegetative state, including even nutrition and hydration in many instances.[99]

One possibility would be to treat as dead a person who has permanently lost consciousness.[21,60,88,136,159] It has been proposed that people should be allowed to choose their own definition of death and to include the cessation of higher brain function as one option.[199]

Organ Donation

In cases of brain death (and perhaps in the future in cases of permanent vegetative state), the patient's organs can be available for transplants. The advances currently being made are reflected in the rising numbers of transplants (now about 20,000/year[71]) and rising rates of organ and donor survival. Although the number of transplant candidates is increasing, donor numbers remain essentially constant.[128] Many people awaiting a heart or a liver die every day.

As of January 31, 1995, there were 37,873 patients on waiting lists.[180] Cadaver donors remain at about 4,000 each year, even though more potential donors exist.[61,128]

There have also been limits placed with regard to recipients of these scarce resources. The University of California, San Diego, and Stanford University both refused to accept a Down's syndrome patient for a heart/lung transplant but were criticized for this decision,[86] and indeed the transplant was performed.

A special problem is the need for pediatric organs. Since 1983, the use of cyclosporin for immunosuppression has eliminated the devastating side effects of impairment of mental and physical development from high-dose steroids used previously, and thus made transplantation a more attractive option for children with a need for a new organ. Some organs for transplantation for children must be size-matched, particularly the heart. It has been estimated that there are up to 1,000 newborns each year in the U.S. with hypoplastic left heart syndrome or endocardial fibroelastosis who might benefit from heart transplants. There are between 500 and 600 infants each year with biliary atresia or congenital metabolic disorders who might benefit from liver transplants, although adult livers might be split and used in infants. As for kidneys, infants can undergo dialysis until they are fully grown and may use adult organs, so the need is not quite as critical.[28] But 30% to 50% of the children registered to receive transplanted organs will die while awaiting them. Therefore, matched donors must be identified and utilized.[28,136,156]

According to the model Uniform Anatomical Gift Act (UAGA) of 1968 and adopted by all states by 1972, the patient has the right to direct donation in advance, as do the next of kin or other guardians. Most states have places on their driver's licenses to indicate this desire, but the cards are not generally accepted as absolute proof of current desire without consent of next of kin.

The Federal Omnibus Budget Reconciliation Act of 1986[2] requires hospitals, as a condition of receiving Medicare and Medicaid funds, to have "written protocols for the identification of potential donors that assure that families of potential donors are made aware of the option of organ or tissue donation." The revised model UAGA of 1987 includes provisions for "routine inquiry" of patients at admission if they would wish to be an organ donor and "required request" to ensure that providers approach the families of patients who suffer brain death about donation. Accreditation by the Joint Commission of Accreditation and Hospital Organization also requires identification and referral of potential donors. Most states have enacted such laws. Unfortunately, the laws and rules as written have not been very effective, apparently because of the reluctance of families to donate.[180] Many states have "implied consent" laws that authorize a medical examiner performing an autopsy to remove the corneas for transplant unless the family makes a specific objection.[18,21,115,191,200]

The use of non-heart-beating cadaver donors is being explored. The University of Pittsburgh has developed a protocol in which terminally ill patients who elect to have life-sustaining treatment stopped and who wish to donate organs are taken into an operating room, treatment is stopped, and their organs retrieved if they do not breathe and their heart stops in a defined period. This may increase the donor pool by 20% to 25%. A review of the evolution of this protocol, its status, the experience with it, and critiques about it have been published.[117,204]

Given the need for organs for transplantation, the shortage of which now leads to the death of thousands of people every year in the U.S., it would be helpful to redefine death so that patients in a permanent vegetative state could be considered for organ donation.

There have been many proposals to increase the availability of organs, including improvement in donor identification and care, more effective contact with donor families, universal checking for donor cards, and public education. In a recent survey, 33% of families approved donation, but 10% of donors were not identified, 17% of families were not asked, and 36% of families denied requests. A strategy of improved procedures in hospitals to identify patients and assure patients are asked, improved techniques for asking, and better education efforts to assure people talk about their desires with their families would be helpful.[62] Other suggested solutions include presumed consent, mandated decision-making, and rewarded gifting,[39,40,166,167,181,183,198] but none are universally acceptable.[48,180] Perhaps most logical, given the primacy of the individual and the high incidence of the expressed desire to donate, is mandated choice.[181]

END-OF-LIFE DECISIONS FOR PERSONS NEVER COMPETENT

The Fetus

In general, based on the mother's autonomy and best interests, and favoring an actual and independent life over a potential and dependent one, the mother's wishes are respected, even if her use of substances such as alcohol or other drugs, or failure to attend to her own health problems, such as diabetes, compromises the development of her fetus. (As of this writing, however, a mother in Wisconsin is being charged for drinking alcohol while pregnant and a pregnant mother in South Carolina is being prosecuted for illegal drug addiction.) This also holds true for situations in which a mother cannot make a decision (e.g., if she is unconscious), in which case her well being will be placed ahead of that of her baby. The American College of Obstetricians and Gynecologists supports this position. Legally, the liberty interest and privacy usually have been considered paramount.[99] However, mothers have been prosecuted for abuse and courts have ordered cesarean sections in critical situations for the fetus (arguing the risk to the mother was small). The law is still evolving, but may eventually require the physician to seek court clarification in conflicts.[69] Before birth, since the fetus is part of her body, the mother legally has exclusive decision-making power. After birth, this infant is considered the shared product of the parents, who then share their authority.

In terms of abortion, several parties have interests. The fetus likely would have an interest in living if it is healthy and might expect a socially satisfying life, although perhaps not if it could expect a burdensome life. Definitions of satisfying and burdensome are, of course, controversial.[186] The mother has an interest in controlling her own life as she feels is most appropriate, but she may need to be protected from making a poor decision. Society has a need to protect the mother's rights and to avoid the burden of an impaired child or one without parental support, but it also needs to protect the vulnerable. Resolution of these interests is at times difficult and must be individualized to some extent.

To the majority of citizens, the absolute sanctity of life is a contestable value. If human life were inherently sacred, the fetus would need to be protected except to save the life of the mother. But its rights are balanced against the rights of the mother, other relatives, and society, and so are limited. Since a mother has rights of privacy and self-determination, she is generally not forced to assume risk for the fetus. Her rights are considered to supersede the rights of her fetus, even to the point of aborting it. She is also considered to be in the best position to choose when an abortion is appropriate.[13] On the other hand, it has been argued that there is a point at which the fetus has sufficient potential to become a human being to warrant protection and thus to have rights which can compete with the mother's. Several stages in development might be considered. However, the stage currently believed to be significant is viability (the ability to survive *ex utero*), which occurs at about 23-24 weeks.

The current legal rules regarding abortion are based on a constitutional rights argument and were embodied by the U.S. Supreme Court decision (*Roe v. Wade*[168]) in which it was decided that the privacy rights of the mother allowed her to obtain an abortion and that a fetus was not a full legal person with rights until viability in the third trimester.[13,71,96,99] Currently, a mother can generally obtain an abortion in the first trimester without justifying her reasons, there are some limitations in some states in the second trimester, and there are marked restrictions in the third trimester.[89]

Abortion is common in the U.S. Almost 60% of the six million pregnancies a year in the U.S. are unintended (either mistimed or, more importantly, unwanted). Of the 3.6 million unintended pregnancies, 1.5 million per year are terminated by abortion (about one-third as many as live births). The ratio is 2 to 4 times higher than that of other industrialized countries. Almost one in five women will have an abortion in

her lifetime. Yet abortion has been marginalized in medical practice and remains outside the mainstream in health care delivery.[91] The details of the situation have been analyzed in depth by a recent Institute of Medicine study which emphasized the importance of developing an effective strategy to prevent unwanted conceptions.[32]

In some states, right-to-die laws are suspended for pregnant women, while in many others there is silence. However, in New Jersey the pregnant woman retains the right to make advance directives.[99]

In the circumstance of a pregnant woman who is brain dead or in a permanent vegetative state, the question arises as to when it is appropriate to maintain somatic functions so that the fetus can mature sufficiently to be viable. To try to decide this question requires consideration of philosophical and legal principles. Management of the patient and her pregnancy on behalf of the fetus may be elected, if the mother previously has expressed this desire. If the wishes of the mother are not known, the decisions should be made by the father of the fetus and with consideration of the fetus's best interests based on quality of life. Presumably, the father would have the right to request or refuse support, but there is no known case in which a conflict between a physician and a husband has occurred, and this issue has not been tested in court. There have been cases in which an unmarried father's wishes have been honored ahead of those of a next-of-kin.[72]

Under these circumstances, the chief consideration is assurance of fetal well-being. Deterioration of fetal status, with or without observable contributing maternal factors, may precipitate the need for delivery.[22,72] If the problem is related to complications affecting the mother, these should be treated in order to avoid early delivery. There has been a case of a pregnant woman in the permanent vegetative state who was successfully supported for 28 weeks until the birth of her baby.[173]

The Anencephalic

A related issue is the status of anencephalics, including the question as to how to treat them and whether they can become organ donors.[13,49, 74,93,94,136,169,178,195] Excellent reviews are available on the subject of anencephaly.[87,100,125,126,136,149]

The Medical Task Force on Anencephaly[136] defines this condition as "a congenital absence of a major portion of the brain, skull and scalp, with its genesis in the first month of gestation." The fibrovascular covering of remaining neural tissue is called the "area cerebrovasculosa." At times there may be a thin epithelial membrane. The neural tissue may contain remnants of a variety of brain structures. The diencephalon may be present, and development of the rhombencephalon is usually normal. In more severe cases, the spinal cord is an unclosed ribbon of neural tissue. The base of the skull is usually malformed, and the vertebral arches may be unclosed. There may be anomalies of other structures in the head including the face and eyes.[20] Typically there is no neck, so that the face and chest form an essentially continuous plane. The distal optic nerves are present but end blindly in the area cerebrovasculosa. Other organ systems or parts of the body may be anomalous, small, or underdeveloped.[147] Because of the unique appearance of this anomaly, the diagnosis is usually obvious.[125,126,136]

It is thought that there are up to 5 times as many anencephalics who die in utero as are born alive. Of those anencephalics who are born, two-thirds are stillborn. However, many of these deaths may be due to trauma to the unprotected brain during the birth process and might be avoided if delivered via cesarean section.[177]

The functions of anencephalics born alive include breathing, swallowing, primitive reflexes, and a variety of movements which at times are quite complex.[136] Brain function is related to the severity of the anomalies and secondary destruction, and may vary considerably. It may also vary with gestational age, which is often less than full term, averaging 33 weeks. The causes of death include respiratory or cardiac failure, endocrine dysfunction, and infections.[132,178]

There are two strategies for early detection of anencephaly: 1) sampling maternal blood and/or amniotic fluid for a variety of substances which appear in increased or decreased amounts in anencephaly; and 2) ultrasonographic imaging of the fetus to visualize the anomaly.[100,136] In the U.S. today only 20% of pregnant women are screened, but in 95% of instances when an anencephalic fetus is found, an abortion is performed.

There is almost universal agreement that if the condition is detected in utero, abortion has a central role (even in the third trimester).[46,187] This is because the mother's interests, namely to avoid a birth of a dying child without the possibility of personhood and for her own mental health, have priority compared to those of the fetus, which has no real interest in living.

In the absence of abortion, there is the question of how to treat an anencephalic born alive, since it will only survive for a few days without vigorous support. Most believe an anencephalic does not have and will never have any true experience, and therefore that it has no interest in living. Death will not cause it harm, and thus there is no reason to support such a patient. Callahan[36] states that death in circumstances in which one does not have the ability to function mentally is a lesser evil than living. Also, since the infant has no cortex, there is no consciousness and therefore no potential for suffering if not treated. Using best-interest criteria, it may be decided that it is not proper to treat.[13,96,195]

On the other hand, there is the question of what to do if care is requested. *In the Matter of Baby K*[107] documents a mother's demands for support which resulted in survival for 20 months, this being the record. This case, which was heard in a trial court and in a U.S. Court of Appeals and was refused review by the U.S. Supreme Court, has raised major issues about anencephalics in particular as well as the physician's obligation to provide futile care in general. The courts decided that an anencephalic was not brain dead; that based on prior antidiscrimination legislation, it should be protected; and that a parent had the right to demand care.[10] This decision indicates the need for public discussion about anencephalics if physicians are to have guidelines and authority to be able to discontinue care in these circumstances.[9,121]

Improvements in transplantation have resulted in the possibility of using the organs of anencephalics who are born alive to benefit children who would otherwise die. On the surface it would seem obvious that since there are infants with fatal conditions who require size-matched organs and who will die without them, and since anencephalics are easy to diagnose, are not conscious and never will be and therefore have no interest in living, and are expected to die rapidly without treatment, it would be appropriate to harvest organs from them. Organ donation by anencephalics also involves the rights of parents to determine the fate of their children. It has been argued that parents may derive psychological benefit from donation in these circumstances. On the other hand, it has been suggested that anencephalic fetuses have certain rights and that using them for the benefit of others is inappropriate (going against the Kantian "categorical imperative" which forbids the use of humans as means), that to use this group of individuals as organ donors would desensitize health care providers to killing, and that this would open the flood gates for reclassifying other groups of individuals so their organs might be used.[21,114]

In fact, organs have been harvested from anencephalic patients since 1967 using a variety of approaches.[111,136] According to a 1990 report,[136] there have been 80 anencephalics from 25 institutions from whom organs were retrieved. In the 41 cases where organs were used, the only strategy that appeared to provide a good chance to retrieve viable organs was immediate maximal support and harvesting. If anencephalics were supported vigorously until their organs were removed, they obviously could be used successfully as donors. This experience demonstrates the need to publically discuss the possibility of maximal support from birth and promote harvesting. (Delivery by cesarean section might prevent early death due to secondary damage to the brain, but it is thought to impose too great a maternal risk to be acceptable.)

However, courts have ruled that anencephalics are not brain dead, and since beating heart donors must be brain dead, they cannot become donors. The case of Theresa Ann Campo Pearson (*In re T.A.C.P.*[106]) illustrates this problem. The parents of an anencephalic child wanted to donate her organs. The case was heard by a trial court in Florida, the Florida District Court of Appeals, and the Florida Supreme Court. It was noted that the child did not meet the criteria of brain death. Arguing that the legislature had recently refused to reclassify anencephalics for the purpose of organ donation and that there

was no obvious consensus for doing this, the courts refused to allow donation.[92] Therefore, as in the case of patients in a permanent vegetative state, although anencephalics are not believed to require aggressive care, they are not treated as if they are dead. This may require defining a new legal status for them, either declaring them dead or creating an exemption for the purpose of donation.[11,15,49,74,94,113,136,169,178,192,195]

The Council on Ethical and Judicial Affairs of the AMA traditionally opined that organs could be retrieved from anencephalics only after they became brain dead, revised that opinion in 1994 to permit retrieval from anencephalics while still living, and then, because of questions of whether anencephalics might have consciousness and whether the condition could always be diagnosed accurately, rescinded this change.[54,82,160] The American Academy of Pediatrics in 1992 stated that one should follow current laws.[185] At this time, there is a moratorium on harvesting organs from anencephalics. It has been stated that attempts at premature action could jeopardize the entire transplant endeavor.[10,77]

A nationwide discussion is necessary to resolve this issue. It has been argued that what is needed are policies and practices, informed consent from families, review of all cases by research or ethics committees containing community representatives, and that institutions doing this should accumulate data and share their experience in order to develop acceptable public policy.[56]

The Infant

Another question is how to care for an infant who is unlikely to survive or will probably have severe disabilities. About 200,000 infants born annually (6%) require intensive care due to several factors: a birth weight of <2500 gm; congenital anomalies; problems from diseases of the mother such as diabetes mellitus, drug abuse, or acquired immunodeficiency syndrome; gastrointestinal problems; or infections. These 6% of newborns account for one-half of hospital costs for all newborns. Many of these infants will not survive or will have significant handicaps.[139] It is believed by some that death may not be the ultimate harm to befall such an infant, and that a life of suffering may be worse and may also adversely affect the infant's family.[89]

Currently, over 10% of such patients are not undergoing treatment,[14] but the extent of care varies depending partially on the type of hospital, and no societal norms have been established. Since an infant is not able to make decisions, the decision-making authority is given to the parents who presumably have the best interests of the child at heart and will be responsible. Using best-interest criteria as defined by the parents, the parents in consultation with the physician may make the decision to withhold care.[13,52,96,195] Issues to be considered by the family include the certainty of the prognosis, the possibility that there may be some new treatment discovered to correct the problem, or whether the mental or physical deficit is severe enough to truly make life not worthwhile to the patient and to the family. The question of family and society support may also be important.[19,195] Indeed, the interests of the child, family members, and society may conflict. It is the rightful role of the physician to act as patient's advocate. If necessary, the decision to withdraw or withhold care can be delayed. An infant care review committee can be involved in problematic cases as a forum and for overseeing.

Public awareness of the subject of withholding treatment began in the 1970s when information about this practice at several institutions was made public. "Pro-life" advocates and advocates for the disabled promoted the issue, utilizing the Federal Rehabilitation Act of 1973.[1] A series of executive orders (Baby Doe regulations[3]) were issued during President Ronald Reagan's administration mandating care for all infants no matter what their disabilities and prognosis. Eventually the courts invalidated these rules (*Bowen v. American Hospital Association*[30]). In 1984, the U.S. Congress passed the Child Abuse Prevention and Treatment Act of 1984,[47] which required treatment unless the infant was permanently comatose or the treatment was futile and inhumane. Enforcement was delegated to the states. In general, these laws have not been enforced aggressively, and no physician has been found liable for withholding or withdrawing care. In 1986, the Redwood County Court in Minnesota approved withholding treatment of nutrition, hydration, and medications for Lance Steinhaus, a baby in a post-traumatic vegetative state (unpublished trial court decision). But the Child Abuse Prevention and Treatment Act of 1984, which has been incorporated by almost all states, has theoretically diminished the power of parents and physicians, placing more authority in the courts. In addition, in 1994 the U.S. Court of Appeals of the Fourth Circuit required a hospital to provide care for an anencephalic child,[107] a precedent which obliged the physician to provide futile care.[89,139]

On the other hand, the parents may not agree with the physician's recommendation for useful treatment, particularly in a handicapped child, or the parents may abandon the child. In this instance, the state has an interest in preserving life and protecting the vulnerable. In such cases, the physician may request to have a guardian appointed for the child.[65]

The Older Child/Adolescent

The older child presents similar but more complex issues. On the one hand, the parents presumably know the child's best interests and should have the right to rear the child in the manner they decide is best. On the other hand, the child, being vulnerable, deserves the protection of the state. In addition, the child may be capable of expressing wishes contrary to those of the parents.

When minors have understanding and maturity, they should be involved in decision-making.[51,52] The American Academy of Pediatrics suggests a comprehensive discussion of the issues, emphasizing the need to consider benefits of treatment versus burdens of treatment and to obtain informed consent from the family (or surrogate) and assent from the child, to consider their values, to obtain consultation for problem situations, to develop policies in hospitals to deal with such issues, and to minimize court involvement.[51,52] The issues are: 1) at what point do children have the perspective, experience, and judgment, and therefore the right to make their own decisions; and 2) how to deal with conflicts that may arise.

Some minors may be legally emancipated,

and thus completely responsible for their own decisions. Marriage, pregnancy or parenthood, self-support/living alone, military service, or court declaration can lead to emancipation. Others (e.g., perhaps if they are 14 years old) may have decision-making capability ("mature minors") but are not emancipated. Those seeking treatment for sexually transmitted disease, pregnancy, or drug and alcohol abuse often are given decision-making status by state statute.[46] There is the practical issue of maintaining privacy and confidentiality if one is to win the trust of a child. A complicating factor is when parents are paying medical bills. One can work with the child and discuss whether to consult with the parents concerning the child's medical care.[21,191]

The Adult

An adult patient who was never competent still maintains the right not to be subjected to inappropriate care. This was established in Massachusetts in *Superintendent of Belchertown State School v. Saikewicz*,[189] in which the Massachusetts Supreme Court permitted refusal of life-sustaining care for a retarded man on a best-interests standard. Issues to be considered might be patient age, pain associated with therapy and ability to cooperate, and the chances for success.[99] That decisions must respect moral and legal rights and be based on a best interest test was confirmed (*In re Storar*[105]). There are many other such cases.[154] Indeed, based on justice in an era of limited resources and the newly formulated communitarian ethics and the burdens that individuals may place on their society, it can be argued that, in futile situations, continuing care is inappropriate.

THE POLITICAL AND INSTITUTIONAL FRAMEWORK FOR SOLUTIONS

The resolution of these problems requires reconsideration of the political foundations of the country. The founding documents provide the guidance required:

We hold these truths to be self-evident, that all men are created equal, that they are endowed by their Creator with certain unalienable Rights, that among these are Life, Liberty and the pursuit of Happiness. That to secure these rights, Governments are instituted among Men, deriving their just powers from the consent of the governed. . . .

Declaration of Independence, 1776

We the people of the United States, in Order to form a more perfect Union, establish Justice, insure domestic Tranquility, provide for the common defense, promote the general Welfare, and secure the Blessings of Liberty to ourselves and our Posterity, do ordain and establish this Constitution for the United States of America.

Constitution of the United States, 1787

It is important to keep in mind that the United States was from its inception a heterogeneous culture encompassing different philosophical systems which might be in conflict on specific issues. However, the emphasis on freedom and tolerance provides the political processes and our tradition of the rule of law provides a framework for resolving controversial issues.

The social contract of our country is the Constitution of the United States, including its amendments, specifically the Fifth and Fourteenth Amendments, which guarantee equal protection and due process.[96] It is also the U.S. Supreme Court's interpretation of the Constitution which ultimately determines how a constitutional issue will be resolved.

There are advantages and disadvantages to our political system. Theoretically, it can respond to new conditions and to the evolving will of the citizenry but is sufficiently constrained to preserve the values imbedded in it. The elements required for good policy making—collecting full and objective information, applying well-considered criteria, following a rigorous and fair process, impartial decision making, and accountability[90]—are known and can be applied in our government. The disadvantages relate to both the processes and to the people involved in them, including their limitations and the forces that influence them. It has been argued that government action is too easily swayed by political pressure, that the participants are often not well versed on the issues, that the venue is too far removed from the actual situation, and that family privacy is violated. In addition, these systems depend on the people who operate and participate in them acting in ways that are moral, intelligent, and tolerant, which has often been shown not to be the case.

Three types of institutions—legislative, judicial, and executive—control the form and substance of our society (specifically medical care) and mandate what the physician must do.[21] They create policy "that is legally binding or at least has persuasive form in law."[90] The flow of this process is related to the balance of forces of restraint, activism, and mediation, which have been described in detail with regard to decisions at the end of life.[99]

The legislature may be in the best position to make policy. It has a mandate to do this, has great resources to develop information, and is accountable. However, it is sensitive to political pressure and may operate with a limited perspective. The legislative process can be slow, costly, and difficult to adjust as innovations occur. Since many laws are mandated at the state level, the process can be fragmented and inconsistent. However, there tends to be convergence of policy, driven by legislatures which are "policy innovators" (e.g., California, New York, New Jersey, Michigan, Massachusetts, and Pennsylvania) and aided by the model laws prepared by the National Conference of Commissioners on Uniform State Laws.[99]

The judicial branch can fairly rapidly affect consideration of an issue. In addition, there tends to be a diffusion of policy led by trend-setting courts, particularly in California, New Jersey, New York, and Massachusetts.[19] However, the judicial process is intended to be interpretive and takes place in an adversarial setting which may consider only limited issues and not all of the many factors which play on the entire problem. In addition, in the "rush to judgment," precedents may be established which are less than thoughtful or comprehensive. Judges may not be well qualified to make medical policy and may not be accountable. Certainly, if all medical decisions had to be resolved by courts or other legal mechanisms, the system would be completely unworkable. Current court involvement in more than 100 right-to-die cases indicates not only problems with the legislative system but

also the current failure of private decision-making.[19,99] However, the courts may be the poorest of the three branches for making policy.

The executive branch can be objective and has immense resources. It has access to information. The executive can establish rules rapidly, but this may be done in a fairly arbitrary fashion with political bias. The executive branch can also establish a national forum. The Congressional Office of Technology Assessment, at the request of U.S. Senators Mark Hatfield, Edward Kennedy, and Dennis DeConcini, presented a background paper entitled "Biomedical Ethics in U.S. Public Policy" in 1993. The paper noted the helpfulness of prior federal bodies and the advantages of a well-funded centralized national forum, and made specific suggestions about the factors to be considered in developing one.[196] The prior federal bodies and their strengths and weaknesses were also reviewed in detail in a recent book from the Institute of Medicine, together with a discussion of the possibilities of establishing a permanent deliberative body or a series of commissions with a specific mandate and a mechanism for monitoring current needs presented.[33] It has been said that such a forum could be useful in facilitating accommodations on the controversies in dying and death.[13]

In an October 1995 executive order, President Bill Clinton authorized a National Bioethics Advisory Board of 15 members to advise government entities; he gave governmental departments and agencies involved in human research 120 days to carry out reviews of their procedures and send this information to the Board.[80] Because of its limited role, the effectiveness of this Board has been questioned.[112] The members of the Board were named starting on July 19, 1996, and its first meeting held on October 4; initially it was given a 2-year mandate. Its chairman is Harold Shapiro, an economist and president of Princeton University; other members include James Childress, a University of Virginia bioethicist; David Cox, a Stanford University geneticist; and Alexander Capron, a University of Southern California expert in medical law.[109] The Board will initially study the various federal agencies' rules for the protection of human research subjects and the management and use of genetic information. The panel may decide future topics for consideration, and Congress and the public may make suggestions. Criteria for choosing topics will include the urgency of the issue and its relationship to the activities and interests of the federal government.[83] However, the concern is that this Board will find it inadvisable to confront controversial issues concerning decisions at the end of life.

CONCLUSIONS

Public moral reasoning is needed to resolve ethical quandaries created by evolving technologies and complicated by the diverse values of individuals in our heterogenous society. It has and should continue to take place at community, state and national levels by a variety of types of groups including theological, academic, professional, and governmental bodies. Descriptions and criteria for such groups and their activities have been reported.[33] Deliberations should take place as close as possible to the locus of action. Some issues affect all the citizenry, and would best be considered in a national forum.

Unfortunately, neither the current process nor the people involved in it have yet solved many of the problems of end of life decisions. Political leadership has not been effective in confronting controversial issues in legislative bodies in a timely fashion, so that much of the law involving decisions at the end of life has been made by default in the courts. The situation is changing, and in recent years many laws concerning right-to-die decisions have been created, although many are half measures or in conflict with other state laws, and much remains to be done, particularly with regard to controversial issues such as physician-assisted death.[99]

Thus, the best answer would seem to lie in the U.S. Congress developing comprehensive law to deal with decisions at the end of life, ideally through efforts by enlightened national leaders but more realistically after evolution of a national consensus, which will be a slow and piecemeal process. It is hoped that this process will be helped by the newly created National Bioethics Advisory Board.

REFERENCES

1. 29 USC §794
2. 42 USC §1220b-8 (a) (1) (A)
3. 45 CFR §84.55
4. 79 F3d 790 (9th Cir), *cert granted*, 117 SCt 37 (1996)
5. American Academy of Neurology: Position of the American Academy of Neurology on certain aspects of the care and management of the persistent vegetative state patient. **Neurology 39:**125-126, 1989
6. American College of Surgeons: Statement of the American College of Surgeons on Advance Directives by patients. "Do not resuscitate" in the operating room. **Bull Am Coll Surg 79:**29, 1994
7. Anderson JA, Gregory DR: Patients and the process of dying, in American College of Legal Medicine (ed): **Legal Medicine. Legal Dynamics of Medical Encounters.** 2nd ed. St Louis, Mo: CV Mosby, 1991, pp 364-385
8. Anderson KL: Jury acquits Kevorkian in 2nd assisted-suicide trial. **The Dominion Post.** March 9, 1996, p 8A
9. Angell M: After Quinlan: the dilemma of the persistent vegetative state. N Engl J Med **330:**1524-1525, 1994
10. Annas GJ: Asking the courts to set the standard of emergency care—the case of Baby K. N Engl J Med **330:**1542-1545, 1994
11. Annas GJ: Death by prescription. The Oregon initiative. N Engl J Med **331:**1240-1243, 1994
12. Annas GJ: The promised end—constitutional aspects of physician-assisted suicide. N Engl J Med **335:**683-687, 1996
13. Annas GJ: **Standard of Care. The Law of American Bioethics.** New York, NY: Oxford University Press, 1993
14. Anspach RR: **Deciding Who Lives. Fateful Choices in the Intensive-Care Nursery.** Berkeley, Calif: University of California Press, 1993
15. Ashwal S, Schneider S: Pediatric brain death: current perspectives. **Adv Pediatr 38:**181-202, 1991
16. Bachman JG, Alcser KH, Doukas DJ, et al: Attitudes of Michigan physicians and the public toward legalizing physician-assisted suicide and voluntary euthanasia. N Engl J Med **334:**303-309, 1996
17. *Barber v Superior Court*, 195 Cal Rptr 484 (Cal App 1983)
18. Berger AS: **Dying and Death in Law and Medicine. A Forensic Primer for Health and Legal Professionals.** Westport, Conn: Praeger, 1993
19. Berger AS, Berger J (eds): **To Die or Not to Die? Cross-Disciplinary, Cultural, and Legal Perspectives on the Right to Choose Death.** New York, NY: Praeger, 1990
20. Bernardo AI, Kirsch LS, Brownstein S: Ocular anomalies in anencephaly: a clinicopathological study of 11 globes. **Can J Ophthalmol 26:**257-263, 1991
21. Bernat JL: **Ethical Issues in Neurology.** Boston, Mass: Butterworth-Heinemann, 1994
22. Bernstein IM, Watson M, Simmons GM, et al: Maternal brain death and prolonged fetal survival. **Obstet Gynecol 74:**434-437, 1989
23. Bianco EA: Consent to treatment, in American College of Legal Medicine (ed): **Legal Medicine. Legal Dynamics of Medical Encounters.** 2nd ed. St Louis, Mo: CV Mosby, 1991
24. Binstock RH, Post SG, Whitehouse PJ (eds): **Dementia and Aging. Ethics, Values, and Policy Choices.** Baltimore, Md: Johns Hopkins University

Press, 1992, pp 216-226

25. Bisbing SB: Competency and capacity, in American College of Legal Medicine (ed): **Legal Medicine. Legal Dynamics of Medical Encounters.** 2nd ed. St Louis, Mo: CV Mosby, 1991, pp 128-136

26. Black PM: Conceptual and practical issues in the declaration of death by brain criteria. **Neurosurg Clin North Am 2:**493-501, 1991

27. Bongar B (ed): **Suicide. Guidelines for Assessment, Management and Treatment.** New York, NY: Oxford University Press, 1992

28. Botkin JR: Anencephalic infants as organ donors. **Pediatrics 82:**250-256, 1988

29. *Bouvia v Superior Court*, 225 Cal Rptr 297 (Cal App 1986)

30. *Bowen v American Hospital Association*, 476 US 610, SCt 2101 (1986)

31. Brock DW: **Life and Death. Philosophical Essays in Biomedical Ethics.** Cambridge, Engl: Cambridge University Press, 1993

32. Brown SS, Eisenberg L: Unintended pregnancy and the well-being of children and families. **JAMA 274:** 1332, 1995

33. Bulger RE, Bobby EM, Fineberg HV (eds): **Society's Choices. Social and Ethical Decision Making in Biomedicine.** Washington, DC: National Academy Press, 1995

34. Callahan D: Controlling the costs of health care for the elderly—fair means and foul. **N Engl J Med 335:** 744-746, 1996

35. Callahan D: Terminating life-sustaining treatment of the demented. **Hastings Cent Rep 25:**25-31, 1995

36. Callahan D: **The Troubled Dream of Life. Living With Mortality.** New York, NY: Simon & Schuster, 1993

37. Callahan D, White M: The legalization of physician-assisted suicide: creating a regulatory Potemkin Village. **U Richmond Law Rev 30:**1-83, 1996

38. Cantor NL: **Advance Directives and the Pursuit of Death with Dignity.** Bloomington, Ind: Indiana University Press, 1993

39. Caplan A, Siminoff L, Arnold R, et al: Increasing organ and tissue donation: what are the obstacles, what are our options?, in: **The Surgeon General's Workshop on Increasing Organ Donation. Background Papers.** Washington, DC: US Department of Health and Human Services, 1991, pp 199-232

40. Caplan AL, Virnig B: Is altruism enough? Required request and the donation of cadaver organs and tissues in the United States. **Crit Care Clin 6:** 1007-1018, 1990

41. Capron AM: Constitutionalizing death. **Hastings Cent Rep 25:**23-24, 1995

42. Capron AM: Liberty, equality, death! **Hastings Cent Rep 26:**23-24, 1996

43. Capron AM: Sledding in Oregon. **Hastings Cent Rep 25:**34-35, 1995

44. Castaneda CJ: Agonizing over the right to die. **USA TODAY.** July 7, 1996, p 4A

45. Castaneda CJ: Oregon's assisted suicide law a "catalyst" for 12 other states. **USA TODAY.** Mar 9, 1995, p 8A

46. Chervenak FA, Farley MA, Walters L, et al: When is termination of pregnancy during the third trimester morally justifiable? **N Engl J Med 310:**501-504, 1984

47. Child Abuse Amendments of 1984, Pub L No.

98-457 (1984), codified at 42 USC §§5101-5115, *amended,* 110 Stat 3063 (Oct 3, 1996)

48. Childress JF: The gift of life: ethical issues in organ transplantation. **Bull Am Coll Surg 81:**8-22, 1996

49. Churchill LR, Pinkus RLB: The use of anencephalic organs: historical and ethical dimensions. **Milbank Q 68:**147-169, 1990

50. Cohen JS, Fihn SD, Boyko EJ, et al: Attitudes toward assisted suicide and euthanasia among physicians in Washington state. **N Engl J Med 331:**89-94, 1994

51. Committee on Bioethics, American Academy of Pediatrics: Guidelines on forgoing life-sustaining medical treatment. **Pediatrics 93:**532-536, 1994

52. Committee on Bioethics, American Academy of Pediatrics: Informed consent, parental permission, and assent in pediatric practice. **Pediatrics 95:** 314-317, 1995

53. Cotton P: Rational suicide: no longer "crazy"? **JAMA 270:**797, 1993

54. Council on Ethical and Judicial Affairs, American Medical Association: The use of anencephalic neonates as organ donors. **JAMA 273:**1614-1618, 1995

55. Council on Scientific Affairs, American Medical Association: Good care of the dying patient. **JAMA 275:**474-478, 1996

56. Cranford RE: Anencephalic infants as organ donors. **Transplant Proc 24:**2218-2220, 1992

57. *Cruzan v Harmon*, 760 SW2d 408 (Mo 1988), *aff'd* sub nom *Cruzan v Director*, Missouri Department of Health, 497 US 261 (1990)

58. Cugliari AM, Miller T, Sobal J: Factors promoting completion of advance directives in the hospital. **Arch Intern Med 155:**1893-1898, 1995

59. Cundiff D: **Euthanasia is Not the Answer. A Hospice Physician's View.** Totowa, NJ: Humana Press, 1992

60. Dagi TF: Death-defining acts: historical and cultural observations on the end of life, in Kaufman HH (ed): **Pediatric Brain Death and Organ/Tissue Retrieval: Medical, Ethical, and Legal Aspects.** New York, NY: Plenum Press, 1989, pp 1-30

61. Darby JM, Stein K, Grenvik A, et al: Approach to management of the heartbeating "brain dead" organ donor. **JAMA 261:**2222-2228, 1989

62. DeJong W, Drachman J, Gortmaker SL, et al: Options for increasing organ donation: the potential role of financial incentives, standardized hospital procedures, and public education to promote family discussion. **Milbank Q 73:**463-479, 1995

63. de Villiers JC: Pitfalls and problems in the diagnosis of cerebral death. **Prog Neurol Surg 13:**180-202, 1990

64. Dresser R: Still troubled. In re Martin. **Hastings Cent Rep 26:**21-22, 1996

65. Dubler N, Nimmons D: **Ethics on Call. Taking Charge of Life-and-Death Choices in Today's Health Care System.** New York, NY: Vintage Books, 1993

66. Dutch doctor free after prosecution proves murder case. **Am Med News.** Dec 4, 1995, p 4

67. Dutch group favors distancing doctors from euthanasia. **Am Med News.** Sept 11, 1995, p 7

68. Dworkin RM: **Life's Dominion. An Argument About Abortion, Euthanasia, and Individual Freedom.** New York, NY: Alfred A Knopf, 1993

69. Emanuel EJ: Cost savings at the end of life. What do the data show? **JAMA 275:**1907-1914, 1996

70. Emanuel L: Structured advance planning. Is it finally time for physician action and reimbursement? **JAMA 274:**501-503, 1995

71. Evans RW, Orians CE, Ascher NL: The potential supply of organ donors. An assessment of the efficiency of organ procurement efforts in the United States. **JAMA 267:**239-246, 1992

72. Field DR, Gates EA, Creasy RK, et al: Maternal brain death during pregnancy. Medical and ethical issues. **JAMA 260:**816-822, 1988

73. Fins JJ, Bacchetta MD: Framing the physician-assisted suicide and voluntary active euthanasia debate: The role of deontology, consequentialism, and clinical pragmatism. **J Am Geriatr Soc 43:** 563-568, 1995

74. Fost N: Removing organs from anencephalic infants: ethical and legal considerations. **Clin Perinatol 16:**331-337, 1989

75. Gatz M (ed): **Emerging Issues in Mental Health and Aging.** Washington, DC: American Psychological Association, 1995

76. Gianelli DM: AMA assisted-suicide task force to study futile care. **Am Med News.** Oct 2, 1995, p 7

77. Gianelli DM: AMA organ donor opinion sparks ethics debate. **Am Med News.** July 25, 1994, pp 1, 8

78. Gianelli DM: Assisted-suicide measure fails in New Mexico; AMA opposed it. **Am Med News.** Mar 20, 1995, pp 3, 21

79. Gianelli DM: Assisted suicide showdown headed to high court? **Am Med News.** Aug 21, 1995, pp 1, 6, 7

80. Gianelli DM: Bioethics Advisory Commission gets final OK. **Am Med News.** Oct 23, 1995, p 9

81. Gianelli DM: End-of-life debate moves to Congress. **Am Med News.** May 13, 1996, pp 3, 9

82. Gianelli DM: Ethics council reverses stand on anencephalic organ donors. **Am Med News.** Dec 25, 1995, p 3

83. Gianelli DM: New bioethics panel to study genetics, research subjects. **Am Med News.** Aug 26, 1996, p 8

84. Gianelli DM: States weight assisted suicide. AMA launches more aggressive action to fight trend. **Am Med News.** Feb 27, 1995, pp 1, 24

85. Gianelli DM: Support for assisted suicide. **Am Med News.** Mar 25, 1996, pp 1, 17

86. Gianelli DM: Transplant denied: careful use of scarce organs, or discrimination? **Am Med News.** Sept 18, 1995, pp 3, 27

87. Giroud A: Anencephaly, in Vinken PJ, Bruyn GW (eds): **Handbook of Clinical Neurology. Vol 30: Congenital Malformations of the Brain and Skull. Part I.** New York, NY: Amsterdam-North Holland, 1970, pp 173-208

88. Glick HR: **The Right to Die. Policy Innovation and Its Consequences.** New York, NY: Columbia University Press, 1992

89. Goldworth A, Silverman W, Stevenson DK, et al (eds): **Ethics and Perinatology.** New York, NY: Oxford Press, 1995

90. Gostin LO: Informed consent, cultural sensitivity, and respect for persons. **JAMA 274:**844-845, 1995

91. Gottlieb BR: Sounding Board. Abortion—1995. **N Engl J Med 332:**532-533, 1995

92. Hanley RA: *In re T.A.C.P.* **Issues Law Med 9:**65-68, 1993

93. Hastings Center (ed): **Guidelines on the Termination of Life-Sustaining Treatment and the Care of the Dying.** Bloomington, Ind: Indiana University Press, 1987

94. Hastings Center Report. **Hastings Cent Rep 18:** 5-33, 1988

95. Haverkate I, van der Wal G: Policies on medical decisions concerning the end of life in Dutch health care institutions. **JAMA 275:**435-439, 1996

96. Heifetz MD: **Easier Said Than Done. Moral Decisions in Medical Uncertainty.** Buffalo, NY: Prometheus Books, 1992

97. Hendin H: Assisted suicide, euthanasia, and suicide prevention: the implications of the Dutch experience. **Suicide Life Threat Behav 25:**193-204, 1995

98. Hill CS Jr: When will adequate pain treatment be the norm? **JAMA 274:**1881-1882, 1995

99. Hoefler JM, Kamoic BE: **Deathright: Culture, Medicine, Politics, and the Right to Die.** Boulder, Colo: Westview Press, 1994

100. Hoffman HJ, Epstein F (eds): **Disorders of the Developing Nervous System: Diagnosis and Treatment.** Boston: Blackwell Scientific, 1986

101. Infants' euthanasia sets off new Dutch debate. **Am Med News.** Jan 1, 1996, p 4

102. *In re Conroy,* 486 A2d 1209 (NJ 1985)

103. *In re Martin,* 538 NW2d 399 (Mich 1995), *cert denied,* 116 SCt 912 (1996)

104. *In re Quinlan,* 355 A2d 647, *cert denied* sub nom *Garger v New Jersey,* 429 US 922 (1976)

105. *In re Storar,* 420 NE2d 64 (NY), *cert denied,* 454 US 858 (1981)

106. *In re T.A.C.P.,* 609 So2d 588 (Fla 1992)

107. *In the matter of Baby K,* 832 F Supp 1022 (ED Va 1993) aff'd, 16 F3d 590 (4th Cir), *cert denied,* 115 SCt 91 (1994)

108. Jecker NS: Physician-assisted death in the Netherlands and the United States: ethical and cultural aspects of health policy development. **J Am Geriatr Soc 42:**672-678, 1994

109. Kaiser J: Bioethics panel. **Science 273:**583, 1996

110. Kamisar Y: Are laws against assisted suicide unconstitutional? **Hastings Cent Rep 23:**32-41, 1993

111. Kantrowitz A, Haller JD, Joos H, et al: Transplantation of the heart in an infant and an adult. **Am J Cardiol 22:**782-790, 1968

112. Katz J: Do we need another advisory commission on human experimentation? **Hastings Cent Rep 25:** 29-31, 1995

113. Kaufman HH (ed): **Pediatric Brain Death and Organ/Tissue Retrieval. Medical, Ethical, and Legal Aspects.** New York, NY: Plenum Press, 1989

114. Kaufman HH, Bodensteiner J, Simmons GM Jr, et al: Anencephaly, in McComb G, Venes J (eds): **Neural Tube Defects, Vol 1.** Park Ridge, Ill: American Association of Neurological Surgeons (In press)

115. Kaufman HH, Brick J, Frick M: Brain death, in Youmans JR (ed): **Neurological Surgery.** 4th ed. Philadelphia, Pa: WB Saunders, 1996, pp 439-451

116. Kaufman HH, Lynn J: Brain death. **Neurosurgery 19:**850-856, 1986

117. Kennedy Institute of Ethics: **Kennedy Inst Ethics J 3:**103-278, 1993

118. Kirchner JT: AIDS and suicide. **J Fam Pract 41:** 493-496, 1995

119. Kohrmann MH, Spivak BS: Brain death in infants:

sensitivity and specificity of current criteria. **Pediatr Neurol 6:**47-50, 1990

120. Kramer AM: Health care for elderly persons—myths and realities. **N Engl J Med 332:**1027-1029, 1995

121. LaPuma J: Managed care: raising new issues. **1996 Medical and Health Annual. Encyclopedia Brittanica.** Chicago, Ill: Encyclopedia Brittanica, 1995, pp 348-351

122. Law, Medicine and Health Care: Medical futility. **Law Med Health Care 20:**307-339, 1992

123. *Lee v State of Oregon*, 891 F Supp 1429 (D Ore 1995)

124. Lee MA, Nelson HD, Tilden VP, et al: Legalizing assisted suicide—views of physicians in Oregon. **N Engl J Med 334:**310-315, 1996

125. Lemire RJ: Anencephaly, in Vinken PJ, Bruyn GW, Klawans HL, et al (eds): **Handbook of Clinical Neurology. Vol 50: Malformations.** New York, NY: Amsterdam-North Holland, 1987, pp 71-95

126. Lemire RJ, Beckwith JB, Warkany J (eds): **Anencephaly.** New York, NY: Raven Press, 1978

127. Levinsky NG: The purpose of advance medical planning—autonomy for patients or limitation of care. **N Engl J Med 335:**741-743, 1996

128. Levy D: Matchmaking at the heart of transplant process. **USA TODAY.** Oct 19, 1995, p 6D

129. Lewin T: Ignoring "right to die directives," medical community is being sued. **New York Times.** June 2, 1996, pp 1, 14

130. Lynn J: Brain death: historical perspectives and current concerns, in Kaufman HH (ed): **Pediatric Brain Death and Organ/Tissue Retrieval. Medical, Ethical and Legal Aspects.** New York, NY: Plenum Press, 1989, pp 65-72

131. Lynn J: Caring at the end of our lives. **N Engl J Med 335:**201-202, 1996

132. McAbee G, Sherman J, Canas JA, et al: Prolonged survival of two anencephalic infants. **Am J Perinatol 10:**175-177, 1993

133. McCann RM, Hall WJ, Groth-Juncker A: Comfort care for terminally ill patients. The appropriate use of nutrition and hydration. **JAMA 272:**1263-1266, 1994

134. McCue JD: The naturalness of dying. **JAMA 273:**1039-1043, 1995

135. Medical Consultants on the Diagnosis of Death: Guidelines for the determination of death. Report of the Medical Consultants on the Diagnosis of Death to the President's Commission for the Study of Ethical Problems in Medicine and Biomedical and Behavioral Research. **JAMA 246:**2184-2186, 1981

136. Medical Task Force on Anencephaly: The infant with anencephaly. **N Engl J Med 322:**669-674, 1990

137. Meisel A: The legal consensus about foregoing life-sustaining treatment: its status and its prospects. **Kennedy Inst Ethics J 2:**309-345, 1993

138. Mejia RE, Pollack MM: Variability in brain death determination practices in children. **JAMA 274:**550-553, 1995

139. Merrick JC: Critically ill newborns and the law: the American experience. **J Legal Med 16:**189-209, 1995

140. Miller FG, Brody H: Professional integrity and physician-assisted death. **Hastings Cent Rep 25:**8-17, 1995

141. Miller FG, Quill TE, Brody H, et al: Regulating physician-assisted death. **N Engl J Med 331:**119-123, 1994

142. Misbin R: **Euthanasia. The Good of the Patient—The Good of Society.** Frederick, Md: University Publishing Group, 1992

143. Momeyer R: Does physician assisted suicide violate the integrity of medicine? **J Med Philos 20:**13-24, 1995

144. Moody HR: **Ethics in an Aging Society.** Baltimore, Md: Johns Hopkins University Press, 1992

145. Multi-society Task Force on PVS: Medical aspects of the persistent vegetative state. Parts 1 and 2. **N Engl J Med 330:**1499-1508, 1572-1579, 1994

146. Murray TH: Aid-in-dying: society's dilemma. **1996 Medical and Health Annual. Encyclopedia Brittanica.** Chicago, Ill: Encyclopedia Brittanica, 1995, pp 345-351

147. Naeye RL, Blanc WA: Organ and body growth in anencephaly. A quantitative, morphological study. **Arch Pathol 91:**140-147, 1971

148. Nelson JL: Critical interests and sources of familial decision-making authority for incapacitated patients. **J Law Med Ethics 23:**143-148, 1995

149. Nolan K: Anencephalic infants: a source of controversy. **Hastings Cent Rep 18:**5, 1988

150. Nuutinen LS, Alahuhta SM, Heikkinen JE: Nutrition during ten-week life support with successful fetal outcome in a case with fatal maternal brain damage. **JPEN J Parenter Enteral Nutr 13:**432-435, 1989

151. Oregon Death With Dignity Act, Ballot Measure 16, adopted November 1994

152. Orentlicher D: The legalization of physician-assisted suicide. **N Engl J Med 335:**663-667, 1996

153. Pallis C: Brainstem death: the evolution of a concept. **Semin Thorac Cardiovasc Surg 2:**135-152, 1990

154. Paris JJ, Poorman M: "Playing God" and the removal of life-prolonging therapy. **J Med Philos 20:**403-418, 1995

155. Parisi JE, Kim RC, Collins GH, et al: Brain death with prolonged somatic survival. **N Engl J Med 306:**14-16, 1982

156. Peabody JL, Emery JR, Ashwal S: Experience with anencephalic infants as prospective organ donors. **N Engl J Med 321:**344-350, 1989

157. Pellegrino ED: Compassion needs reason too. **JAMA 270:**874-875, 1993

158. *People v Eulo*, 472 NE2d 286 (NY 1984)

159. Pernick MS: Back from the grave: recurring controversies over defining and diagnosing death in history, in Zaner RM (ed): **Death: Beyond Whole-Brain Criteria.** Boston, Mass: Kluwer Academic, 1988, pp 17-24

160. Plows CW: Reconsideration of AMA opinion on anencephalic neonates as organ donors. **JAMA 275:**443-444, 1996

161. President's Commission for the Study of Ethical Problems in Medicine and Biomedical and Behavioral Research (ed): **Defining Death: A Report on the Medical, Legal, and Ethical Issues in the Determination of Death.** Washington, DC: US Government Printing Office, 1981

162. Purves D: Book review of Dennett DC: **Consciousness Explained, 1991.** Science 257:1291-1292, 1992

163. Quill TE: **Death and Dignity. Making Choices and**

Taking Charge. New York, NY: WW Norton & Co, 1993

164. *Quill v Vacco*, 80 F3d 716 (2nd Cir), *cert granted*, 117 SCt 36 (1996)

165. Reilly BM, Magnussen CR, Ross J, et al: Can we talk? Inpatient discussions about advance directives in a community hospital. **Arch Intern Med 154:** 2299-2308, 1994

166. Rivers EP, Buse SM, Bivins BA, et al: Organ and tissue procurement in the acute care setting: principles and practice—part 1. **Ann Emerg Med 19:**78-85, 1990

167. Rivers EP, Buse SM, Bivins BA, et al: Organ and tissue procurement in the acute care setting: principles and practice—part 2. **Ann Emerg Med 19:**193-200, 1990

168. *Roe v Wade*, 410 US 113 (1973)

169. Rothenberg LS: The anencephalic neonate and brain death: an international review of medical, ethical, and legal issues. **Transplant Proc 22:**1037-1039, 1990

170. Rowe JW: Health care myths at the end of life. **Bull Am Coll Surg 81:**11-18, 1996

171. Rubin SM, Strull WM, Fialkow MF, et al: Increasing the completion of the durable power of attorney for health care. A randomized, controlled trial. **JAMA 271:**209-212, 1994

172. Ryan CJ, Kaye M: Euthanasia in Australia—The Northern Territory Rights of the Terminally Ill Act. **N Engl J Med 334:**326-328, 1996

173. Sampson MB, Petersen LP: Post-traumatic coma during pregnancy. **Obstet Gynecol (Suppl) 53:**2-3, 1979

174. *Satz v Perlmutter*, 362 So2d 160 (Fla App 1978), *aff'd*, 379 So2d 359 (Fla 1980)

175. Schrode KE: Life in limbo: revising policies for permanently unconscious patients. **Houston Law Rev 31:**1609-1668, 1995

176. Sedler RA: The Constitution and hastening inevitable death. **Hastings Cent Rep 23:**20-25, 1993

177. Shewmon DA: Anencephaly: selected medical aspects. **Hastings Cent Rep 18:**11-19, 1988

178. Shewmon DA, Capron AM, Peacock WJ, et al: The use of anencephalic infants as organ sources. A critique. **JAMA 261:**1773-1781, 1989

179. Silverman HJ, Tuma P, Schaeffer MH, et al: Implementation of the patient self-determination act in a hospital setting. An initial evaluation. **Arch Intern Med 155:**502-510, 1995

180. Siminoff LA, Arnold RM, Caplan AL, et al: Public policy governing organ and tissue procurement in the United States. Results from the National Organ and Tissue Procurement Study. **Ann Intern Med 123:**10-17, 1995

181. Spital A: Mandated choice: a plan to increase public commitment to organ donation. **JAMA 273:** 504-506, 1995

182. Spital A: Mandated choice for organ donation. **JAMA 274:**942, 1995

183. Spital A: The shortage of organs for transplantation: where do we go from here? **N Engl J Med 325:** 1243-1246, 1991

184. *State v Fiero*, 603 P2d 74 (Ariz 1979)

185. Steinberg A, Katz E, Sprung CL: Commentary: Use of anencephalic infants as organ donors. **Crit Care Med 21:**1787-1790, 1993

186. Steinbock B, McClamrock R: When is birth unfair to the child? **Hastings Cent Rep 24:**15-21, 1994

187. Strong C: An ethical framework for managing fetal anomalies in the third trimester. **Clin Obstet Gynecol 35:**792-802, 1992

188. Sullivan MD, Youngner SJ: Depression, competence, and the right to refuse lifesaving medical treatment. **Am J Psychiatry 151:**971-978, 1994

189. *Superintendent of Belchertown State School v Saikewicz*, 370 NE2d 417 (Mass 1977)

190. Tarasaka JM: Consent and informed consent, in Tarasaka JM: **Legal Guide for Physicians.** White Plains, NY: AHAB Press, 1995, pp 6.01-6.100 [1], 6.01-6.100 [3]

191. Tarasaka JM: Death, withholding/withdrawing life support, no code orders and physician assisted suicide, in Tarasaka JM: **Legal Guide for Physicians.** White Plains, NY: AHAB Press, 1995

192. Task Force for the Determination of Brain Death in Children: Guidelines for the determination of brain death in children. **Arch Neurol 44:**587-588, 1987; **Ann Neurol 21:**616-617, 1987; **Pediatr Neurol 3:**242-243, 1987; **Pediatrics 80:**298-300, 1987

193. Teno JM, Hill TP, O'Connor MA (eds): Advance care planning. Priorities for ethical and empirical research. **Hastings Cent Rep (Suppl) 24:**S1-S36, 1994

194. Truog RD: "Do-not-resuscitate" orders during anesthesia and surgery. **Anesthesiology 74:**606-608, 1991

195. Urofsky MI: **Letting Go; Death, Dying & the Law.** New York, NY: Macmillan, 1993

196. US Congress, Office of Technology Assessment: **Biomedical Ethics in U.S. Public Policy—Background Paper.** Washington, DC: US Government Printing Office, 1993 (OTA-BP-BBS-105)

197. van der Maas PJ, Pijnenborg L, van Delden JJM: Changes in Dutch opinions on active euthanasia, 1966 through 1991. **JAMA 273:**1411-1414, 1995

198. Veatch RM: Routine inquiry about organ donation—an alternative to presumed consent. **N Engl J Med 325:**1246-1249, 1991

199. Veatch RM: The impending collapse of the whole-brain definition of death. **Hastings Cent Rep 23:** 18-24, 1993

200. Weedn VW: Donor and donee patients, in American College of Legal Medicine (ed): **Legal Medicine. Legal Dynamics of Medical Encounters.** 2nd ed. St. Louis, Mo: CV Mosby, 1991, pp 386-407

201. Wekesser C (ed): **Euthanasia: Opposing Viewpoints**. San Diego, Calif: Greenhaven Press, 1995, 214 pp

202. Wenger NS, Oye RK, Bellamy PE, et al: Prior capacity of patients lacking decision making ability early in hospitalization. Implications for advance directive administration. **J Gen Intern Med 9:**539-543, 1994

203. Winslow GR, Walters JW (eds): **Facing Limits. Ethics and Health Care for the Elderly.** Boulder, Colo: Westview Press, 1993

204. Youngner SJ, Arnold RM: Ethical, psychosocial, and public policy implications of procuring organs from non-heart-beating cadaver donors. **JAMA 269:** 2769-2774, 1993

CHAPTER 7

MENTAL AND EMOTIONAL COMPETENCE

ROBERT W. KEEFOVER, MD

The American legal system assumes that individuals possess the capacity to freely choose their objectives and to direct their behavior accordingly. Provisions are made, however, for circumstances in which medical or psychological conditions impair a person's ability to accurately perceive environmental stimuli, to evaluate the meaning and significance of these perceptions, to organize his/her thoughts, and to respond appropriately. Even when these primary intellectual functions remain intact, certain disorders of motivation and impulse control may limit a person's ability to conform his/her behavior to legal standards. This chapter examines the legal principles pertaining to such mentally incapacitated individuals. The specific focus here is on those aspects of competency that are most relevant to the practice of medicine: informed consent, involuntary treatment, medical decision-making by proxies, hospitalization by commitment, and criminal competency.

THE CAPACITY TO EXERCISE RESPONSIBILITY

As illustrated in Table 1, a number of neuropsychiatric conditions may negatively affect a person's level of responsiveness, orientation and concentration, mood and motivation, impulse control, insight and judgment, memory capacity, expressive language capabilities, perceptual abilities, and stress or provocation tolerance. Some of these disorders, primarily those with a neurological basis, can also diminish receptive language capabilities, intellectual capacity, visuospatial performance, and praxis abilities. When one or more such impairments renders a person incapable of acting appropriately with respect to the best interests of him/herself or others, the judicial system must determine whether or not that person's individual rights and/or level of accountability under the law can and should be limited (i.e., the extent to which the individual is competent to exercise responsibility).

Clearly, not all mentally or emotionally ill patients are incompetent; just as with innocence and guilt, competence must be presumed until incompetence is proven. Further, because individuals are seldom incompetent in all things at all times, a determination of competency usually is temporally and situationally specific.[5] Since it is only through adjudication that competency status can be determined, the role of the physician in this process is essentially to substantiate the presence, nature, and cause of a mental disorder, and to advise the court in these matters.

TABLE 1
EXAMPLES OF MENTAL AND EMOTIONAL DISORDERS POTENTIALLY INFLUENCING COMPETENCY STATUS

Psychiatric Illnesses

Affective Disorders
    Depression
    Bipolar affective disorder
Anxiety Disorders
    Obsessive-compulsive disorder
    Post-traumatic stress disorder
Characterological Disorders
    Disruptive behavior disorders
        Attention deficit disorder
        Conduct disorder
        Oppositional-defiant disorder
    Personality disorders
        Paranoid
        Antisocial
        Borderline
Dissociative Disorders
    Multiple personality disorder
    Fugue
    Psychogenic amnesia
    Depersonalization disorder

Impulse Control Disorders
    Intermittent explosive disorder
    Kleptomania
    Pyromania
Paraphilias
    Exhibitionism
    Pedophilia
    Voyeurism
    Necrophilia
Psychotic Disorders
    Schizophrenic spectrum
    Delusional disorder
    Bipolar affective disorder
    Brief reactive psychosis
Substance-Induced
    Alcohol

Neurological Illnesses

Acute Confusional States/Delirium
    (e.g., metabolic disturbances, toxins)
Brain Masses
    (e.g., tumors)
Central Nervous System Infections
    (e.g., abscess, cryptococcosis, HIV (human
        immunodeficiency virus))
Dementia
    (e.g., Alzheimer's disease, Pick's disease)
Epilepsy

Head Injury
Mental Retardation
Sleep Disorders
    REM (rapid eye movement)
        behavior disorder
    Narcolepsy
    Somnambulism
    Sleep apnea
Stroke
Tourette's Syndrome

At the most general level, there are two types of competency, civil and criminal. In both instances, the relevant legal concerns are: 1) whether the individual is able to understand the nature of the problem with which he/she is confronted; 2) if the individual fully comprehends all decision options; 3) can the individual appreciate the potential consequences of choosing a given alternative; and 4) whether he/she can act in consonance with his/her decision. The difference between civil and criminal competence hinges primarily on whether the decisions for which an individual is to be held accountable have resulted in violations of the law.

CIVIL COMPETENCY

Civil competency refers to a person's capacity to make appropriate decisions concerning a broad range of personal issues (e.g., to marry, make a will, and enter into a contract); legal standards for determining civil competency vary according to the function in question. This hierarchy of capacities acknowledges that individuals may be competent for certain functions but not for others. For example, a person may be competent to have a will prepared, but may lack the capacity to manage his/her current financial affairs; the underlying principle here being that a will takes effect only after death, while financial mismanagement can negatively affect the person during life.

In the medical setting, issues pertaining to civil competency typically arise within the context of a patient's inability to make informed decisions about treatment. In some cases (e.g., if the patient is in a coma), it will be obvious that he/she cannot participate in this process. In others, however, the patient's capacity to rationally consider his/her therapeutic options may be less clear. In either circumstance, the physician who proceeds with treatment without the approval of the patient or his/her legal proxy may be committing a tort offense (civil wrong against the individual) or even criminal assault and battery. Civil competency, therefore, becomes relevant for doctors when they are seeking informed consent, considering involuntary treatment or hospitalization, or honoring medical decisions made on behalf of the patient by others.

Informed Consent for Medical Treatment

The doctrine of informed consent is based on two legal principles: self-determination and the fiduciary relationship that exists between a physician and a patient. The first is founded on common law and derives from an individual's constitutional right to privacy. The second reflects an assumption that the doctor possesses special knowledge of the patient's physical condition while the patient is helpless regarding his/her condition.[38] Simply stated, the physician has a responsibility to inform the patient thoroughly regarding his/her illness and all available treatments, so that the patient can make a rational decision about whether or not to undergo a given therapy.

It should be noted here that tort law traditionally has recognized the necessity to sometimes provide emergency care when patients are unable to participate in the medical decision-making process.[41] Just what constitutes an emergency may not always be clear, but when a patient is so critically ill that he/she is incapable of providing consent[23] and crisis precludes taking time to appoint or seek out a guardian, the decision to render treatment without the patient's explicit permission is legally defensible.

Litigation concerning failure to obtain informed consent is likely to center around three important questions: 1) did the physician actively seek voluntary informed consent; 2) was the patient informed sufficiently to make a reasonable decision; and 3) did the patient's mental state allow him/her to comprehend his/her plight and make a rational choice about receiving or refusing treatment (i.e., was he/she competent to give consent)? The physician generally addresses the first two of these questions by applying the so-called "reasonable man" standard. That is, consent is sought and obtained only after fully disclosing to the patient all the information that a reasonable person would need in order to make an informed decision about a procedure or treatment.[38] If the doctor feels that a patient's emotional state is so tenuous that full disclosure of the medical predicament would be counter-therapeutic, the "therapeutic privilege" may be exercised and certain details withheld from the patient.[23] In some jurisdictions, however, the court may interpret this as an implicit and arbitrary determination by the doctor that the patient was in fact mentally or emotionally incompetent. Therefore, the invocation of therapeutic privilege should be very carefully considered and only exercised with the full knowledge and approval of a close relative.[44]

The third question posed above concerns whether the patient was a "reasonable man" (i.e., whether he was in fact competent to consent to treatment) at the time he gave permission. While the law may assume competence until incompetence is proven,[17] physicians cannot make that assumption. In treating a consenting, but essentially incompetent, patient, the physician may be as culpable as would be the case in treating a mentally competent patient who refused treatment.[38] Both actions may represent negligence[41] in obtaining "informed" consent. In questionable cases, therefore, it is important that doctors substantiate their reasons for believing a patient to be competent of informed consent before proceeding with treatment.

Unfortunately, physicians will find no clear standard against which to measure their "bedside" determination of a patient's competence to provide informed consent. Often, however, the legal test for competency has been the same one used to establish capacity to execute an agreement; the individual must be of sufficient reason to understand the nature, terms, and effect of the agreement.[17] Given this, a prudent course of action is to document that the assessment included several key elements, including the patient's ability to: 1) know that there are choices; 2) make a reasonable choice; 3) express a rationale for that choice; and 4) understand the risks and benefits of all treatment alternatives. Regarding the last of these, it is not enough that the individual exhibits an "ability" to understand: the physician should also substantiate the patient's true comprehension of these issues.[35]

In addition to coma, in which case a proxy decision-maker may be necessary (see below), a person's capacity to provide informed consent may be compromised by a wide variety of other mental or emotional disturbances. Prominent among these are intellectual deficiency, acquired cognitive impairment, psychosis, and impulse dyscontrol. Therefore, it is prudent to enlist the expertise of other professionals in determining a patient's competence in this regard.[14,16] Obviously, every effort should be made to communicate consent-related information to the patient in a manner that takes into account his/her intellectual capacities and cultural background. Further, repeated exposure to the material may enhance comprehension of its meaning. Finally, frequent reassessment of the patient can reveal that competence has been restored with effective treatment or with the elimination of barriers such as psychoactive medications. In such cases, the individual may be able to reassume decision-making responsibility from that point on in the course of the illness.[14]

Involuntary Treatment

As is implied in the doctrine of informed consent, a competent patient may reject any and all interventions. This entitlement is founded on the right to privacy guaranteed under the United States Bill of Rights.[38,41] Indeed, while failure to obtain voluntary informed consent may represent negligence, treatment of a patient who has specifically withheld consent (i.e., refused treatment) can be considered battery. Both actions are tort offenses, but the latter is viewed as intentional and the former is not.[41]

It is also the case that an individual's right to refuse needed medical therapy may be overridden on the basis of mental incompetence.[41] Thus, when a patient's unwillingness to give informed consent is believed to be due to an incapacitation of intellectual or emotional faculties, the physician may be obligated to administer treatment against the patient's will. This course of action not only requires that the patient's incompetence be legally established, but also that some other person be appointed to serve as the patient's proxy decision-maker (i.e., a guardian who can provide informed consent on behalf of the patient). Although the general concept of guardianship will be discussed in greater detail below, it is appropriate to mention here that the process is initiated in different ways from one jurisdiction to another, so that physicians will probably want to seek consultation with a psychiatrist, the local community mental health center, or the hospital lawyer in most cases.

Involuntary Hospitalization (Commitment)

Involuntary hospitalization may or may not be viewed simply as one form of involuntary treatment. In any event, most physicians recognize "commitment" as the process by which individuals who are mentally disturbed, who are dangerous to self and others, and who refuse needed treatment are confined to a hospital against their will. While it is the psychiatrist who most often is involved in such situations, non-psychiatric physicians may also be called upon to initiate, or at least participate in, commitment proceedings. Given the impact an involuntary hospitalization may have on a patient's life and the physician's own lack of formal training in this regard, non-psychiatrists are often uneasy about when involuntary commitment is called for, the procedures that must be followed when initiating the process, and the legal obligations or liabilities associated with participation in a "commitment."

The theoretical basis for commitment lies in two legal concepts: parens patriae and the police power of the state.[8,39,42] In the first case, the state functions as parent and, therefore, has a responsibility to provide for those who are unable to care for themselves or otherwise insure their own well-being. The second concept relates to the state's obligation to protect its citizens from individuals who may endanger them. While earlier local codes tended to emphasize the doctrine of parens patriae, dangerousness to self and others has more recently become the primary focus.[39]

In the past, involuntary hospitalization was widely viewed as an act of compassion. However, with the successful introduction of antipsychotic medications in the mid-1950s and the resulting decline in asylum patient populations, the commitment of mentally ill patients to a hospital has not only become less necessary but also less acceptable in the eyes of many people. Fueled by legislative concerns over the costs of operating state asylums, increasing public sensitivity to individual human rights, and at least according to some, a growing "anti-psychiatrist" movement,[8] lawmakers in many states have been prevailed upon to consider the total abolition of involuntary commitment laws. Although this rather ambitious goal has not been realized, the current availability of a comprehensive federally-funded community mental health center system has led many to conclude that hospitalization is avoidable.[39] The result has been that in many states substantially more stringent commitment laws have been passed, placing almost total emphasis on patient rights and the concept of hospitalization as a last resort. In some cases, these changes have greatly complicated the process.

In contrast to other forms of involuntary treatment, the principle legal question posed in a commitment proceeding considers whether or not the patient should be involuntarily confined to a hospital. Furthermore, it is usually psychiatric hospitalization that is being considered: the illness demanding medical attention is the same illness suspected of impairing the patient's ability to consider and appropriately act on his/ her condition. Not surprisingly, while few physicians would hesitate to seek involuntary hospitalization for a psychotic and uncooperative patient who presents with a basilar skull fracture, the need for commitment may seem less clear if serious injury has not yet been sustained during the patient's nightly nude strolls along busy freeways. The physician's reluctance to act in the latter scenario may stem in part from a perception that psychiatric hospitalization equates with imprisonment or that psychiatric treatment is largely ineffective.[39]

In addition to personal attitudes and examination findings, several other factors may influence the physician's decision to seek commitment. Prominent among these is the fact that information concerning the patient's recent mental state and behavior must often be obtained from family members, friends, or representatives of social agencies. These individuals, the petitioners, usually are acting out of a genuine concern for the patient's welfare but also may have a more personal stake in the matter. In an estimated 5% of cases, the petitioner fears harm at the hands of the patient. In another 25%, these individuals may be seeking relief from the responsibility of providing care.[39] While allegations that patients have been "railroaded" into the hospital are largely unfounded,[39] physicians can hardly avoid skepticism regarding the motives of some petitioners. In any case, these individuals have taken a significant step in asking that someone be "locked up for their own good" and are seldom comfortable with any other outcome.

In view of these external pressures and the "heavy-handedness" that involuntary hospitalization represents, it is disconcerting that legal guidelines concerning a physician's obligation to initiate or facilitate commitment proceedings are somewhat ambiguous. Although doctors, particularly psychiatrists, clearly have a legal obligation to arrange for the restraint and observation of those patients whose mental or emotional state makes them a threat to their own well-being,[13] the clinician's responsibilities to those who may be targeted for violence by a patient are less well-defined. Further, given the margin of error associated with predicting future behavior, one may ask how any physician, especially a non-psychiatrist, can be expected to know when a patient's potential for suicide or overt aggression justifies enforced confinement.

The widely cited *Tarasoff* decision in California[45] firmly established one of the clinician's responsibilities regarding potentially violent patients: mental health professionals who are privy to the specific aggressive intentions of their patients have an obligation to warn potential victims. In a rehearing of the case,[46] the court further maintained that therapists have a duty to "protect" potential victims. While that does not necessarily mean that they are required to involuntarily hospitalize or otherwise forcibly detain potentially aggressive individuals, it suggests that these actions would be appropriate in many cases. Most courts, however, have not been inclined to hold physicians accountable for protecting the potential victims of violent patients.[4]

In the absence of specific guidelines concerning a physician's obligation to detain potentially self-injurious or violent patients, it is helpful to bear in mind that commitment serves first and foremost to facilitate a more deliberate and sophisticated evaluation of the individual's mental state. This being so, it is probably better to err on the side of caution by seeking commitment in the face of nagging doubt. Thoughtful consideration of the patient's long-term well-being can make the decision clearer.

Physicians, especially non-psychiatrists, seldom are found negligent in failing to commit. Tort liability is not, however, out of the question. Given the disgruntlement that can be expected of family, friends, or agencies who may have sought the patient's hospitalization prior to some tragedy and the fact that, in some cases, the risk for self-harm or endangering others may have been patently obvious, it is probable that some action against the physician may be considered. If so, careful documentation that a reasonable examination was attempted and that due consideration of the problem was undertaken should provide an adequate defense.

By the same token, tort liability for physicians who initiate or participate in commitment proceedings also appears to be limited. When legal action is brought against the committing physician, it is usually based on charges of: 1) malicious prosecution; 2) false imprisonment; 3) assault and battery; or 4) violation of civil rights. In most cases, however, the physician is considered a witness of the court and is immune from such actions. Further, charges related to these activities are often rejected, even when gross negligence may have been involved, because the process frequently occurs in an emergency setting where a physician-patient relationship was never established. Still, physicians have lost such cases because they "did not utilize the minimal skill required to effectuate the process."[13]

The discussion thus far has focused on why and when a physician should consider seeking the commitment of a patient. The question of how this can be accomplished will now be considered. Unfortunately, only general guidelines can be provided here, since the manner in which an involuntary commitment must proceed is determined primarily by state statute[48] and varies widely with the location in which it occurs. It follows that any physician whose practice is likely to require even occasional involvement in such proceedings should become acquainted with pertinent local laws. Table 2 illustrates some of the more important features of the hospital commitment process for the 50 states and the District of Columbia; however, it does not reflect the intricacies that often are involved.

The first step leading to commitment is, by definition, taken by someone other than the identified patient: this individual is the "petitioner" referred to above. In many states, the petitioner may be anyone who has a reason to believe the action is necessary. In others, the law restricts this function to specific individuals: family members, guardians, law enforcement officials, physicians, mental health professionals, public facility and social service administrators, or the court itself. Often, the nature of the commitment (emergency or non-emergent) determines who may initiate the process. Particularly in the case of an emergency, it is typically only a designated mental health professional or public official who may actuate commitment, since this often involves forcible apprehension and hospitalization without judicial review.[48] In some states, emergency physicians are among those designated to serve in this capacity.

The acceptable justifications for commitment also vary with the circumstances under which the process is initiated. In those states providing for non-judicial emergency commitments, it is virtually always necessary that the patient's behavior constitutes a threat, either to self or others, before this type of confinement can be effected.[48] In non-emergent commitments, the presence of a mental illness in need of treatment may be all that is required. Some states even regard substance abuse as a basis for commitment (Table 2).

Probably the major point of divergence in commitment statutes from one state to another lies in who the petitioner must convince in order to successfully achieve the involuntary hospitalization of a patient. That is, who is authorized to determine the significance of the evidence presented in support of commitment and then make the decision to proceed with hospitalization or divert the patient to care in a less restrictive environment. In some states, especially when emergency hospitalization is being sought, this can be the family doctor or an emergency room physician. In others, however, the decision can only be made by specifically designated professionals (e.g., a psychiatrist or other mental health expert). In states with still more restrictive commitment laws, even in emergency cases, only a judge or court appointee (e.g., a mental hygiene commissioner) may order apprehension and make the determination after holding an adversarial hearing. When this is so, the petitioner's evidence typically must be evaluated by a mental health professional who then offers testimony regarding the necessity for commitment.

State commitment statutes also differ in terms of how long a patient may be detained following apprehension before a decision regarding formal or "full" commitment is rendered. As shown in Table 2, periods of evaluation confinement range from hours to days. These time limits do not represent the maximum duration of a full commitment, but rather refer to the length of time a patient may be detained before a determination is made regarding the need for extended confinement. Whether or not the latter is necessary often depends on the results of an in-hospital evaluation conducted by professionals at the admitting hospital, and their decision may or may not require judicial sanction. Once a "full" commitment has been ordered, involuntary hospitalization is likely to extend for weeks to years, although periodic reconsideration of the patient's need for confinement is usually mandated.[48]

Involuntary Hospitalization vs. Involuntary Treatment

Although seldom a concern for non-psychiatrists, it should be noted that even patients who are committed to a hospital may retain the right to refuse treatment. This is particularly true for psychiatric patients and is based primarily on concerns that neuroleptic medications and electroconvulsive therapy ("shock treatments") may have disabling and enduring side effects.[41] Unless the issue is specifically addressed during commitment proceedings, the patient's competency to consent to medical treatment will not have been adjudicated at the time of confinement. Assumed to be competent, he/she may therefore refuse the very care that could hasten release from involuntary hospitalization. In this regard, the courts seem to be caught in the middle of a struggle between advocates for patient rights and those who are more concerned with the patient's medical needs.[2]

Guardianship (Proxy Decision-Makers)

When a person in need of medical care is incapable of providing informed consent, the decision to accept or reject treatment can be made by another individual acting on his/her behalf. Examples of persons for whom this may be necessary include a child, a comatose patient, or a mentally incompetent individual. In the case of children, this function is virtually always performed by parents or other legally recognized custodians. Therefore, only guardianship for the latter two categories of patients will be discussed here.

The concept of guardianship extends back to Roman times and is based on the principle that society has an obligation to provide for the security of an individual's property should he/she become unable to manage personal affairs.[15] Guardians may be appointed because of physi-

TABLE 2
Hospital Commitment Procedures by State*

State Confinement	Who Petitions / Initiates Hospitalized Evaluation and Continued Commitment	Evaluation Time	Who Evaluates
Alabama ‡	Anyone	7 days	Physician, MHP
Alaska	Anyone	72 hrs	Two MHPs
Arizona	Anyone may ask the court to hospitalize patient	24 hrs	Physician, psychologist
Arkansas †	Anyone	72 hrs	Physician
California †	Anyone	14 days	Qualified professional
Colorado †	Police, MHP	72 hrs	Physician, psychologist
Connecticut ‡	Anyone	7 days	Psychiatrist & another physician
Delaware	Psychiatrist	3 days	Hospital staff
Dist. of Columbia †	Police, physician, psychologist, Dept. Health & Human Services	48 hrs	Hospital staff
Florida	Court, police, MHP	72 hrs	Physician, psychologist
Georgia	Physician	24 hrs	Psychiatrist, psychologist
Hawaii †	Anyone may ask the court to hospitalize patient	5 days	Physician
Idaho	Court, family, friend, guardian, police (with certification by physician or MHP)	72 hrs	Court-appointed psychiatrist and another physician or MHP
Illinois	Anyone 18 years or older	7 days	Physician, psychologist, qualified examiner
Indiana †	Family, friend, police (with certification by physician)	90 hrs	Physician
Iowa	Anyone	48 hrs	Physician
Kansas †	Anyone may ask the court to hospitalize patient	3 days	State hospital staff
Kentucky	Court, family, friend, guardian, police, MHP	24 hrs	Physician & another MHP
Louisiana †	Any responsible person (with certification by coroner and physician)	15 days	Hospital staff
Maine †	Anyone (with certification by physician or psychologist)	18 hrs	Judge
Maryland †	Anyone (with certification by one physician and another physician or psychologist)	12 hrs	Hospital staff
Massachusetts †	Physician, police	10 days	Physician, psychologist
Michigan	Anyone	24 hrs	Physician, psychologist
Minnesota †	Health officer, police	72 hrs	Medical officer on duty
Mississippi †	Anyone	24 hrs	Physician & another physician or psychologist
Missouri	Anyone	96 hrs	MHP
Montana †	Anyone may ask the court to hospitalize patient	5 days	Court (with advice from MHP)
Nebraska †	Anyone	36 hrs	Physician, psychologist
Nevada †	Family, guardian, MHP, physician, psychologist, police	72 hrs	Physician and another physician or psychologist

TABLE 2 (cont'd)

HOSPITAL COMMITMENT PROCEDURES BY STATE*

State Confinement	Who Petitions / Initiates Hospitalized Evaluation and Continued Commitment	Evaluation Time	Who Evaluates
New Hampshire †	Any responsible person	3 days	Psychiatrist
New Jersey	Family, guardian, corrections/ police/welfare administrator	20 days	Physician
New Mexico	Physician, police, psychologist	30 days	Physician, psychologist
New York	Cohabitant, family, public or charitable residence administrator (with certification by designated MHP)	72 hrs	Physician
North Carolina	Anyone	24 hrs	Physician, psychologist
North Dakota	Anyone	24 hrs	MHP
Ohio	Health/parole/police official, physician, psychologist	24 hrs	Hospital staff
Oklahoma †	Physician, psychologist	28 days	Physician, psychologist
Oregon ‡	Any two persons, health officer, magistrate	12 hrs	Physician
Pennsylvania †	Physician	2 hrs	Physician
Rhode Island †	Physician	24 hrs	Physician
South Carolina †	Anyone (with certification by physician)	24 hrs	Physician
South Dakota †‡	Anyone	24 hrs	MHP, physician
Tennessee †	Family, health/hospital/police/ welfare official, physician, psychologist (with certification by two MHPs)	varies	Hospital staff
Texas ‡	Anyone	24 hrs	Physician
Utah	Anyone (with certification by physician)	24 hrs	Physician
Vermont	Anyone may ask the court to hospitalize patient (with certification by physician)	none	Court
Virginia	Anyone	48 hrs	Physician, psychologist
Washington	Anyone	24 hrs	Physician
West Virginia †	Anyone may ask the court to hospitalize patient (with certification by physician or psychologist)	3 days	Hospital staff
Wisconsin ‡	Three adults (at least one having personal knowledge of patient's behavior) may ask the court to hospitalize patient	72 hrs	Physician and another physician or psychologist
Wyoming †	Anyone (with certification by MHP)	7 days	Court-appointed examiner

*MHP = mental health professional (psychiatrist, psychologist, psychiatric nurse, social worker, certified counselors).
† Commitment specifically requires danger to self or others.
‡ Specifically excludes commitments based on mental disturbance secondary to substance abuse alone.

cal as well as mental incapacitation and, while plenary guardianship may involve comprehensive decision-making authority, often it is either financial (i.e., a conservatorship) or medical functions that are covered by the appointment. Similar delineations of responsibility may be specified when one competent person gives another person the "power of attorney" to act on his/her behalf only in defined circumstances. The question in the medical setting, of course, specifically concerns who may legally make vicarious treatment judgments on behalf of a mentally or emotionally impaired individual.

Two legal standards are applicable to decision-making by a surrogate: "substituted judgment" and "best interest." In the first case, the proxy's decisions are those the principal would likely have made if capable of doing so. In the second case, the proxy essentially acts as a parent and chooses according to personal perceptions of what ultimately will benefit the ward.

Neither of these standards is flawless. The substituted judgment standard becomes problematic when the principal either has never been competent or has never been in a position to consider a decision similar to that with which the proxy is currently confronted. The "basic interest" concept, however, encourages decisions that are made on the premise that optimal medical results are of overriding importance, even when this is achieved at the expense of individual autonomy.[15] In practical terms, there may be little difference between decisions made in accordance with one standard or the other since, in either case, the factors influencing the process are mediated by the intellectual faculties and personality traits of the surrogate decision-maker.[15]

In the not-too-distant past, doctors routinely exercised a prerogative to make medical decisions on behalf of mentally incapacitated patients. Today, however, it is more likely to be an attorney who executes this responsibility. Similarly, many physicians traditionally assumed that a patient's next-of-kin could function satisfactorily as a surrogate decision-maker.[19] In reality, however, guardianship is usually assigned in accordance with state statute[40] rather than on the basis of kinship. Even though family members often are in a position to know what the patient would probably decide, courts occasionally have found perfectly competent and well-intended

relatives unacceptable as surrogate decision-makers.[20] Finally, the patient should not be forgotten when a surrogate decision-maker is being sought. Even though he/she may be unable to rationally consider medical options, the individual's preference regarding a guardian may be obtainable.[14]

Although many physicians welcome being relieved of the responsibility for making unilateral treatment decisions for their incompetent patients, others resent the intrusion of medically naive individuals into their practice. For those in this latter group, it is particularly frustrating that the process of finding an appropriate guardian sometimes delays the provision of needed care. This scenario has become increasingly common in recent years because of reluctance on the part of otherwise qualified individuals to serve as guardians. Geographic or functional detachment, concerns over legal ramifications, and interpersonal conflicts are among the reasons why family members frequently decline this responsibility. The court may choose to expedite the process by appointing an attorney to serve as guardian. However, the increased demand for such services on behalf of indigent clients has also diminished the enthusiasm of lawyers to act in this capacity.[15]

CRIMINAL COMPETENCY

Criminal competence refers to an individual's mental capacities within the context of his/her apprehension, detainment, trial, conviction, sentencing, and punishment for crimes committed against others. Here, the physician serves almost exclusively to facilitate the conveyance of justice; his/her primary function is to examine the accused individual in order to elicit and formulate medical findings for the legal system.[31] The court may want to know whether or not the accused suffers from a mental illness and how his/her incapacities relate to applicable legal standards.[31] As is the case with civil competence, criminal competency is not a global concept. Therefore, the accused must be evaluated with specific regard to capacity concerning several issues. These include competence to: 1) acknowledge "Miranda rights" at the time of apprehension; 2) stand trial; and 3) assume criminal responsibility. Each is a different question; depending on which is being addressed, the examiner may be required to determine the individual's mental or emotional competency either retrospectively or in the here and now.

Competence to Waive Miranda Rights

When taken into custody, a person who is suspected of committing a crime must be advised that he/she is entitled to legal counsel before providing any information of a potentially incriminating nature. Once given this so-called Miranda warning,[25] the suspect may remain completely silent until the case has been discussed with a lawyer. Obviously, if an individual's "Miranda rights" are to be meaningful, the suspect must be able to: 1) comprehend the notification he/she is given of them; 2) consider the significance of any information provided; and 3) inhibit personal expression of potentially damaging statements. Although this has not constituted a significant problem for the courts, it remains possible that a person who has waived Miranda rights will subsequently be determined to have been incompetent to do so and that this will become an issue during adjudication.[10]

Competence to Stand Trial

The process of being tried and sentenced for alleged criminal behavior cannot be a passive experience for the accused individual. Active participation is required at least in the courtroom, if not on the witness stand. Consequently, a requirement that the defendant be present in both mind and body has evolved from English common law of the 1700s prohibiting the trial of an individual "in absentia."[35] When there is doubt about whether the defendant's mental state at the time of the hearing renders him/her absent in mind, competency to stand trial must be determined before the trial can proceed.[30]

It is important for physicians to recognize that this is a precise question. In many cases, courts fail to specify the type of information being sought and the reasons for requesting a

mental status evaluation. Consequently, the examiner's report back to the court may inappropriately focus solely on the presence or absence of mental illness and/or the need for hospitalization. In response to such feedback, the court may commit the accused individual to a psychiatric facility for treatment of an indefinite duration without further consideration of the right to trial.[34] Cases in which unconvicted defendants remained hospital-confined for the rest of their lives have been documented.[17,43] This clearly represents a gross violation of the defendant's rights as an individual and may well be a more untoward outcome than would have resulted had he/she been found guilty.

The so-called "Dusky test"[12] is used to determine competence to stand trial. In essence, this Supreme Court–approved standard requires that the defendant be oriented to time and place, have some recognition of events, have sufficient ability to consult a lawyer with a reasonable degree of rational understanding, and have a rational and factual understanding of the proceedings against him/her. In evaluating the defendant's competence to stand trial, an examining physician should address the individual's ability to: 1) evaluate legal defense options; 2) establish a client/attorney relationship; 3) assist in planning a defense strategy; 4) evaluate the roles of the participants in the trial; 5) comprehend basic courtroom procedures; 6) comprehend the charges that have been lodged against him/her; 7) understand the nature and severity of the possible penalties for the alleged crime; 8) understand the possible outcomes of the trial; 9) challenge the assertions of witnesses who testify against him/her; 10) provide relevant testimony on his/her own behalf; and 11) behave appropriately in the courtroom. In conducting such assessments, physicians may find it useful to refer to one of the checklists or rating scales that have been developed around issues such as these.[22,34] One instrument of this type is shown as an example in Figure 1.

Defendants found incompetent to take part in a trial usually are held for psychiatric evaluation in order to determine their treatment potential. If treatment is likely to restore the capacity to participate in pending legal proceedings, the defendant may then be hospitalized until appropriate care re-establishes compe-

COMPETENCY TO STAND TRIAL ASSESSMENT INSTRUMENT

Degree of Incapacity	Total	Severe	Moderate	Mild	None	Unratable
1. Appraisal of available legal defenses	1	2	3	4	5	6
2. Unmanageable behavior	1	2	3	4	5	6
3. Quality of relating to attorney	1	2	3	4	5	6
4. Planning of legal strategy, including guilty plea to lesser charges where pertinent	1	2	3	4	5	6
5. Appraisal of role of:						
a. Defense counsel	1	2	3	4	5	6
b. Prosecuting attorney	1	2	3	4	5	6
c. Judge	1	2	3	4	5	6
d. Jury	1	2	3	4	5	6
e. Defendant	1	2	3	4	5	6
f. Witnesses	1	2	3	4	5	6
6. Understanding of court procedure	1	2	3	4	5	6
7. Appreciation of charges	1	2	3	4	5	6
8. Appreciation of range and nature of possible penalties	1	2	3	4	5	6
9. Appraisal of likely outcome	1	2	3	4	5	6
10. Capacity to disclose to attorney available pertinent facts surrounding the offense including the defendant's movements, timing, mental state, and actions at the time of the offense	1	2	3	4	5	6
11. Capacity to realistically challenge prosecution witnesses	1	2	3	4	5	6
12. Capacity to testify relevantly	1	2	3	4	5	6
13. Self-defeating v. self-serving motivation (legal sense)	1	2	3	4	5	6

Examinee: _____   Examiner: _____

Date:_____

Figure 1: Form used to assess a person's competency to stand trial. (Reproduced from McGarry et al[22])

tency. While the process appears straightforward, that is not always the case. For example, some jurisdictions require not only that the defendant be mentally competent but also free of psychoactive drugs before the trial continues. An individual whose mental illness has been stabilized through the use of psychiatric medications may, therefore, be considered only "synthetically sane" and not truly competent.[33,50]

Competence to be Held Criminally Responsible

When there is doubt, U.S. citizens are constitutionally entitled to an evaluation that seeks to determine their mental competence at the time of the alleged crime.[1] The results of this assessment may influence either the verdict handed down (e.g., "not guilty by reason of insanity") or the sentence rendered. Legal concerns over whether an accused individual should be held responsible for commission of a crime are based on two centuries-old doctrines, "actus reus" (the crime must have been voluntarily committed) and "mens rea" (criminal behavior must have been intended). Regarding the latter, it is understood that an individual who suffers from one of several mental disorders may have been incapable of forming an intent to commit the crime in question. Lacking the capacity to form criminal intent, the defendant may not be found criminally responsible.[6] When first-degree murder is charged, the defense may also argue that the defendant was incapable of the "premeditation" requirement for that conviction.[28]

Since 1843, the basic standard for establishing the absence of guilt by reason of insanity has been the so-called "M'Naghten" rule or test. Concerned over the court's acquittal of a delusional Scotsman named Daniel M'Naghten, who had been accused of murdering a prominent citizen's secretary, England's House of Lords sought an explanation for this unexpected decision from the Chief Justice in the trial. In response, the Judge opined that a defendant may be judged not guilty by reason of insanity when it can be shown that at the time the crime was committed, the accused party was suffering from a disease of the mind that impaired reasoning to the extent that he did not know the nature and quality of the act, or that it was wrong.

Shortly after its introduction into American courts 7 years later, the rule came under intense criticism from many who felt that it was too narrow. That is, it failed to protect those who, while not psychotic, were unable to control their impulses and emotions. Such individuals were said to suffer from "moral insanity." These concerns were taken into account in 1962, when the American Law Institute drafted its Model Penal Code. That document states that "A person is not responsible for criminal conduct if at the time of such conduct as a result of mental disease or mental defect, he lacks substantial capacity either to appreciate the criminality of his conduct or to conform his conduct to the requirements of law."[6] In other words, the American Law Institute standard added the test of "inability to conform behavior to legal standards" to the M'Naghten test. It is virtually always one or the other of these two standards that is applied when a court seeks to determine criminal responsibility.

Given the above, two factors must be taken into account when evaluating an accused individual for competency to be held criminally responsible: the ability to understand right from wrong (either intellectually or emotionally) and the ability to direct one's behavior in accordance with that understanding. Of the disorders listed in Table 1, it is those of psychiatric origin that are most often the focus of these evaluations.[32] This may be due in part to the fact that, as a category of illness, they are relatively more prevalent in the population at large. For example, schizophrenia, the basis for two out of three mental incompetence acquittals,[29] and "mania" (i.e., bipolar affective disorder) are found in a combined 2% of the population.[18,27] In addition to being fairly prevalent, many major psychiatric disorders are chronic and impair both understanding and impulse control over extended periods of time. As a rule, however, they feature few verifiable lesions or physical findings and can be difficult to demonstrate convincingly to a court.

Some neuropsychiatric illnesses feature symptoms that are so bizarre that they seem to stretch the bounds of credibility. Obsessive-compulsive disorder and Tourette's syndrome are illustrative examples of these maladies. In both disorders, patients may be aware that some behaviors they feel compelled to display are inappropriate or even violate the law, but they are incapable of restraining the urge to exhibit them nonetheless. For example, they may impulsively touch members of the opposite sex in intimate places or utter obscene comments. Disorders such as these challenge the premise that cognitive appreciation of the wrongness of an act establishes competency to be held responsible for it, the essence of the M'Naghten test. Little research has been conducted on this topic, but there is evidence to suggest that the level of insight obsessive-compulsive disorder patients have into the irrationality of their compulsions correlates poorly with their ability to exert volitional control over them.[36] Still, when the court applies a standard for criminal responsibility that excludes the "volitional prong" contained in the American Law Institute standard mentioned earlier, disorders like these are not likely to represent an effective defense.

Psychiatric illnesses that feature few overt alterations in mental function and yet often result in criminal behavior deserve particular mention here. Easily the most important among these is the antisocial personality disorder (APD). The term "personality disorder" refers to an enduring, inflexible, and pervasive pattern of perceiving and responding to experiences in ways that cause significant distress or impairment in daily functioning.[3] In a sense then, personality disordered patients are "ill" because they are who they are, a proposition that can be understandably difficult for many, including the judiciary, to appreciate.

"Anti-social personality disorder" is the specific diagnosis currently applied to adults who chronically fail to conform to social norms and repeatedly perform acts that are grounds for arrest.[3] The older terms "psychopath"[9] and "sociopath" essentially refer to the same clinical phenomenon.[47] According to the American Law Institute Model Penal Code, conditions that manifest only as chronic criminality should not be included under the term "mental disorder."[26] However, among the clinical features of APD leading psychiatrists to conclude that these individuals are ill are an apparent lack of anxiety, an inability to experience depression, and a pervasive impulsivity.[3,47] These character traits notwithstanding, within the context of a trial, it seems fair to ask whether the accused exhibits criminal behavior because he/she has an APD or whether APD has been diagnosed simply because the person repeatedly commits crimes. Even if a judge or jury is willing to accept the first premise and concedes that this mitigates the defendant's responsibility for the crime in question, the fact that patients with APD are generally believed to be incorrigible and incapable of learning from experience may compel the court to seek some form of confinement. Indeed, these individuals can become more treatment-responsive when incarcerated or otherwise immobilized.[47]

As with APD, patients diagnosed with posttraumatic stress disorder (PTSD) seldom demonstrate overt signs of mental or emotional pathology. Although they are somewhat less inclined to engage in criminal activity, the symptoms associated with this condition can have serious legal implications.[21] PTSD was not formalized as a diagnostic entity until 1980, when it became apparent that many Vietnam War veterans were experiencing serious and enduring psychiatric problems. Thus, while war-related psychological disorders are hardly a new phenomenon, PTSD per se is strongly associated with the Vietnam conflict. Of particular relevance to this discussion are reports that 50% of all Vietnam veterans have suffered from PTSD[49] and that 25% have been convicted of a crime.[37]

In reviewing cases involving the PTSD defense, Marciniak[21] points out that because the disorder is presumed to result from a traumatic event, the defendant's behavior before and after the precipitating incident or circumstance can be compared. This being so, diminished responsibility on the basis of PTSD may be an easier argument to present in court than is true for APD. Other factors in a given case, however, may limit the effectiveness of the PTSD defense. For example, when the crime in question was nonviolent in nature and committed repeatedly or over an extended period, courts accepting a "not guilty by reason of insanity" verdict only when the defendant lacked the capacity to appreciate the nature, quality, and wrongfulness of his/her actions may consider the PTSD argument irrelevant.[21]

When PTSD is a pertinent issue in a criminal case, several guidelines may be followed in establishing the nature of the relationship between the disorder and the offense: 1) PTSD-associated symptoms such as interpersonal difficulties and substance abuse should be considered only "mitigating factors" rather than excuses for the defendant's conduct; 2) the crime in question should recreate, in a psychologically meaningful way, elements of the traumatic stressor that presumably brought on PTSD; and 3) the events or circumstances surrounding the crime should have the potential to realistically or symbolically force the defendant to face unresolved psychological conflicts.[21]

In contrast to most psychiatric illnesses, neurological disorders often are objectively demonstrable. Some, however, present their own special problems when the physician is trying to relate them to the commission of a crime. Seizure disorders are prime examples of such neurological conditions because they cause only transient alterations in mental status interposed with long periods of perfectly normal functioning. The evaluating physician must not only confirm the presence and character of a seizure disorder, but must also attempt to determine retrospectively whether or not the accused was impaired by an ictal event or by post-ictal confusion when the crime with which he/she is charged was committed. Even when this question can be satisfactorily answered, the possibility that the individual's vulnerability to seizures was heightened as a consequence of semi-volitional behaviors such as substance abuse or medication noncompliance may also have to be addressed. When the crime in question involves violence, Delgado-Escueta et al[11] suggest that the evaluation be conducted by a neurologist with special competence in seizure disorders. Further, they suggest that aggressive/violent behaviors during ictus be documented using video-monitored electroencephalographic recordings and that such behaviors be confirmed as having been a feature of the defendant's past seizure history.[11]

In addition to "not guilty by reason of insanity," some courts have yet another verdict option when defendants are determined to have been mentally or emotionally incompetent at the time of their criminal activities. During the drafting of the American Law Institute Model Penal Code, at least one consultant argued that attempts to define insanity for the purpose of determining criminal responsibility should be abandoned and that assessments of mental competence should only be used to determine ability to stand trial or to inform the judge at the time of sentencing.[6]

It is implied in the above proposition that a defendant would be tried in the usual manner, with evidence regarding mental incapacities at the time of the alleged crime having little or no bearing on whether the finding is guilty or not guilty. If he/she then is proven guilty but is believed to have been mentally or emotionally disturbed when the crime was committed, the guilty verdict might be qualified with an acknowledgment that some mental affliction played an influential role (i.e., he/she is guilty of the crime but was mentally ill when it occurred). The latter conclusion might then be taken into account when the judge attempts to render a sentence appropriate to the circumstance (e.g., hospitalization vs. imprisonment). In 1975, Michigan became the first of a growing number of states to provide for a sentence of "guilty but mentally ill."[24] Although this trial outcome seems reasonable in that it acknowledges that the defendant did indeed engage in criminal behavior, it marginalizes the long-established principle of mens rea or criminal intent with regard to guilt.

SUMMARY

An individual's constitutional right to autonomy and privacy are to one degree or another withdrawn when he/she is legally declared incapable of assuming personal or even criminal responsibility. It is therefore appropriate that, in the final analysis, decisions concerning mental and emotional competency are made in court and not at the bedside. Still, the role played by physicians in these deliberations is important and should not be approached casually. The fact that legal processes are adversarial in nature and focus as much on rules and precedent as on medical principles can disorient doctors. While the foregoing discussion provides only a basic introduction to the issues involved, it will hopefully serve to diminish physicians' anxieties and thereby enhance their effectiveness in these proceedings.

REFERENCES

1. *Ake v Oklahoma*, 470 US 68 (1985)
2. American Psychiatric Association, Committee on Nomenclature and Statistics: **Diagnostic and Statistical Manual of Mental Disorders.** 4th ed. Washington, DC: American Psychiatric Association, 1994
3. Applebaum PS: The right to refuse treatment with antipsychotic medications: retrospect and prospect. **Am J Psychiatry 145:**413-419, 1988
4. Beck JC: Current status of the duty to protect, in Beck JC (ed): **Confidentiality Versus the Duty to Protect: Foreseeable Harm in the Practice of Psychiatry.** Washington, DC: American Psychiatric Press, 1990, pp 9-21
5. Brody J: Organization of the cerebral cortex. **Comp Neurol 102:**511-556, 1955
6. Bromberg W: By reason of insanity, in: **The Uses of Psychiatry in the Law: A Clinical View of Forensic Psychiatry.** Westport, Conn: Quorum Books, 1979,

pp 39-65

7. Bursten B: The psychiatrist-witness and legal guilt. **Am J Psychiatry 139:**784-788, 1982

8. Chodoff P: The case for involuntary hospitalization of the mentally ill. **Am J Psychiatry 133:**496-501, 1976

9. Cleckley HM: Psychopathic states, in Arieti S (ed): **American Handbook of Psychiatry.** New York, NY: International Universities, 1959

10. *Colorado v Connelly*, 147 US 157 (1986)

11. Delgado-Escueta AV, Mattson RH, King L, et al: The nature of aggression during epileptic seizures. **N Engl J Med 305:**711-716, 1981

12. *Dusky v United States*, 363 US 402 (1960)

13. Fishalow SE: The tort liability of the psychiatrist. **Bull Am Acad Psychiatry Law 3:**191-230, 1975

14. Fleming C, Momim ZA, Brensilver JM, et al: How to determine decisional capacity in critically ill patients. **J Crit Illness 122:**422-429, 1995

15. Gutheil TG, Bursztajn HJ, Brodsky A, et al: **Decision Making in Psychiatry and the Law.** Baltimore, Md: Williams & Wilkins, 1991

16. Hafemeister TL, Sales BD: Interdisciplinary evaluations for guardianship conservatorships. **Law Human Behavior 8:**335-354, 1984

17. Hess JH Jr, Thomas HE: Incompetency to stand trial: procedures, results, and problems. **Am J Psychiatry 119:**713-720, 1963

18. Karno M, Norquist GS: Schizophrenia: Epidemiology, in Kaplan HI, Sadock BJ (eds): **Comprehensive Textbook of Psychiatry.** 5th ed. Baltimore, Md: Williams & Wilkins, 1989, pp 699-705

19. Krasik EB: The role of the family in medical decision making for incompetent adult patients. **U Pitt Law Rev 48:**539-618, 1987

20. Lo B, Rouse F, Dornbrand L: Family decision making on trial. Who decides for incompetent patients? **N Engl J Med 322:**1228-1232, 1990

21. Marciniak RD: Implications to forensic psychiatry of post-traumatic stress disorder: a review. **Milit Med 151:**434-151, 1986

22. McGarry AL, Curran WJ, Lipsitt PD, et al: **Competency to Stand Trial and Mental Illness: Final Report from the Laboratory of Community Psychiatry, Harvard Medical School.** Washington DC: US Government Printing Office, 1973 (DHEW Publication No. (HSM) 73-9105)

23. Meisel A, Roth LH, Lidz CW: Toward a model of the legal doctrine of informed consent. **Am J Psychiatry 134:**285-289, 1977

24. Mich Pub Acts 180 (codified at Mich Comp Laws §768.36 (1982)) (1974)

25. *Miranda v Arizona*, 384 US 436 (1966)

26. **Model Penal Code, Proposed Official Draft.** Philadelphia, Pa: American Law Institute, 1962

27. Mollica RF: Mood disorders: epidemiology, in Kaplan HI, Sadock BJ (eds): **Comprehensive Textbook of Psychiatry.** 5th ed. Baltimore, Md: Williams &

Wilkins, 1989, pp 859-867

28. Morse SJ: Diminished capacity: a moral and legal conundrum. **Int J Law Psychiatry 2:**271-298, 1979

29. Pasewark RA, Pantle ML, Steadman HJ: Characteristics and disposition of persons found not guilty by reason of insanity in New York State, 1971-1976. **Am J Psychiatry 136:**655-660, 1979

30. *Pate v Robinson*, 383 US 375, 378 (1966)

31. Rachlin S: **Legal Encroachment on Psychiatric Practice.** San Francisco, Calif: Jossey-Bass, 1985

32. Reich J, Wells J: Psychiatric diagnosis and competency to stand trial. **Compr Psychiatry 26:**421-432, 1985

33. Rivinus TM: Psychiatric effects of the anticonvulsive regimens. **J Clin Psychopharmacol 2:**165-192, 1982

34. Robey A: Criteria for competency to stand trial: a checklist for psychiatrists. **Am J Psychiatry 122:** 616-623, 1965

35. Roth LH, Meisel A, Lidz CW: Tests of competency to consent to treatment. **Am J Psychiatry 134:**279-284, 1977

36. Rotter M, Goodman W: The relationship between insight and control in obsessive-compulsive disorder: implications for the insanity defense. **Bull Am Acad Psychiatry Law 21:**245-252, 1993

37. Shultz CR: Trauma, crime, and the affirmative defense. **Colorado Law Rev 11:**2401-2403, 1982

38. Simon RI: **Clinical Psychiatry and the Law.** 2nd ed. Washington, DC: American Psychiatric Press, 1992

39. Slovenko R: Criminal justice procedures in civil commitment. **Hosp Comm Psychiatry 28:**817-826, 1977

40. Solnick PB: Proxy consent for incompetent nonterminally ill adult patients. **J Legislative Med 6:**1-49, 1985

41. Stone AA: The right to refuse treatment. Why psychiatrists should and can make it work. **Arch Gen Psychiatry 38:**358-362, 1981

42. Stone AA: The right to treatment and the psychiatric establishment. **Psychiatric Annals 4:**21-42, 1974

43. Student Note: Incompetency to stand trial. **Harvard Law Rev 81:**454-473, 1967

44. Student Note: Informed consent and the dying patient. **Yale Law J 83:**1632-1664, 1974

45. *Tarasoff v The Regents of the University of California*, 13 Cal 3d 177, 118 Cal Rptr 129, 529 P2d 553 (1974)

46. *Tarasoff v The Regents of the University of California*, 17 Cal 3d 425, 131 Cal Rptr 14, 551 P2d 334 (1976)

47. Vaillant GE: Sociopathy as a human process. A viewpoint. **Arch Gen Psychiatry 32:**178-183, 1975

48. Van Duizend R, McGraw BD, Keilitz I: An overview of state involuntary civil commitment statutes. **Mental Disabilities Law Reporter 8:**328-335, 1984

49. Walker JI, Cavenar JO Jr: Vietnam veterans. Their problems continue. **J Nerv Ment Dis 170:**174-180, 1982

50. Winick BJ: Psychotrophic medication and competence to stand trial. **Am Bar Found Res J 1977:** 769-816, 1977

CHAPTER 8

REPRODUCTIVE HEALTH, WOMEN, AND THE LAW

MARK GIBSON, MD, AND JOYCE McCONNELL, JD, LLM

In this chapter, the legal underpinning protecting privacy in reproductive health care is reviewed. The legal status of a woman's right to control her reproductive status through contraception and abortion will provide a framework for this discussion. During the last several decades, there has been an evolution toward support for autonomy regarding a woman's reproductive health care followed by a retrenchment due to the influence of competing interests.

The personal and sensitive matters of reproductive and sexual choice involving the privacy of the individual in American society have been carefully examined by the courts and are a principal focus of health care in women for a great portion of their lives. Here, the legal status of individual choice and privacy is a paramount, if often silent, underpinning of the relationship between the provider and the patient, the information they share, and the choices available to them.

Whether a woman may act autonomously to prevent or to terminate a pregnancy has been the subject of more than a quarter century of United States Supreme Court jurisprudence. During these years, the court has balanced the interests of the states, husbands, biological fathers, and fetuses against the privacy rights of women. For women and their physicians, the outcome of this judicial balancing often means that physicians are limited in the care they may legally provide their patients.

Tracing the evolution of woman's privacy rights, including the right to contracept to prevent a pregnancy and to abort to terminate a pregnancy, reveals that these rights expand and contract depending on the weight the Court gives to other interests.

CONTRACEPTION

In 1965, in *Griswold v. Connecticut*[6] the Supreme Court invalidated a state statute criminalizing the use of contraception by married persons. In this, the Court focused not on a woman's autonomous privacy rights, but on the privacy afforded the "intimate relation of husband and wife and their physician's role in one aspect of that relation."[7] The Court found that the First Amendment and other amendments in the U.S. Bill of Rights "create zones of privacy," one of which is the privacy due a marital couple.[8]

Seven years later, in *Eisenstadt v. Baird*,[5] the Court struck down a Massachusetts statute that permitted physicians and pharmacists to dispense contraceptives to married persons only.

The Court held that the statute discriminated against unmarried persons. Again, however, the Court focused its attention not on a woman's privacy rights, but rather on the rights of unmarried persons to contracept. When the Court weighed the interests of unmarried persons against the interests of the state in controlling premarital sex and health, the Court responded that a married couple consists of two individuals and that, to have meaning, the right to privacy must be an individual right.

Since *Griswold*, the rights of adults to seek and receive family planning care have become an ingrained and accepted part of health care practice and policy. However, there is still a question about how to deal with adolescents ("minors"), who attain full reproductive capacity long before they attain a status in the law allowing them full autonomy. The simultaneous concern for the rising birth rate and society's discomfort with the sexual mores and behaviors of the young have created an ambivalent legal environment for the provision of reproductive health services to minors.

Society's difficulty in dealing with the sexuality of young women has resulted in focusing the discourse on women's reproductive care primarily on adult women. However, young women, particularly those who are sexually active, need health care providers and policymakers to acknowledge the necessity for reproductive health care. Since the law provides adult women reproductive privacy and freedom to consent to health care, theoretically it promises the same to a minor.[3] Practically, however, it provides minor young women little reproductive privacy (and virtually removes the right to consent to terminate a pregnancy). Thus, it is a female's age, not need, that impedes an adolescent's ability to access health care without parental knowledge and consent. In most states, it is a law that an adolescent under the age of majority (18 years old) must have parental consent to obtain health care. Unfortunately, this places sexually active adolescents and their health care providers in the position of legal uncertainty.

How does the law reconcile the parental consent requirements with individual privacy rights to contracept guaranteed by the U.S. Constitution? It balances parental responsibility to provide health care for a minor child against the constitutional right to contracept and finds that parental consent burdens the adolescent's right to a permissible degree. Thus, states are free to burden the reproductive rights of adolescents with parental consent requirements. This presents a dilemma for the health care provider who recognizes an adolescent's need for reproductive care, her need for privacy, and the degree to which parental consent may interfere with both.

Since the majority of adolescents are sexually active before they turn 18 years old, they need and want reproductive care. The United States leads developed nations in its prevalence of teenage pregnancy. Sexually transmitted diseases, including human immunodeficiency virus/acquired immunodeficiency syndrome, are disturbingly common among American youth. Thus it may be that these outcomes are in part a consequence of the legal environment in which reproductive health care is not made available to minors, so that the proposition that the social climate permitting legal impediments to such care is a fundamental issue.

In the face of need, physicians familiar with the general rule that minors cannot consent to their own health care nonetheless may treat minors without parental consent. Are physicians recklessly risking legal liability? The answer is no, because all jurisdictions, either through common law or legislative enactment, acknowledge exceptions to the general rule.

In the common law there are two such exceptions: the emancipated minor and the mature minor.[1] The emancipated minor exception permits a minor to consent to medical care if: 1) she no longer lives with her parents, and 2) she manages her own affairs.[1] The mature minor exception is less restrictive, allowing the physician to accept consent of the minor when she is mature enough to comprehend the nature and consequences of a medical procedure and its alternatives.[4]

Legislatures typically adopt exceptions based on the status of the minor or the minor's health.[1] The status exceptions are not unlike the common law. They embody the common law concepts of the independent or mature minor and reflect commonly accepted acts of independence: marrying, joining the armed services, and giving birth to a baby. Exceptions based on the minor's health also acknowledge public health policy. For example, a common exception allows for treatment of venereal disease. Here, the state legislatures recognize the potential for requirements for parental consent to deter minors from seeking such treatment and determine that the cost of an untreated individual to society is so great that the parental right to consent to a minor child's health care must give way to protecting the public health.[2]

For the adolescent and the health care provider, the exceptions created by the common law and legislative actions still leave inconsistencies as to when the health care provider may treat without parental consent. One common exception illustrates this problem well: in many jurisdictions, once a minor gives birth to a child, the minor is emancipated and may consent to her own health care. However, during pregnancy and prior to giving birth, she remains unemancipated and must obtain parental consent for medical care. In states where minors are not emancipated upon the birth of a child, the adolescent mother is in the anomalous position of having the right to consent to her child's health care, but not her own. These and other examples indicate inconsistencies in the law.

ABORTION

There is perhaps no issue in contemporary society more ethically complex and more divisive than termination of pregnancy. An individual's position regarding this reproductive health choice is generally viewed as "all or none," and a vast gap appears to exist between those who advocate for such procedures as fundamental to and symbolic of the full expression of female autonomy and those who view them as a societal license for mass homicide. The profound and deep feelings held by the most vocal advocates of both positions appear not to allow comprehension of or compassion toward the views of those with opposing positions. Yet this is an issue with shades of gray that extend as shadows beginning with the simple, inescapable fact that the biological interdependence of the maternal-fetal unit may place two individuals, one developing and one actual, in mortal opposition.

There is no doubt that pregnancy itself is a risk to a woman's health and life. Each year,

mortality among women in developing countries due to pregnancy reaches several per hundred and is due to a variety of causes such as hemorrhage, infection, eclampsia, and thromboembolic complications. Modern health and medicine have lowered these figures dramatically in advanced societies but have not eliminated them. For example, the statistical probability of maternal death in randomly selected pregnancies among women in Uganda is 1.1%, but in the United States is 0.008%. Women may face lifelong consequences of nonfatal complications due to gestation or childbirth. Finally, the burden of a child itself may compromise life for the mother, causing depletion of critical resources for herself or for her existing children. Each one of these concerns may be used as justification to terminate a pregnancy "to save the mother's life." Even among vocal opponents of abortion, this escape clause is accepted. An example would be the case of the woman with Eisenmenger's syndrome, with left to right shunt, where maternal mortality even with optimal care still approaches 50%. Indeed, most legislative exceptions do not specify the level of probability required to justify abortion, as will be discussed.

Moreover, modern humanistic philosophy does not view life simply as an all-or-none issue, but also as a matter of quality. Thus, to a humanist, survival is only the first of many elements of life to be valued and protected. The argument for abortion would hold that critical elements of the pregnant woman's well-being as well as the ultimate quality of life envisioned for the fetus deserve the protection of the choice to terminate a pregnancy—that these qualitative issues take precedence over concern for fetal life per se. Although this humanistic analysis may be criticized by opponents of abortion, its proponents can point out that such rationalization is commonly applied to the taking of human life in wars waged against societies with ideologies held to devalue life or constrain its full, free expression.

The second major argument concerns the possibility of current societal and legal sanctions to terminate pregnancy if there is expected to be impairment of length or quality of life of the fetus. The covering term, "fetal developmental anomalies," is used to encompass a broad range of possibilities that defy simplistic categorization. The extent of genetic and anomaly screening in the U.S., and the application of this to the termination of pregnancy, is extensive. Termination for abnormalities of the fetus ranges from those performed for clearly lethal anomalies, such as anencephaly, to those performed for conditions limiting intellectual development (Down syndrome) or even simply limited height and impaired reproductive potential (Turner's syndrome).

Thus, the sociocultural division on the issue of pregnancy termination is neither so wide nor so clear when these extremes of maternal and fetal considerations are examined. Although termination of pregnancy to save a mother's life or to avert futile birth of an infant with conditions incompatible with life is opposed by some (most notably, the Roman Catholic Church), there is generally consensus on the moral and ethical rightness of such actions. By way of contrast, there are few supporters of other criteria such as the termination of pregnancy for reasons such as gender selection or the use of termination of pregnancy as a routine mode of family planning. Whether or not the opponents and proponents of abortion rights acknowledge it, their area of contention is often in the ill-defined middle ground. More often than not, were they to listen, they would find themselves in agreement regarding the extreme cases used to support their respective positions.

While both *Griswold* and *Eisenstadt* pertain to persons, male or female, they were essential for the passage of *Roe v. Wade* in 1973 and its more specific guarantee of a woman's constitutional protected liberty interest in including the right to terminate her pregnancy.[10] *Roe* represents the highest point of women's autonomy reached to date, yet even it does not provide absolute autonomy. For, according to the Court, the states have a legitimate interest in regulating abortions depending on the stage of pregnancy, and increasingly so as pregnancy and fetal development advances. From this interest grew the Court's familiar trimester framework. Thus, a woman's autonomy is greatest during the first trimester, when state law is not permitted to interfere with the decision of a woman and her doctor regarding abortion. In the second trimester, the court allowed regulation, but with limitations. In the third trimester, the court did not restrict in any way the regulation by states of abortion providing that the health of the mother is not at stake.

Since *Roe,* the rights of women to receive and their physicians to provide medical treatment have eroded. The Supreme Court abandoned the strict trimester framework in *Planned Parenthood of Southeastern Pennsylvania v. Casey* and adopted a more flexible approach.[9] According to the restrictions imposed by the state of Pennsylvania in *Casey:* 1) a woman had to give informed consent to the abortion procedure; 2) a woman had to receive certain information 24 hours before the procedure; 3) a minor had to obtain informed consent of one parent or through judicial bypass; and 4) a woman had to notify her husband of her intent to terminate the pregnancy. The Supreme Court in *Casey* found all restrictions, except the last, to be constitutional.

These four criteria erode physician-patient autonomy in several critical regards. First, although the essential content of *Roe* as regards the right of a woman to terminate pregnancy before viability was preserved, the trimester framework was rejected. Noting that advances in medical technology had at the same time extended the practical limit of pregnancy termination procedures and lowered the gestational age of extrauterine viability, the Court held that it could not adhere strictly to the trimester framework. In effect, the Court embraced a more biologically and medically founded view that fetal development occurs as a continuum and that medical technology bearing on the fetus is continuously changing.

Second, the Court allowed the interests of the state to ensure a period of deliberation prior to the procedure. This arbitrarily determined interval, regardless of duration, appears to be founded on the assumption on the one hand that a woman's decision regarding termination of pregnancy is implicitly ill-considered, and on the other hand, that the physician and the patient themselves are not capable of determining when extension of the time to settle on the abortion decision is needed. Whether the law is meant to imply incompetence, venality, avarice, or other vices or shortcomings among physicians and women is of less consequence than the validation of the intrusion of state regulation in and of itself.

Third, the content of information provided to the patient specified in the Pennsylvania law was upheld by the Court. Here, in effect, is established a remarkable precedent for the inclusion of the voice of the state in the details of physician-patient communication. Again encountered is the implication that the state's interest in the welfare of the fetus justifies regulation of the woman's medical treatment that implies incompetence or ill motive on the part of her physician. Together these stipulations regulate and demean the exchange of information between the physician and the patient and subject a woman's autonomy to new restrictions; the court held that restrictions to this extent may be permitted because they do not create an "undue burden," on the woman's decision or the physician's treatment.

Fourth, while young women under the age of 18 years have the same constitutional rights as adult women in matters of reproduction, this right is limited by the rights of parents to consent to medical care for minor children.[3] Thus, the states may substantially burden the pregnant adolescent's right to terminate her pregnancy without violating the Constitution. States place great stock in protecting the rights of parents to decide what they believe to be in the best interests of their children. In many jurisdictions, young women seeking to terminate pregnancies must obtain parental consent or obtain a judicial declaration that they are mature enough to make the decision on their own and that there are justifiable reasons for not obtaining parental consent. Although cumbersome for the patient and her provider, this decision does provide for a constitutional judicial bypass to parental consent requirements. In fact, either parental consent or judicial bypass may constitute daunting obstacles to the young woman abruptly faced with decisions that will affect the

rest of her life. As upheld in *Carey*, these obstacles represent the imprint of the state's interest in the welfare of the unborn on the autonomy of a woman in the most intimate and momentous decision she may make.

Fifth, as to a woman's obligation to notify her husband, the Court concluded that, while a husband has an important interest in the fetus, that interest cannot trump that of the woman who must biologically bear the child. If the court had not found that the woman's interest outweighed her husband's, a physician, no matter what she or he believed best for the patient, could not have legally terminated the pregnancy without evidence that the patient notified her husband. In the case of a woman whose intentions to abort are shared and supported by her spouse, this stipulation is of little consequence. In circumstances where problems in the marital relationship might otherwise exclude the husband's awareness of the pregnancy and its termination or where in fact they are a principal reason for the decision to abort, it could be argued that a woman's autonomy is considerably burdened by the law.

REFERENCES

1. Batterman N: Under age: a minor's right to consent to health care. **Touro Law Rev 10:**637, 641, 1994
2. Batterman N: Under age: a minor's right to consent to health care. **Touro Law Rev 10:**640, 1994
3. *Carey v. Population Services International*, 431 US 678 (1977)
4. Cohn R: Minor's right to consent to medical care. **Medical Trial Tech Q.** 1985, pp 286, 290 (citing *Bakker v. Welch*, 144 Mich 632, 108 NW94 (1906))
5. *Eisenstadt v. Baird*, 405 US 438 (1972)
6. *Griswold v. Connecticut*, 381 US 479 (1965)
7. *Griswold v. Connecticut*, 381 US at 482
8. *Griswold v. Connecticut*, 381 US at 484
9. *Planned Parenthood of Southeastern Pennsylvania v Casey*, 505 US 533 (1992)
10. *Roe v Wade*, 419 US 113 (1973)

Chapter 9

Legal Aspects of Alcohol and Drug Testing

Janet M. Williams, MD, FACEP

Physicians are frequently called upon to perform blood alcohol testing on potentially intoxicated motorists for both medical and legal purposes. Many states have enacted "DUI" (driving under the influence) laws that define intoxication based on blood alcohol concentration (but not drug concentration). Therefore, issues of patient consent for alcohol testing and release of information are of paramount importance, and failure to obtain proper consents places the physician at risk of adverse legal ramifications. Laws regarding the taking of blood samples for alcohol testing vary from state to state. Similarly, what constitutes technical battery by a physician who performs a test at the request of police but without the patient's consent varies across the United States. Physicians should familiarize themselves with the laws in the states in which they practice. It would be helpful for physicians to develop written protocols at their institutions about how to comply with state regulations and have these reviewed by their legal counsels.

Testing of Breath or Urine for Legal Reasons

The statutes of some states dictate that a mo-

torist on a public road, who is licensed and cognizant of the laws regarding driving, has consented by implication to undergo blood alcohol testing ("implied consent").[4] In implied consent, patient consent is inferred by the actions of the patient, without written agreement. If a law enforcement officer suspects a motorist to be under the influence of alcohol, the driver may be asked to undergo analysis of urine or breath (not blood) samples by implied consent. In such cases, it is usually up to law enforcement personnel to perform or arrange for testing of urine and breath samples. Note that in some states without implied consent, a person may refuse to take such tests.

Blood Alcohol and Drug Testing When Medically Indicated

When the Patient Consents (Does Not Refuse)

Quite often, drug and alcohol levels are obtained during the medical evaluation of a patient. Although the presence of drugs and alco-

TABLE 1

EXAMPLE OF WEST VIRGINIA UNIVERSITY'S POLICY ON ALCOHOL TESTING

Policy

West Virginia University Hospitals (WVUH) will cooperate, upon request of the police, in taking blood samples from consenting patients for use in determining blood alcohol levels.

Procedure

1. **Who May Request Testing**

   Any physician with hospital privileges may order alcohol testing. In addition, the following law enforcement officers (only) may request that alcohol testing be performed:

   a) A member of the West Virginia State Police.

   b) A sheriff or deputy sheriff of *any* West Virginia county.

   c) A member of *any* West Virginia city police department.

   d) Any other duly authorized public law enforcement officer.

   If there is any doubt as to the identity, credentials, or affiliation of the law enforcement officer, hospital personnel should ask to see identification and/or credentials and document this in the chart prior to performing testing.

   If the request is made by an out-of-state law enforcement officer, the patient must consent in writing to the test.

2. **Who May Test**

   The withdrawal of blood for alcohol analysis can only be performed by the following hospital personnel:

   a) A doctor of medicine or osteopathy.

   b) A registered nurse.

   c) A trained medical laboratory staff person.

3. **When Testing Can Occur**

   Hospital personnel can draw blood for alcohol analysis when ordered by a *physician.* However, the accepted hospital personnel may only draw blood for alcohol analysis when ordered by a *law enforcement officer* under the following conditions. All three should be documented in the chart:

   a) The request is from an approved law enforcement officer (see Section 1 above).

   b) The patient is under arrest at the time of the request. (If in doubt, ask the officers with a witness present.)

   c) The patient does not refuse to allow the test to be administered.

   The requesting police officer must sign the permit in all cases.

4. **Consent**

   a) Consent is implied for blood alcohol analysis requested by West Virginia police if the preceding procedures are followed. However, while no consent need be obtained, if the patient expresses in *any manner* a reluctance to have the test, implied consent by the patient is invalid and the blood test should *not* be administered. (This should also be documented.)

   b) Consent is *not* implied for requests by out-of-state officers. The patient must consent in writing to testing.

---

hol can be detected in urine samples, quantitative testing requires sampling of blood. (Drug testing is confounded by lack of defined urine levels for intoxication.) In the case of an intoxicated patient, blood testing may usually be performed as part of the medical evaluation by implied consent as long as the patient voluntarily submits to the evaluation. The patient must be made aware of the tests to be performed, but is not required to consent verbally or in writing.

The appropriate policy and procedure in effect at the given facility must be strictly followed in order to preserve probative matter. Table 1 illustrates an example of one medical facility's policy on alcohol testing (West Virginia University policy). Such policies and procedures dictate how the sample should be drawn, including the use of standard venipuncture technique and use of a nonalcoholic antiseptic to cleanse the skin. The sample(s) must be properly labeled and the proper chain of custody must be maintained for the evidence to be considered legally admissible. A chain of custody consists of documenting and witnessing the handling and possession of evidence from when it was initially obtained until submitted as evidence in court. If the chain of custody cannot be shown, evidence such as a blood alcohol levels may be subject to exclusion in court.

TABLE 1 (cont'd)

EXAMPLE OF WEST VIRGINIA UNIVERSITY'S POLICY ON ALCOHOL TESTING

c) While a patient under arrest may refuse a blood alcohol test, a urine or breath test may not be refused. The law enforcement officer may order a urine or breath test if the blood test is refused; however, WVUH does not perform urine or breath testing for alcohol. If the law enforcement officer requests one of these alternative tests, he or she must make other arrangements to have the testing performed. (This is not the responsibility of hospital personnel.)

d) If an officer is observed using physical force to make the patient consent and/or submit to the test, the test will not be conducted.

5. **Method of Testing**
The following restrictions apply to drawing blood alcohol levels:
a) Accepted medical practices must be used.
b) An unused sterile needle and vessel must be used.
c) A nonalcoholic antiseptic must be used to clean the skin before venipuncture.

6. **Patient Requests**
A patient may also request testing of his/her own blood, breath, or urine within 2 hours of being taken into custody or presenting at the hospital or emer-

gency department in addition to requests by the law enforcement officer.

7. **Payment**
A reasonable fee may be charged to the city or county if a law enforcement officer requests a test or to the patient if he/she requests the test.
a) If a state or county officer requests the test, the bill for testing should be submitted to the county where the arrest was made.
b) If the patient or physician requests the test, the bill should be submitted to the patient.

8. **Results of Testing**
Testing results should be reported to:
a) The attending physician and/or resident *and* recorded in the chart. (No matter who orders the test.)
b) The requesting law enforcement officer. (Only if he/she requested the test.)
c) The patient if he/she requests the results. (No matter who orders the test.)

9. **Chain of Custody**
A form will be used to establish a chain of custody for samples to be tested for alcohol.

When the Patient Does Not Consent

If the patient expresses any reluctance to have the test performed, implied consent by the patient is invalid and the blood test may not be performed. Physical force to make the patient consent and/or submit to a test is not acceptable practice in any state.[2]

When the Patient is Unconscious

The physician should always evaluate the patient in an emergency situation as medically indicated. In *Breithaupt v. Abram,*[1] the U.S. Supreme Court granted immunity to practitioners who obtain blood samples from unconscious patients. According to this ruling, the physician may proceed with blood drawing and testing under the doctrine of implied consent in an unconscious patient who is in medical jeopardy

and physically unable to give consent. A physician who has acted in good faith in the evaluation and care of a patient is extremely unlikely to be found liable for battery.[5] In addition, such evidence is admissible in court.

Release of Information Obtained for Medical Reasons

It is not uncommon for law enforcement personnel to be present in the emergency department after injured motorists are brought to the hospital. The police may request information regarding a patient such as, "How drunk is he, doc?" As a rule, the physician should not divulge specific information to any outside party unless there is a reporting statute which overrides the physician's obligation of patient confidentiality. General information related to the patient's condition and admission status may be shared in most cases.

All information contained in the medical record, including test results, is confidential. This ethical principle applies to computerized medical records as well. Disclosure of information or the records themselves to unauthorized persons without the patient's written consent can result in liability on the part of the physician. This requirement of confidentiality is expected of the entire medical staff, including nurses, technicians, office clerks, and other ancillary personnel.[2]

According to the courts and legislatures, ownership of medical records is shared by two parties. The medical record itself in the physical sense is owned by the health care provider or practice, while the information contained within the records is considered property of the patient. Thus, medical information may be released under two conditions: with written informed authorization by the patient, or when there is a subpoena or court order. Failure to release confidential information in the face of a court order may result in imprisonment for contempt of court. On the other hand, it is not appropriate for the physician to notify legal authorities of positive tests for alcohol or illegal drugs, although this issue is being reconsidered in some jurisdictions.

Blood Alcohol and Drug Testing When Not Medically Indicated but Requested by Police

When the Patient Consents

The physician may be asked by the police to perform alcohol and/or drug testing. In such cases, physicians should comply with the statutes specific for the state in which they practice. If a law enforcement officer has a court order for blood testing to be performed and the patient consents, the physician should proceed with the testing. Without a state statute and/or court order, a physician is not obligated to act upon a police request for blood testing. In the absence of a state law, a physician even if acting in good faith upon a police request must be cog-nizant of the potential liability for battery. A technical battery occurs if a physician orders a test (blood alcohol level) which is not medically necessary for diagnosis and treatment. This holds true even if other blood tests such as an admission panel are being performed.

When the Conscious Patient Does Not Consent

Two cases define the power of the government to invade the body (including venipuncture) of a conscious patient without consent in order to obtain incriminating evidence. In *Rochin v. California*,[2] the court rejected obtaining gastric samples by the use of physical force and "methods too close to the rack and screw." However, in *Schmerber v. California*,[3] the court ruled that blood alcohol testing in a patient who verbally, but not physically, resisted was admissible, but not necessarily permitted as a matter of medical ethics.

Some states have enacted laws to guide law enforcement officers as well as health care practitioners in such cases. In Florida, a law enforcement officer may use "reasonable force" to obtain a blood sample on a motorist if the officer has probable cause to believe that a motorist is under the influence of drugs or alcohol and if the motorist has caused the death or near death of a human being.[6] The state statutes and policies and the procedures in effect at the particular facility must be strictly adhered to in order to preserve the evidence.

If the patient is unconscious, testing is medically indicated.

References

1. *Breithaupt v Abram*, 352 US 432 (1957)
2. *Rochin v California*, LM 290, 342 US 165 (1952)
3. *Schmerber v California*, 384 US 757 (1966)
4. Siegel DM: Consent and refusal of treatment, in Rice MM (ed): **Emergency Medicine Clinics of North America: Medical-Legal Issues, XI**. Philadelphia, Pa: WB Saunders, Nov 1993, Vol 4, p 834
5. Siegel DM, Henry G: **Emergency Medicine Risk Management: A Comprehensive Review**. Dallas, Tex: American College of Emergency Physicians, 1991, pp 185-190
6. Taraska JM: **Legal Guide for Physicians**. White Plains, NY: AHAB Press, 1995, pp 5.1–5.43

CHAPTER 10

The Legal System and Unintentional Injury

Carolyn B. Reynolds, MD, and Mark A. Reynolds, MD

Scope of the Problem

Unintentional injuries are a health problem of profound national significance. In 1993, approximately 14% of all Americans visited an emergency department because of an injury. Of the 90.3 million emergency department visits in 1993, 36.5 million (40%) were due to injury-related problems[9] (95% were related to unintentional injury and 5% to intentional injury). The treatment of unintentional injuries accounted for 3.9% of all ambulatory care visits in 1993.[8] Injuries resulted in approximately 2.72 million admissions, about 9% of all admissions to short-term hospitals in 1993.[3] Unintentional injuries were the primary cause of 4% of all deaths reported regardless of age (a total of 90,523 deaths in 1993).[3] In persons aged 1 through 44 years, unintentional injuries were the number one cause of death and in 1993 resulted in a total of 47,299 deaths in this age group.[3]

Broadly termed, an unintentional injury is any inadvertent outcome from the application of an external agent that results in short- or long-term disability. The agents of injury include kinetic, thermal, electrical, or radiant energy, as well as toxic chemical compounds. The time frame for the development of these adverse consequences is usually very brief, an interval measured in milliseconds to minutes. However, some authors include the chronic and subacute consequences of prolonged exposure to toxins when defining the term "injury." In this broad usage of the term, "unintentional injury" could be expanded to include the long-term damage due to many commonly abused substances, such as tobacco and alcohol, and the effects of environmental toxins.

The severity of injury is largely a function of the amount of energy that is transferred to the victim. The majority of the injuries that result in a visit to an emergency department are due to relatively low energy transfer, but the greatest mortality, morbidity, and disability, and therefore the greatest cost to society, is found in that subgroup of individuals subjected to high-energy transfer. Motor-vehicle crashes are the most common source of high-energy transfer. Injuries secondary to motor-vehicle crashes resulted in 10.9% of all emergency department visits but accounted for 46.28% of all injury-related fatalities in 1993.[3]

APPROACH TO THE PROBLEM

The interaction between the legal system and the incidence, occurrence, and response to unintentional injury is an extensive subject. In a broad historical sense, much of the work of government has been to promote a safe and tranquil environment for the populace. Much of the infrastructure of society represents an accretion of rules over decades and centuries that are designed to promote "domestic tranquillity" and a safe environment. In the 19th century, city planning initiatives were implemented that provided a guarantee of safe and pure water supplies and the efficient management of sewage; these initiatives had the single greatest impact on public health in history. The institution of uniform traffic codes and regulations in the late 19th century and early 20th century allowed the planning and building of roads that could be used by motorized vehicles with relative safety. Building and product code regulations ensured the safe management and distribution of potentially very dangerous materials and energies.

The interaction between the problem of unintentional injury and the legal system is complex. The modes of interaction can be categorized in a number of ways (e.g., whether the law that is applied is statutory or civil in nature, the kind of temporal relationship the law has with the injurious event, and the element contributing to the injurious event that the law addresses).

William Haddon was the first to conceptualize the problem of unintentional injury from an epidemiological viewpoint. Haddon described the injurious event in terms of the interaction of the host, agent, and environment, and he placed this interaction within a temporal framework of preinjury, injury, and postinjury. This conceptualization provided an organizational framework for the analysis of injury. The efforts of Haddon and others have resulted in a shift in the paradigm with which the occurrence of injury or "accidents" was perceived. Prior to this time, an unintentional event that resulted in injury was considered to be a behavioral problem. People were "accident-prone." The person or persons involved were at fault. There was a failure of vigilance. The conceptual framework that was developed by Haddon and promoted by consumer advocates such as Ralph Nader provided a far more complex and useful approach to the problem of injury. "Accidents" were not just a personal problem. "Accidents" had real, tangible, and identifiable environmental antecedents. These antecedents could be identified and modified. The environment in which the injurious event took place could be analyzed from an epidemiological perspective. Environmental factors could be seen as vectors for the transmission of the injurious forces. Behavioral or host factors could be conceptualized as modifying susceptibility to these environmental vectors of injury. These factors could be modified to reduce the risks of the occurrence of an injurious event. For example, highways could be designed and constructed with an eye to reducing the risk of future injury. Concrete walls and posts could be constructed to dissipate the kinetic energies of impact over time and space. Vehicles could be designed and constructed to absorb the energies and prolong the application of these kinetic forces to a degree that would be tolerable for the "appropriately packaged" human occupant. At the point of impact, the injurious energies could be modulated in real and measurable ways by seat belts and air bags. Programs could be instituted to identify, isolate, and promote laws to negatively reinforce behaviors that increased personal susceptibility to the environmental mediators of injury. Programs could be instituted to promote the creation of institutions and services that would ameliorate the effects of the injury and salvage the injured. This paradigm made it possible to design and evaluate injury control strategies in an objective and scientific fashion. Haddon's work provided the basis for the many effective regulatory strategies that have been implemented by federal and state government during the past three decades.

The civil and statutory components of the legal system and their interactions can be analyzed using Haddon's conceptualization. Statutory regulations have been designed that ameliorate the effect of injury in each of its phases. Laws have been designed to reduce the likelihood of an injurious event occurring. Laws and regulations have been implemented to reduce the effect of an injurious event when it does happen. Postinjury mechanisms (e.g., emergency medical services and regional trauma systems) have been designed and mandated in order to salvage as much life and function as possible after the injurious event has occurred. Criminal and civil (tort and product liability) issues may also be raised in the postinjury phase, thus driving the system to new and perhaps more effective laws to regulate the antecedents of injury. During the past three decades, federal regulatory agencies have had a major impact on the environmental elements of Haddon's conceptualization of the "disease" of unintentional injury. These regulatory bodies were developed in the recognition that a proactive and intelligently directed governmental policy could significantly reduce the likelihood of injury. A series of laws were enacted in the 1960s and 1970s that created a number of federal agencies that have approached the problem from many different directions.

Prevention of injury is the major goal in injury control. The legal system plays a crucial role in injury prevention because it can effectively manipulate individual behaviors. Federally mandated programs implemented to reduce the risk of occurrence of an injurious event have been directed at each of the factors that interact in the production of an injurious event.

BEHAVIORAL MODIFICATION

Traditionally, the approach to modifying the human element has been directed at education and efforts to "convince" the populace to act in a safer manner. Many educational and public information programs have been implemented in an attempt to modify the behavior of the public at risk. Unfortunately, these programs have had little, if any, measurable impact. Factors that mitigate against this approach to the problem include: 1) failure to communicate the message to the population at risk; 2) failure to convince the population that does hear the message; and 3) failure to modify behavior of that segment of the population that does hear the message and is unconvinced by it.

Enforcement of legally mandated behaviors is far more effective in reducing the incidence of injury. Effective initiatives to decrease motor-vehicle accidents include mandated speed limits, seat restraint laws, and helmet laws, as well as laws restricting persons from driving after ingesting alcohol. However, these laws have limitations and are frequently difficult to enforce in a uniform fashion. A number of identifiable factors affect compliance with injury-prevention laws: 1) the required behavior must conform to an individual's usual pattern in order to be effective; 2) a high probability of detection and conviction must motivate the individual to comply with the law; 3) compliance with the law must not interfere with an individual's comfort and convenience; and 4) enforcement officials cannot allow any exceptions from compliance. Violations of mandated behaviors must be easily identifiable and subsequent convictions must be swift and severe. The most crucial factor compelling compliance with injury-reduction legislation is the likelihood of being caught.

Although shown by research to be effective (vide infra), there are opponents to these legislated behavioral controls. The opponents cite a number of arguments against injury-prevention laws. They claim that the laws are not effective in reducing injury. Further, they contend that an onerous and intrusive governmental restriction of individual liberties on a large proportion of the populace in order to reduce the incidence of injury for a small fraction of the population does not justify the cost of the legislation and its enforcement. These arguments have had variable impact depending upon the law and the population covered by the legislation. Very few would argue against the use of child restraints in children under 4 years of age. However, many fail to see the societal benefit of imposing helmet laws on adult motorcyclists when no one but the cyclist is at risk.

HIGHWAY SAFETY

In the early 1960s, the problem of highway mortality became a major priority. In 1964, 48,000 persons died on the highways of the nation. This reflected a 10% increase from the previous year. In 1965, hearings by the United States Congress were held on the issue of highway safety. It was determined during the course of these hearings that significant negligence existed on the part of both industry and government. During this same year, Ralph Nader published *Unsafe at Any Speed*. This book documented the breadth of the problem and the degree of culpability of both the automobile industry and the traffic safety establishment. By 1966, President Lyndon Johnson characterized the problem of highway deaths as second only to the Vietnam War. Johnson suggested national traffic safety legislation to require the establishment of motor-vehicle standards, provide for state grants to aid in the development of safety programs, and fund traffic safety research. By August 1966, Congress had passed a series of motor-vehicle standards bills. These became the Highway and Motor Vehicle Safety Act of 1966.[10]

Also passed in 1966 was the National Traffic and Motor Vehicle Safety Act, which established the National Traffic Safety Agency in the Department of Commerce. In addition, this Act required minimum safety standards for motor vehicles and equipment, authorized research and development, and expanded the National Driver Register of individuals whose licenses had been denied, terminated, or withdrawn. According to the Act, each standard was required to be practical, meet the need for motor-vehicle safety, and to be phrased in objective terms. In prescribing standards, the Secretary was required to consider: 1) relevant available motor-vehicle safety data; 2) whether the proposed standard was appropriate for the particular motor vehicle or equipment for which it was prescribed; and 3) the extent to which the standard contributed to carrying out the purposes of the Act.[8] The Act was designed to provide a coordinated national highway safety program through financial assistance to the states. Under this Act, the states were required to establish highway safety programs in accordance with federal standards.[1]

Under the direction of William Haddon, the National Traffic Safety Bureau established a total of 43 motor-vehicle standards (covering vehicle accident prevention and passenger protection) and 18 highway safety standards (covering vehicle inspection, registration, motorcycle safety, driver education, traffic laws and records, accident investigation and reporting, pupil transportation, and police traffic services).[1] These initiatives have resulted in a great improvement in the health and well-being of the American populace.

Laws regulating the speed of vehicles are among the earliest that attempted to control the factors that affect traffic safety. In 1901, the state of Connecticut imposed a speed limit on motorized vehicles of 12 mph in urbanized areas and 15 mph on rural roads.[1]

Speed

Speed is one of the fundamental factors that govern the forces unleashed in a motor-vehicle crash. According to data from the Fatal Accident Reporting System, in 1990 "driving too fast for conditions or in excess of the speed limits" represented approximately 20% of all reported "driver factors" that contributed to fatal crashes. Approximately 34% of all "driver factors" are speed-related.

Speed contributes to the problem of traffic safety via two primary mechanisms: physical and traumatic. The physical consequences of excessive speed are due to the general physics of motion: 1) Greater distances are covered per unit time, so there is less time to react to an obstacle and the vehicle has a longer stopping distance. 2) The vehicle and occupants possess greater kinetic energy and momentum, so there is difficulty negotiating turns. The traumatic consequences of excessive speed are the result of the release of inordinate amounts of energy at the time of impact. Excessive speed results in a greater probability of a crash occurring and in a greater potential for death and disability if the crash occurs. The probability of death doubles with every 10 mph over 40 mph.

Speed variance is a measure of the distribution of the speeds of vehicles around the mean speed. The probability of collision increases with increasing speed variance. As the speed of the vehicle diverges from the mean, there is a dramatic increase in the closure rates between vehicles and an increase in the frequency of avoidance maneuvers (including lane changes, braking, and passing). These factors result in a dramatic increase in the probability of a collision occurring. As the speed variance of a vehicle exceeds 10 mph, the risk of a crash increases exponentially. Studies have demonstrated that speed variance has a significant correlation with fatal crashes.

Speed-related factors affecting traffic safety and unintentional injury have been addressed by the legal and legislative system in different ways. The most obvious approach is to formulate laws regulating the speed of vehicles. Other approaches include regulation of the design of high-speed highways and other roads as well as regulation of driving behavior. The underlying purpose of all these initiatives is to reduce the velocity of vehicles, reduce the closing speed between vehicles, increase the distance between vehicles, and reduce speed variance and its attendant driving behaviors.

Until 1973, state legislatures determined the maximum highway speed limit for that state. Effective in January 1974, U.S. Congress enacted the national maximum speed limit of 55 mph as part of the Emergency Highway Conservation Act. This was initially intended to serve as a temporary fuel-conservation measure in response to increasing prices of oil because of the oil embargo. However, a special report from the Transportation Research Board of the National Academy of Sciences indicated that the reduced speed limit had resulted in a reduction in highway mortality and had saved 9,100 lives during the first year of its implementation, when miles traveled decreased only 2%. In 1974, there were 45,196 highway fatalities, compared to 54,052 in 1973. This was the greatest single-year decrease in highway deaths since World War II. Acting on this information, Congress made the 55-mph speed limit permanent. By 1983, the average speeds on urban interstate highways had returned to pre-1974 levels, although the average speed on rural roads continued to remain 6 mph below pre-1974 levels. Slipping public support, the resolution of the fuel crisis, the perception that the law was widely disregarded, and an interest in returning control to individual states culminated in 1987 in an amendment to the law which permitted states to raise the speed limit to 65 mph on rural interstate roads. According to the National Highway Traffic Safety Administration (NHTSA), there was a 30% increase in the number of fatalities on rural highways in which the speed limit was increased to 65 mph. There was an estimated increase of 539 fatalities and $900 million in economic costs annually.[3] The NHTSA also reported that of the 6.5 million motor-vehicle crashes reported to state and local police departments in 1990, there were 39,779 fatal crashes with 44,529 fatalities and 3.2 million

injuries. However, overall the fatality rate was 2.1 deaths per 100 million vehicle miles traveled (VMT). This is lower than the rate of 2.51 deaths per 100 million VMT in 1985 and substantially less than the rates throughout the 1960s and 1970s. An analysis of data from the period between 1981 and 1982 demonstrated no significant correlation between the absolute speed of the vehicles involved and the fatality rate, although there was a significant correlation with speed variance.[2] In 1991, the Intermodal Surface Transportation Efficiency Act (ISTEA) allowed the 65-mph speed limits to become permanent.

Safety-Restraint Laws

Safety-restraint laws that applied to children were among the first such laws to be broadly implemented. The first mandatory child safety-restraint use law was implemented in Tennessee in 1978. By 1985, all 50 states had passed legislation requiring the use of safety seats or safety belts for children. These laws reduce injuries to young children by an estimated 8% to 59%, and an estimated 200-300 fatalities are prevented per year. However, motor-vehicle crash-related injuries remain a major cause of disability and death among children in the U.S.

Studies have demonstrated that the effectiveness of safety belts is in the range of 40% to 50% for preventing mortality and in the range of 45% to 55% for preventing severe morbidity. As of February 1994, 48 states had safety-belt laws, and the national average safety-belt use rate was 66%.[6]

In December 1994, 25 states required helmet use for all motorcycle riders, another 22 states required helmet use for certain riders, and only three states had no such requirements. There is considerable evidence that helmet laws result in a significant reduction in the incidence of mortality and disability due to head injury, and thus significant reduction in the cost to society.

Alcohol Consumption

Alcohol consumption and subsequent intoxication have been implicated in over 50% of unintentional injuries caused while driving. This is a result of the dose-related impairment of mentation caused by alcohol ingestion. When the blood alcohol concentration (BAC) level is 0.10 gm/dl or over (the legal limit in many states), alcohol impairs virtually every measurable behavioral skill. A correlation exists between the severity of the accident and the BAC level of the individual injured. Generally, the greater the BAC level of the responsible individual, the more violent and severe the accident. Because of the political impact of groups such as Mothers Against Drunk Driving (MADD), there has been considerable success in recent years in applying legal means to control intoxicated drivers. Only four states do not specify a BAC level that is illegal by definition. Increases in the severity of the legal consequences of inebriation have had a dramatic impact on the overall effectiveness of these laws. In states where the legal drinking age has been increased to 21 years, the number of alcohol-related accidents in the teenage population has been significantly reduced.

Because alcohol plays such an important role in injury, it is crucial that health care professionals recognize alcohol problems in their patients and intervene where indicated. Members of the health care team should refer these patients to the appropriate facility for treatment. The treatment of a patient's alcohol problem is as important as the treatment of their injuries.

Laws mandating risk-reduction behaviors such as seat-belt use, helmet use, and abstinence from alcohol while driving have been demonstrated to be effective in reducing the incidence, severity, and cost of injury. Reduction in these costs is of benefit to society as a whole.

OCCUPATIONAL SAFETY

Approximately 10 million occupational injuries occur in the U.S. annually and result in approximately 9,000 deaths per year. Although the rate of fatal occupational injuries has gradually declined, the rate of nonfatal occupational injuries appears to be increasing. The resulting economic cost of both fatal and nonfatal occupational injuries totals billions of dollars. The multibillion dollar cost of occupational injury affects every American consumer by increasing costs of goods and services. Occupational fatalities often involve motor-vehicle accidents. Other

frequent causes of occupational fatalities are nonhighway vehicular injuries and electrocutions. Specific occupations with high rates of injury include mining, farming, construction, manufacturing, trucking, and warehousing.

A broad area of occupational injury control focuses on environmental control. By mandating workplace monitoring of equipment, practices, physical environment, and employee health and safety programs, agencies such as the Occupational Safety and Health Association (OSHA) and the National Institute for Occupational Safety and Health (NIOSH) have tried to decrease the incidence of occupational injuries. Currently, approximately 48% of all work environments report no injuries annually.

The Occupational Safety and Health Act of 1970 was passed to ensure "so far as possible every working man and woman in the nation safe and healthful-working conditions and to preserve our human resources."[7] The purposes of the Act are quite comprehensive and include the establishment of occupational safety and health standards, carrying out inspections and investigations, ensuring the maintenance of record-keeping by employers on occupational injuries and illnesses, requiring reporting by employers of work-related deaths, and conducting research relating to occupational safety and health.[5] As a result of this legislation, OSHA was created under the Assistant Secretary of Labor for Occupational Safety and Health to enforce the regulations established by the 1970 Act.

Also established by this act was NIOSH. NIOSH is a research agency which is part of the Centers for Disease Control of the U.S. Department of Health and Human Services. The mandate of NIOSH includes: 1) investigation of potentially hazardous working conditions; 2) evaluation of hazards in the workplace; 3) development and dissemination of injury-prevention strategies; and 4) research into the causes and the antecedents of injuries and occupation-related illnesses.

HOUSEHOLD SAFETY

The major causes of unintentional injury in the household include falls, poisoning, fires, and direct physical injury due to product malfunction or mishandling. The home environment lacks the strict control and emphasis on safety imposed upon occupational environments by regulatory agencies. Many of the unintentional injuries that occur in the home environment are due to the victim's inability to recognize the hazard associated with the activity.

The annual unintentional injury rate in the home has been reduced as a result of consumer protection legislation, precedents set by product-liability decisions, and consumer safety education. Examples of protective requirements include the installation of smoke detectors and fire sprinklers in public buildings. Child-protective packaging standards and strict product-labeling requirements illustrate how product liability and tort decisions have helped reduce unintentional injuries from product misuse by driving and directing the regulatory process. National educational programs such as those that address potential lead exposure from paint have reinforced a campaign of recognition of hazards in the household environment.

RECREATIONAL SAFETY

The "recreational" category encompasses all activities outside the home or workplace. Recreational products include children's toys, all-terrain vehicles, bicycles, and watercraft.

CIVIL AND CRIMINAL LAW

The fear of litigation in the complex and extensive domain of product liability law serves to limit unintentional injuries resulting from defective products. The theory of *caveat emptor* ("Let the buyer beware") formed the foundation of early judicial decisions in the U.S. regarding seller liability.[4] However, the evolution of court decisions in the U.S. has led to the modern judicial recognition of the seller's liability based upon both express and implied warranties of high quality merchandise.[11] Law today finds the seller liable for negligence in the manufacture or sale of any product that may inflict substantial harm if defective.

Three theories of possible seller negligence comprise the basis of liability in this area of product law. Theoretically, a seller may be negli-

gent if the product design creates a flaw or if a flawed product goes undiscovered. A manufacturer who fails to exercise reasonable care to avoid and discover unintended dangers occurring in the construction process is subject to liability. The seller's negligence is difficult to prove under this theory unless an obvious product flaw or manufacturing defect exists.

Second, a seller may be liable or negligent in failing to warn or adequately warn consumers of a risk or hazard inherent in the seller's product design. The warning must include any risks related to the intended use as well as the reasonably foreseeable use of the product. No negligence exists if a seller fails to warn of unknown hazards after a diligent search for them.

Third, a seller may be liable if negligently marketing a deceptively designed product. A negligent liable seller would market a product in which the reasonably foreseeable harm as designed outweighed the utility of the product. A product risk-benefit analysis determines the seller's liability in this instance.

The legal system's changing opinion of negligent seller liability in deceptively designed product litigation has curtailed unintentional injury from poorly designed products. A further reduction in unintentional injuries can be expected with the continued expansion of product liability litigation.

Product liability litigation as well as other types of civil litigation often spawn subsequent legislation and regulation. For example, on September 1, 1976, the NHTSA regulated a standard for integrity of automotive fuel systems upon rear-impact accidents. They based this regulation on a theory that it protected "against unreasonable risk of death or injury, was reasonable, practicable and appropriate and met the need for motor-vehicle safety."[11] This regulation directly resulted from the numerous civil cases concerning the Ford Pinto during the early 1970s.

In addition to spawning new federal automobile safety regulations, the "Pinto case" pioneered an area of criminal penalty for product liability. Previously, the type and amount of deterrence achieved to regulate product design rested mainly in civil penalties. Now an emerging new trend in criminal prosecution involves pursuing perpetrators of unintentional injuries with criminal penalties. Successful criminal prosecution of these cases is difficult due to a lack of demonstrable criminal intent by the defendant, which is the key element required for conviction. However, prosecution and conviction have been successful by using another criminal standard of "recklessness." The standard of recklessness requires a substantial breach in the duty of care that all persons must exercise as well as a subjective awareness that the conduct in question creates a risk of harm to others.[5] Criminal conviction of voluntarily intoxicated reckless drivers who cause fatal automobile accidents represents the most successful prosecutions in this emerging front. This front is quickly expanding into other areas of potential reckless behavior such as snow skiing.[4]

REFERENCES

1. Comptroller General of the United States: **Effective-** **ness, Benefits, and Costs of Federal Safety Standards for Protection of Passenger Car Occupants.** July 7, 1976

2. Graves E: 1993—Summary: National hospital discharge survey. **Adv Data 264:**1-16, 1995

3. Hudson GP: Advance report of final mortality statistics. **Monthly Vital Stat Rep 44(7):**1-83, 1996

4. Keeton WP, Dobbs DB, Keeton RE, et al: **Prosser and Keeton on the Law of Torts. 5th ed.** St Paul, Minn: West Publishing Co, 1984, 679 pp

5. Luria D: Death on the highway: reckless driving as murder. **Oregon Law Rev 57:**799-836, 1988

6. National Highway Traffic Safety Administration: **Traffic Safety Facts, 1994: Occupant Protection.** Washington, DC: National Center for Statistics and Analysis, Research and Development, 1994

7. PL 91-596 (1970)

8. Schappert SMA: National ambulatory medical care survey: 1994 summary. **Adv Data 273:**1-20, 1996

9. Stusson B: Summary national hospital ambulatory medical care survey: 1993 Emergency Department Survey. **Adv Data 271:**1-16, 1996

10. Weiner E: **Urban Transportation Planning in the US —A Historical Overview.** Washington, DC: US Department of Transportation, Nov 1992

11. Wheeler ME: Product liability, civil or criminal—the Pinto litigation. **Forum 17:**250-255, 1981

CHAPTER 11

ABUSE, PART A: CHILD ABUSE AND NEGLECT

ELLEN E. HRABOVSKY, MD

Child abuse and neglect is defined as "the physical and mental injury, sexual abuse, negligent treatment or maltreatment of a child under the age of 18 by a person who is responsible for the child's welfare under circumstances which indicate that the child's health or welfare is harmed or threatened thereby"[4] (Public Law No. 100-294). An abused child is any child who sustains physical or mental injury or death due to a non-accidental event or any injury or death at variance with the given history. Caregivers are also guilty of abuse if an act of omission results in injury or death. A neglected child is one who is abandoned or unsupervised, or a child for whom caregivers refuse to give proper subsistence, education, medical or surgical care, or any special care warranted by the health of the child.

Reported child abuse cases number about 1.4 million (or 2% to 3% of the population under age 18 years) annually in the United States and seems to be increasing.[3] Approximately 5% of "mild" injuries and 20% of burns seen in emergency departments are inflicted deliberately. Homicide of children is a steadily increasing problem, as are the more violent forms of child abuse. Child abuse occurs in all levels of society. Emotional and sexual abuse are poorly reported and difficult to document. Firm statistics on neglected children are elusive. However, parents who physically injure their children are often under severe financial and social stress. Drugs and alcohol are more often involved in situations of neglect than in deliberate abuse.

Health care workers who are in contact with children are obligated by state law to report *suspected* child abuse. This includes any physical or mental abuse, wound, injury, or disability that reasonably indicates abuse or neglect of any child under 18 years of age (or a handicapped child under 21 years of age). Individuals, health care workers, or others who report suspected abuse/neglect in good faith are protected from legal consequences by law. The laws vary from state to state but, in general, failure to report a case when there is reasonable suspicion of deliberate injury or neglect may result in civil and criminal liability. The laws may include fines or imprisonment, depending on the nature of the offense. In civil suits, large malpractice settlements have resulted from injury recognized and not reported.[1]

A child protection team established by the hospital is the ideal way to handle and report cases of suspected physical injury. However, institutions in which there is not a large pediatric population or a well-developed child protection team must find other ways of handling and reporting suspected cases of abuse and neglect. If a hospital-based child protection team is not available, the county Child Protective Services managed through the welfare department is the appropriate agency to receive reports. It is essential that some form of Child Protective Services be involved in the investigation and follow-up to allow the treating physicians and other health care personnel to concentrate on the care of the child and the family unit.

The care of the child is the priority of the treating medical team and this team cannot be primarily involved in the investigation, prosecution, or remediation of the child's outside care givers. However, it is incumbent upon the medical team initially treating the injured child to recognize the warning signs of abuse, to preserve and document existing evidence, and to immediately report these concerns.

In some areas, intervention and prevention strategy programs are in place to identify high-risk families. Some child abuse teams are studying these possibilities, but there is little hard data available yet to confirm the efficacy of pre-injury intervention.

EVALUATION

Historical "Red Flags" of Abuse

Certain injuries or injury complexes have historical features which should raise suspicion in the mind of the examiner. A history which is not consistent with the identified injury is the most common "red flag." For example, the toddler who presents with a glove-like pattern of scald on the hands or a stocking pattern on scalded feet did not fall into the tub of hot water.[6]

A history which is inconsistent with the severity of the injury is another warning to suspect a non-accidental cause of that injury. Often a child who has suffered severe, non-accidental injury will reportedly have fallen from the bed, porch, first-floor window, or some other insignificant distance. However, studies correlating distance fallen with severity of injury have

shown that falls from beds, porches, first-floor windows, and other such short heights rarely result in serious injury in children.[2] In 19 cases of reported fatal falls from short distances reviewed by Reiber,[5] 17 were definitely inflicted injury and the other two most likely had a falsified history.

A history that is changed over time or is reported differently by witnessing family members is very suggestive of a non-accidental source of injury. For example, the presenting history of a 2-year-old child who subsequently died of sepsis secondary to a ruptured stomach was that she had rolled off the bed and lost consciousness. The next examiner was told that the child tripped on a toy and bumped her head and then went to sleep and could not be aroused. This resulted in transfer to another institution for pediatric neurosurgical care. Only when faced with the evidence of blood in the stomach and free air in the abdomen did the perpetrator admit to "tapping" the child in the epigastrium with his fist. The false history contributed to a significant delay in making the correct diagnosis and the ultimate death of the child.

A marked delay between the time of injury and seeking care is of concern in the absence of a plausible reason for the delay. A history of frequent or multiple injuries, visits to multiple emergency departments in the area, fractures in unlikely bones for the expected level of activity of the injured child, fractures in children under 2 years of age, and fractures which do not have a rational explanation of the cause are other indicators of non-accidental injury.

In summary, the situations are reportable in instances where the following occur:

1. Discrepancy between physical findings and the caregiver's explanation of injury.

2. Inconsistent and/or changing history obtained from different family members or from the same person over time.

3. Delay in seeking care resulting in increased harm to the child.

4. Fractures without a reasonable explanation of the source of the trauma.

5. History of repeated injury.

6. Multiple wounds/scars of varying age or of identifiable shapes (e.g., belt buckle or hand print).

Interviewing the Maltreated Child

Children as young as age 3 can accurately observe things happening to and around them. However, children ordinarily try to please and will agree with leading questions even when they do not conform to the child's memory. Repeated questions are seen as an indication that the original answer was "wrong." Therefore, the child must be interviewed in a neutral manner, in a supportive environment, and with no suggestion that the interviewer has an agenda.[7]

Children frequently take on responsibility for the abuse to themselves and carry a great deal of guilt. This issue should be addressed directly and early in the interview to assure the child that he/she is not at fault.

The history should be documented in detail as soon as possible, preferably by more than one person.

PHYSICAL EXAMINATION AND DOCUMENTATION

In young children, the diagnosis of abuse is made on physical evidence. A member of the child protection team can provide invaluable assistance in obtaining and properly documenting necessary evidence. In the absence of such assistance, all visible wounds, burns, and scars must be documented photographically. If the general condition of the child (i.e., malnutrition) is of concern, photographs showing the whole child are needed. Color pictures are helpful in recognizing the age of various wounds, but wound detail is better defined in black and white photographs. Pictures obtained using a Polaroid camera give good immediate documentation, but they deteriorate over time and should not be the sole means of photographic documentation. The permanent identifying photographs of the injuries should be obtained using a 35-mm camera. The camera used to take the pictures in the emergency department should ideally be equipped to automatically date and time the pictures. The patient should be identified in the picture with a hospital label containing the patient's name and hospital number. Any radiographs which document injury must be duplicated and preserved as part of the evidence.[4]

MANAGEMENT

The treating physicians must deal with the physical injury as their first priority. If there is real concern that the injury represents either abuse or neglect, admission of the child to the hospital is always appropriate. While the child is in the hospital, a more complete evaluation can be undertaken and the caregivers can be interviewed. If the situation involves extreme circumstances, temporary custody can be obtained for the protection of the child. More often this is an opportunity to identify stresses in the family and begin intervention with home visits, counseling, parenting classes, or even placement of the child in a foster home with monitored visits from the family during the process of remediation.

REFERENCES

1. Fulginiti VA: Violence and children in the United States. **Am J Dis Child 146:**671-672, 1992
2. Lyons TJ, Oates RK: Falling out of bed: a relatively benign occurrence. **Pediatrics 92:**125-127, 1993
3. National Center on Child Abuse and Neglect: **Study Findings: Study of National Incidence and Prevalence of Child Abuse and Neglect.** Washington, DC: US Department of Health and Human Services, 1988
4. Reece RM (ed): **Manual of Emergency Pediatrics.** 4th ed. Philadelphia, Pa: WB Saunders, 1992
5. Reiber GD: Fatal falls in childhood. How far must children fall to sustain fatal head injury? Report of cases and review of the literature. **Am J Forensic Med Pathol 14:**201-207, 1993
6. Rosenberg NM, Marino D: Frequency of suspected abuse/neglect in burn patients. **Pediatr Emerg Care 5:** 219-221, 1989
7. Wissow LS: Child abuse and neglect. **N Engl J Med 332:**1425-1431, 1995

ADDITIONAL READINGS

1. Council on Scientific Affairs, American Medical Association: AMA diagnostic and treatment guidelines concerning child abuse and neglect. **JAMA 254:** 796-800, 1985
2. Helfer RE, Kempe CH (eds): **The Battered Child.** Chicago, Ill: University of Chicago, 1968

CHAPTER 11

ABUSE, PART B: SPOUSE ABUSE

JANET M. WILLIAMS, MD, FACEP

Spouse abuse, or domestic violence, refers to a pattern of behaviors that may include repeated battering, psychological abuse, sexual assault, progressive social isolation, deprivation, and intimidation of a victim by an intimate partner. It involves all age groups as well as all racial, ethnic, religious, educational, and socio-economic classes, and is becoming recognized as a major public health problem in the United States as well as worldwide.[8,11] A wide spectrum of sequelae has been described in victims of spouse abuse, including fatal and nonfatal injury, various medical complaints, drug and alcohol abuse, attempted suicide and other mental illnesses, and miscarriages.[1]

Traditionally, medical care of battered victims has been limited to treating the obvious traumatic and physical manifestations. However, the ethical principle of beneficence requires physicians to "address not only the bodily assault that disease or an injury inflicts but also the psychological, social, even spiritual dimensions of this assault."[3] This section will discuss the various forms of spouse abuse, the magnitude of the problem, when to suspect it in the health care setting, how to diagnose and manage spouse abuse cases, and legal aspects of caring for these patients.

FORMS OF ABUSE

Spouse abuse may manifest in a variety of ways. *Physical abuse* includes victimization through slapping, kicking, choking, restraining, assault with a weapon, and physical abandonment. *Emotional abuse*, through means such as intimidation, threats, and deprivation, often serves as a way for the batterer to exercise control over the victim. *Sexual abuse* includes any form of forced sexual activity or sexual degradation. Although women are more likely than men to be the victims injured in abusive relationships, spouse abuse also includes cases of victimization of husbands and may occur within gay and lesbian relationships as well.

Spouse abuse tends to follow a "cycle of violence" comprising three phases.[8] The first, the "tension-building phase," is characterized by increasing tension, anger, and arguments between the intimate partners. This is followed by the second, the "acute battering phase," which may include battering, sexual abuse, or harmful threats. During the third, the "honeymoon phase," the batterer often apologizes and makes excuses or promises that it will not happen again. Although some women successfully end the relationship after the first cycle of abuse, most abuse is recurrent and escalates in frequency and severity. Nationally, 75% of battered women identified in a medical setting will go on to suffer repeated abuse. Typically, a victim will go through five to seven physical separations from her partner before taking legal steps for protection from the ongoing violence.[6] It is not surprising that victims of this cycle of violence often develop symptoms consistent with post-traumatic stress disorder.

Historical Perspectives

Throughout recorded history, women have been kept subordinated to men in many cultures through a variety of means, such as foot-binding (China), forced seclusion (Middle East), and household supremacy of husbands over wives and children which condoned the use of physical force "as needed" (England and the U.S.). The practice of wife-beating flourished in the U.S. during the colonial period and was actually legalized in 1824. The North Carolina Supreme Court stated: "if no permanent injury has been inflicted, nor malice, cruelty nor dangerous violence shown by the husband, it is better to draw the curtain, shut out public gaze, and leave the parties to forget and forgive."[2]

Social awareness of domestic violence began to grow during the 1960s. The first shelter for abused women was established in London in 1971. Although recent years have shown some development of legislative, social, and therapeutic reform to control and prevent spouse abuse, it is still accepted as a way of life in many subcultures in the U.S. and throughout the world.

Scope of the Problem

Ninety-five percent of the victims of spouse abuse are women, and recent studies have estimated that eight to 12 million women in the U.S. are abused annually by their current or former intimate partners.[1] Domestic violence is thought to be the most under-reported crime according to the Federal Bureau of Investigation.[5] Prevalence studies have estimated that one-fifth to one-third of all women will be physically assaulted by a partner sometime during their lifetime, and the rate of injury to women from battering surpasses that of motor-vehicle crashes, rapes, and muggings combined.[9] Seventy-five percent of these battered women will go on to suffer repeated abuse. More than 50% of all domestic assaults result in injury, with most of these victims requiring hospitalization or emergency care. In fact, 22% to 35% of women seeking emergency medical care do so for symptoms related to abuse.[7] Of the 5,745 women murdered in 1991, over one-half were murdered by a current or former intimate partner.[10] Besides the personal pain and suffering experienced by victims, the economic cost of injury and death due to domestic violence in the U.S. is estimated to exceed $1.7 billion annually.[10]

Demographics

There is no specific demographic, economic, racial, religious, or psychosocial profile which characterizes battered women; however, certain women are known to be at greater risk for abuse. Black women are two to three times more likely to be abused than white women. However, black women are also twice as likely to seek medical care and to report the episode(s) as white women.[9] Domestic violence is thought to be more prevalent in lower socioeconomic groups such as the unemployed and poor working classes. Higher rates of abuse have been noted in relationships in which the woman has a job higher in status than the man's job. Other high-risk characteristics of the abused population include:[1]

- women who are single, separated, or divorced;
- women who are between the ages of 17 and 28 years;
- women who abuse alcohol or drugs;
- women who are pregnant;
- women whose partners are excessively jealous or possessive; and
- mothers of abused children.

When to Suspect Spouse Abuse

There are a variety of barriers to identifying spouse abuse. Many women are reluctant to seek help for fear of retaliation by the abuser or because they are being held captive in an isolated setting without money, outside communication, or transportation. Cultural, ethnic, or religious factors also influence how a woman responds to the abusive relationship. Physicians may avoid inquiring about spouse abuse due to a lack of awareness of the problem or because they feel that their responsibility ends after caring for the objective injury or symptoms at hand.

It is clear that the magnitude of the spouse abuse problem warrants routine screening of all injured as well as noninjured female patients in emergency departments and trauma centers, as well as primary care and mental health settings. Just as a thorough medical history includes assessment of risk factors such as past medical history, smoking, alcohol, and drug use, it should also include questions about violence or abuse in the home. Simple statements or questions may be used to facilitate disclosure such as: "We see many women who have been abused, and help is available," or "Your injuries concern me. Injuries such as these are often caused by abuse. Is this happening to you?"

Health care providers should suspect spouse abuse when the woman's explanation of how an injury occurred does not fit with the clinical picture or if there has been a significant delay in seeking treatment. Injuries during pregnancy should also raise suspicion of abuse. At the time of presentation, an abused woman may exhibit a variety of behavioral signs such as appearing frightened, ashamed, or embarrassed. Many battered women have been labeled with quasi-medical terms such as "hysteria," "hypochondria," and having "vague complaints."

Victims of abuse may present with a variety of noninjury complaints, including chronic pain, psychogenic pain, anxiety, depression, suicidal ideation or gestures, gynecological problems, overuse of alcohol or drugs such as tranquilizers, and/or vague symptoms without evidence of physiological abnormalities. Frequently, the abusive partner will accompany and stay close to the patient as well as dominate the conversation and answer questions which are directed at the victim. An abusive partner's use of control may result in limited access to emergency medical care, noncompliance with medication, missed appointments, and lack of transportation or communication.

CLINICAL FINDINGS

The extent of injuries resulting from spouse abuse ranges from injuries leaving no objective physical findings to severe injury which may result in death. Contusions, lacerations, and abrasions are the most common injuries and are usually located in the central part of the body (i.e., the head, face, neck, breast, and abdomen). Mid-arm injuries are often seen as a result of defensive reflexes. Injuries to areas that are less commonly associated with falls, such as black eyes, injuries to the front teeth, strangulation marks on the neck, weapon injuries, bites, and burns, are suspect. The presence of multiple symmetrical injuries is suggestive of domestic violence, as is evidence of old injuries such as scars and a deviated nasal septum found concurrently with new injuries.

THE HEALTH CARE PROVIDER'S ROLE IN THE PREVENTION AND TREATMENT

The medical community has the responsibility to address spouse abuse through primary and secondary prevention efforts. Primary prevention refers to interventions that are designed to prevent the battering from occurring in the first place, while secondary prevention refers to attempts to minimize the outcome of battering by providing acute medical care and a variety of support services to both the victim and batterer.

Primary Prevention of Spouse Abuse

There are several steps that health care providers can take to practice primary prevention of spouse abuse. First, medical professionals are in a prime position to screen patients to identify those at risk for abuse and to offer appropriate referral options such as support groups, parenting classes, alcohol and drug treatment, and family counseling. It is vital that health care facilities establish and implement model protocols for the early identification and referral of patients at risk for abuse. Second,

TABLE 1

CLASSIFICATION OF BATTERED WOMEN*

Positive:	Injury was attributed to spouse or boyfriend in the medical record of the event.
Probable:	The record reports that the patient was beaten, kicked, hit, punched, but no personal etiology was noted.
Suggestive:	The recorded etiology of the injury did not seem to account adequately for the injury.
Negative:	Nothing in the report of the injury would raise suspicion that the injury was a result of battering.

* Adapted from Flitcraft.[4]

curricula covering spouse abuse and gender bias should be integrated into the professional education, training, and continuing education of health and social service providers. Third, the development and distribution of public information on spouse abuse may serve to increase awareness of the problem and the availability of community resources.

Secondary Prevention and Acute Care of Spouse Abuse Victims

The acute care of an abused victim may be summarized in five steps:

1. Provide a safe environment for the patient. The victim should be assured that she is safe in the health care setting and that all information will be treated confidentially. It is best to interview and examine the patient alone, which may involve asking the potential abuser to leave. This may be achieved by asking all visitors to leave and explained as being a routine part of departmental policy. In cases where the abuser is deemed potentially violent, the hospital security staff should be summoned.

2. Identify battered women through screening and recognition of high-risk characteristics. In order to achieve this goal, health care facilities must develop and implement policies and procedures for identifying, treating, and referring victims of domestic violence. In addition, medical personnel must be aware of

the high-risk indicators for abuse, including common chief complaints, suspicious medical histories, behaviors, and clinical findings. Flitcraft[4] has developed a protocol for identifying and classifying battered women, which is shown in Table 1.

3. Examine, diagnose, and treat all physical as well as emotional injuries. The treatment of life-threatening injuries is top priority. A complete assessment for occult injuries should be performed since many victims of abuse present with multiple injuries both new and old. A number of these patients will also require psychiatric care for depression, suicidal ideation, or other manifestations of severe stress.

4. Document findings accurately. Well-documented medical records are important to provide concrete evidence of violence and abuse, especially in cases going to trial. Records should include basic information such as date and time of arrival, name of person(s) accompanying the victim, chief complaint in the patient's words, complete medical history, relevant social history, and a detailed description of the injuries (e.g., type, number, size, and location), which should be recorded on a body chart. All significant statements made by the patient and companions may be admissible in court, so they should be recorded accurately. The physician should also document whether the explanation of the injuries is appropriate and credible. Results of all diagnostic tests should be recorded. Color

photographs are particularly valuable and require the patient's permission as well as a documentable chain of custody. Photos are best taken prior to treatment, shooting from different angles, and using a ruler to illustrate the size of an injury. At least two photos of every major traumatized area should be taken. The pictures should be marked with the patient's name, the location of the injury, the name of the photographer, and the date.

5. Provide referral to domestic violence support agencies and shelter services. Once a victim of spouse abuse has been identified and all injuries and illnesses have been treated, a number of interventions are possible. The first concern should be for the safety of the woman and her children. The clinician must inquire about a battered woman's safety before she leaves the medical setting. It is vital for health care providers to be aware of community resources that are available to provide safety, advocacy, and support. She should be offered access to a shelter and referred to counseling and to local domestic violence organizations.

Controlling Spouse Abuse: Complex Social Prevention

Although the role of the medical community in addressing the domestic violence epidemic cannot be overstated, a multidisciplinary approach to preventing spouse abuse is required since the problem extends beyond the medical context and has strong roots entwined in our social, cultural, and legal systems. Complex social prevention, which proposes that nonmedical interventions may have the greatest success in controlling spouse abuse, is based on the following six premises:[9]

1. There is a need to determine the *cause* of spouse abuse and to determine which interventions are most effective to prevent it.

2. The fact that spouse abuse is a crime and a health hazard must be given national recognition.

3. The cultural acceptance of violence must be decreased.

4. The position of women in society must be elevated in terms of their social and economic options.

5. Spouse abuse prevention must become a major priority for public health funding.

6. More flexible role models for women and men should be supported.

LEGAL ASPECTS

Until recent years, domestic violence had been viewed by society as being a "private matter" between intimate partners. However, collaborative efforts between law enforcement and social services agencies have begun to impact this problem and support victims of spouse abuse. In most states, police no longer have to witness the abuse to arrest the abuser, regardless of whether the woman files charges. Domestic violence is a crime in all states. Potential criminal actions against batterers include prosecution for assault, aggravated assault, battery, harassment, intimidation, or murder.

Most states do not have explicit laws requiring physicians to report instances of spouse abuse. It is usually the responsibility of the abused person to report the abuse to the proper authorities. A physician should only report abuse with the knowledge and consent of the abused victim. Every state has some form of legislation designed to offer protection to victims of domestic violence. The most common civil action in protecting abused victims is a protective order, injunction, or restraining order. In some states, the court may have authority to order a batterer to leave the home, receive counseling, or take other actions. Police may have authority to arrest abusers who violate protective orders.

REFERENCES

1. American Medical Association: **Diagnostic and Treatment Guidelines on Domestic Violence.** Chicago, Ill: American Medical Association, 1992

2. Calvert R: Criminal and civil liability in husband-wife assaults, in Steinmetz K, Straus M (eds): **Violence in the Family.** New York, NY: Dodd, Mead, 1975, p 9

3. Council on Ethical and Judicial Affairs, American Medical Association: Physicians and domestic violence. Ethical considerations. **JAMA 267:**3190-3193, 1992

4. Flitcraft A: Battered Women: An emergency room epidemiology. New Haven, Conn: Yale School of Medicine, 1977 (MD Thesis)

5. Martin D: The historical roots of domestic violence, in Sonkin DJ (ed): **Domestic Violence on Trial.** New York, NY: Springer Publishing, 1987, pp 3-19

6. Pizzey E: **Scream Quietly or the Neighbors Will Hear.** Hillside, NJ: Enslaw, 1977

7. Randall T: Domestic violence intervention calls for more than treating injuries. **JAMA 264:**939-940, 1990

8. Ross DA: Adult abuse, in Rosen P, Barkin RM (eds): **Emergency Medicine: Concepts and Clinical Practice.** St Louis, Mo: Mosby-Year Book, 1992, pp 2096-2104

9. Stark E, Flitcraft A: Wife abuse in the medical setting: an introduction for health personnel, in Rosenberg M, Fenley MA (eds): **Violence in America: A Public Health Approach.** New York, NY: Oxford University Press, 1991, pp 133-151

10. Straus MA: Medical care costs of intrafamily assault and homicide. **Acad Med 62:**556, 1986

11. Waxweiler RJ, Rosenberg ML, Fenley MA (coordinators): **Injury Control in the 1990s: A National Plan for Action.** Des Plaines, Ill: Association for the Advancement of Automotive Medicine, 1993, pp 35-37

CHAPTER 11

ABUSE, PART C: GERIATRIC ABUSE

GREGORY A. TIMBERLAKE, MD, FACS

Domestic violence is a tragedy of our society that primarily affects three segments of the population: children, spouses (usually women), and the elderly. The realization that domestic violence is a chronic disease has helped clinicians recognize the problem more easily and intervene in situations involving the first two at-risk groups. Much less attention has been paid to the third at-risk population, the elderly. The failure to appreciate and ameliorate this problem is particularly troubling because domestic violence is frequently a chronic disease that is episodic and recurrent. Additionally, with the "graying" of the population, the number of persons at risk likely will increase yearly unless the scope and breadth of the problem are recognized by health care providers and society as a whole. Indeed, in two recent articles reviewing reports of abuse to protective services, between 40% and 63% of the reports involved abuse of elderly persons.[21,41]

This chapter reviews what is known about the extent of the problem of geriatric abuse and neglect. Suggestions are made for clinical evaluation schemes and possible management strategies.

DEFINITIONS AND EPIDEMIOLOGY

What constitutes geriatric abuse? This has been much more difficult to define than child or spouse abuse. Indeed, there is no consensus definition of what constitutes abuse in persons aged 65 years and older. Part of the difficulty stems from the wide variety in forms of abuse and neglect that may exist for the elderly and violate their legal rights, including physical, emotional, psychosocial, sexual, and financial abuse. Another reason why the definition of elder abuse is unclear is the relative lack of attention paid to the problem until recently. Unfortunately, not only are the acts of abuse and neglect varied, but there is no agreement on the definitions of what constitutes elder abuse. As a result, only a broad overview of generally accepted descriptions of different types of elder abuse can be given.[1,5,12,13,20,27,28,45] The earliest case reports of abuse of geriatric patients in the medical literature appeared just over 20 years ago.[3] A search of the *Index Medicus* for a recent 5-year period reveals only 26 articles on elder abuse.[20]

Physical acts of violence are commonly included in all definitions of elder abuse. The most commonly seen acts include slapping, striking, and hitting with hands, fists, feet, or objects. As a result, the abused elderly patient will have bruises, abrasions, sprains, strains, and occasionally fractures, lacerations, burns, or other wounds. In summary, physical abuse implies acts of violence meant to cause physical pain or injury.

Psychosocial and emotional abuse often accompany acts of physical abuse but constitute another category of abuse of older persons. This type of abuse may be defined as acts, usually expressed through verbal utterances, meant to cause psychological or emotional distress. Examples include threats, insults, and other statements meant to demean, humiliate, or infantilize an older adult. Particularly noxious are threats to remove the patients' freedom by institutionalization or abandonment. Although societal norms differ among ethnic groups, any acts that cause substantial distress to the older adult may be considered psychological abuse.[23]

Sexual abuse, while much less commonly included in definitions of elder abuse, may have aspects of both physical and psychological abuse. Although infrequently reported, it may not be infrequent in occurrence.

Financial and legal abuse is often included in descriptions of elder abuse. These acts include any misappropriation of money or property or other material exploitation. Common examples include theft of pension or social security checks, coercion in the signing or changing of wills and other such legal documents, and other enforced changes in the elderly person's financial or other assets for the enrichment of another.

A final aspect of elder abuse is *neglect or failure of the designated caretaker to meet the needs of a dependent older adult.* Neglect of the elderly may either be intentional or unintentional. Intentional neglect is exemplified by caretakers deliberately failing to fulfill their responsibilities in order to punish or harm the person whose care they have been entrusted with. Typical examples include the withholding of food, water, or medication. Unintentional neglect arises as a result of either ignorance on the part of the designated caregiver or that person's genuine inability to provide the needed care. A controversial subset of elder neglect is "self-neglect"

(i.e., an elderly person previously living independently who becomes unable to provide those services necessary for maintenance of physical or psychological health). One particularly difficult subset to identify and assist may be the estimated 2.5 million elderly who have a dependence on alcohol use.[22]

The true incidence and prevalence of elder abuse is unknown, although the indications are that it is increasing. Epidemiological studies carried out in Boston, Canada, and Great Britain revealed overall incidence rates of approximately 3%.[25,34,37] Physical abuse was reported in 2%, psychological abuse in 1%, and neglect in 0.5%. In the Boston study, two-thirds of the abusers were spouses and one-third were adult children.[34] Other studies have estimated the incidence to be as high as 10%, with 4% suffering from moderate to severe acts of abuse.[5,14,43,44] These figures would imply that 1.5 to 2 million elderly are subject to abuse or neglect yearly, yet only 20% of the cases are being reported.[9] In fact, elder abuse may be only slightly less common than child abuse, despite the average state's spending of $22 per child but only $2.90 per aged client for protective services.[21]

Abuse of institutionalized older adults may occur at a much higher rate than that in the general population. One study of nursing home staff, asking them to report acts committed against elderly nursing home residents in the preceding year, found that 10% of nurse's aides reported committing at least one act of physical abuse and 40% at least one act of psychological abuse.[15] In addition, acts of elder abuse may be carried out by other residents or visitors. Inappropriate use of physical or medicinal restraints, isolation of older persons from other residents, staff, or visitors, and failure to respect the decision-making capacity of the elderly all occur in the institutional environment. Concerns over the possibility of widespread abuse and neglect affecting the institutionalized elderly led to the establishment of nursing home ombudsman programs under the Older American Act of 1976 and the establishment of standards for quality of care in nursing homes as part of the Omnibus Budget Reconciliation Act of 1987. The presence of ombudsmen in nursing programs has resulted in increased reporting of abuse, increased substantiation of abuse re-

TABLE 1
RISK FACTORS FOR ABUSE OF THE ELDERLY*

Risk Factor	Mechanism
Poor health and functional impairment in the elderly person	Disability reduces the elderly person's ability to seek help and defend himself or herself
Cognitive impairment in the elderly person	Aggression toward the caregiver and disruptive behavior resulting from dementia may precipitate abuse; higher rates of abuse have been found among patients with dementia
Substance abuse or mental illness on the part of the abuser	Abusers are likely to abuse alcohol or drugs and to have serious mental illness, which in turn leads to abusive behavior
Dependence of the abuser on the victim	Abusers are very likely to depend on the victim financially, for housing, and in other areas; abuse results from attempts by a relative (especially an adult child) to obtain resources from the elderly person
Shared living arrangements	Abuse is much less likely among elderly people living alone; a shared living situation provides greater opportunities for tension and conflict, which generally precede incidents of abuse
External factors causing stress	Stressful life events and continuing financial strain decrease the family's resistance and increase the likelihood of abuse
Social isolation	Elderly people with fewer social contacts are more likely to be victims; isolation reduces the likelihood that abuse will be detected and stopped, and in addition, social support can buffer the effects of stress
History of violence	Particularly among spouses, a history of violence in the relationship may predict abuse in later life

*Reproduced with permission from Lachs MS, Pillemer K: Abuse and neglect of elderly persons. *N Engl J Med* 332:437-443, 1995.[20]

ported, and higher sanction activity.[24] Fortunately, programs have been developed which appear to lessen the risk of recurrent abuse by nursing home personnel.[35,46]

A number of putative risk factors have been identified that may heighten the older person's risk of maltreatment (Table 1). Of these, only cognitive impairment and shared living arrangements with the abuser find strong support in the literature.[1,6,11,15,16,26,36,42] It has been suggested that physical and functional impairment, in the presence of other risk factors, increases an elderly person's vulnerability to abuse because the impairment may diminish their ability to either defend or escape from the situation.[20] Although the presumed frailty of older adults has been suggested as a risk factor in their abuse, no direct relationship has been found between elder abuse and the older person with poor health, functional (but not cognitive) impairment, or dependence on the abuser.[6,26,29,31,33,36] Abusers of the elderly tend to display three characteristics: sub-

stance abuse or mental illness, dependence on the victim financially or for other necessities such as shelter, and a history of violence or antisocial behavior outside the family.[2,32,46]

CLINICAL EVALUATION FOR ELDER ABUSE

All clinicians should inquire of their elderly patients about the possibility of inadequate care or mistreatment in their lives, even in the absence of obvious symptoms of family/caretaker violence. Given the prevalence of elder abuse and the difficulty in identifying asymptomatic family violence, failure to do so may result in failure of the elderly person to thrive in the community. A recent publication from the American Medical Association strongly supports this recommendation.[1] Although this recommendation seems reasonable and prudent, there is little scientific evidence currently available to either support or refute it.[4]

The clinical evaluation of the older adult must begin with obtaining a careful and detailed history from both the patient and any suspected abuser. Several interviewing techniques increase the likelihood of obtaining accurate data. First, both the patient and the suspected abuser must be approached in an empathetic, caring, and nonconfrontational manner. Second, both the patient and the suspected abuser should be interviewed separately and privately. Disparities between information obtained in each interview may be useful in raising the threshold of the interviewer's suspicion that an abuse situation exists. Finally, both should be questioned about specific stressors that may provoke the abuse. This information may assist in evaluating the pattern and frequency of abuse episodes and suggest interventions that may be helpful.

Not uncommonly, abused older adults are reticent to disclose evidence of abuse, particularly in the presence of other patients or health care providers. The interviewer must attempt to gain the patient's trust and confidence; one's own discomfort at asking such questions must be subjugated to the patent's needs. It is often helpful to begin with general questions about the home environment, such as where they live and their perceptions of safety at home or in the neighborhood. Further inquiries can then be made in an attempt to establish who, if anyone, is the responsible caregiver. The interview should then be directed to raise questions about specific instances of maltreatment or neglect that may have occurred.

Similarly, the suspected abuser should be interviewed in private. During this interview, the physician should use a nonconfrontational, nonjudgmental style. Although this may be difficult, valuable information and the opportunity to intervene may be lost if a confrontation is allowed to develop. Again, gaining the interviewee's trust by displaying empathy may be very helpful and can lead to an understanding of the difficulties encountered in caring for the older adult.

On physical examination, several presentations suggest the possibility of elder abuse (Table 2).[18,39] The diagnosis is clear in those patients with obvious physical abuse. As in patients with child abuse, any older adult with multiple injuries in different stages of healing, with neglected injuries, or with vague or implausible explanations for the injuries should have the diagnosis of abuse considered. A patient who is functionally impaired and presents without the designated caretaker, or appears to have malnutrition, lack of hygiene, or neglected medical needs should also be evaluated for the possibility of abuse, neglect, or "self-neglect." Although injury may be the most dramatic marker of abuse, the clinician must be aware that neglect, manifested by malnutrition and dehydration, may be more common.[17]

More subtle forms of neglect and mistreatment often are encountered by the health care provider outside the emergency department. Neglect, psychological abuse, financial abuse, or some combination of these may predominate. Psychological abuse may be difficult to identify and may manifest clinically only as withdrawal, depression, or anxiety.

Although the clinician cannot be expected to perform a detailed assessment of the patient's finances and potential for financial, legal, or material exploitation, the clinician must be alert to clues offered by the patient or suspected abuser. It is also important for the clinician to have some understanding of the patient's financial and social resources to help plan interventions to defuse the abusive situation.

Once the suspicion of elder abuse is raised, the health care provider should embark on a thorough, structured evaluation.[1,18-20,28] An example of one such plan is reproduced in Table 3.[20] A thorough, complete history and physical examination are crucial. Documentation must be detailed and done with the understanding that the medical record may appear in legal proceedings. Particularly important is the performance of a structured mental status examination.[8,30] Dementia or delirium may manifest as cognitive impairment. In its presence, short-term memory loss may render the patient unable to provide an accurate history. Similarly, severe cognitive impairment may compromise the decision-making capacity of the older patient, which must be considered if the patient's consent is necessary before therapeutic interventions are undertaken. Finally, impairment of cognition may itself be a risk factor for abuse.[20]

TABLE 2

CONDITIONS SUGGESTIVE OF
ELDER ABUSE OR NEGLECT[*]

- Delays in seeking medical treatment for injury or illness
- Disparity between older adult and suspected abuser histories
- Implausible or vague explanations for illness or injury
- Frequent exacerbations of chronic diseases despite a medical care plan and adequate resources
- Fearful or withdrawn behavior by the patient
- Inappropriate care giver attitudes
- Signs of physical abuse
- Signs of confinement
- Unexplained malnutrition or dehydration
- Laboratory findings inconsistent with the provided history

[*]Modified from Rathbone-McCuan and Voyles[39] and Lachs and Pillemer.[20]

The effort required to evaluate these patients and their situations can be daunting to the clinician. The health care provider may feel alone in the management of these often difficult and complex problems. It is important to realize that appropriate resources exist in society to help the abused older adult, and it often is only necessary to learn how to gain access to these services to begin to ameliorate the abusive situation. Further, a proper evaluation may require several visits unless there is a life-threatening injury or a risk of imminent danger to the patient. The clinician should obtain information from as many sources as possible. A home visit is ideal and necessary to evaluate the patient and his or her functioning in that environment. If the suspected abuse has been reported to state authorities, then professional staff members from Adult Protective Services will be available and invaluable in assisting the clinician in these evaluations. In may cases, once the potential or real abusive situation has been recognized, steps can be undertaken to remedy the needs of the patient while the formal evaluative and diagnostic process is proceeding. A number of programs and modules for intervention by Adult Protective Services have been described.[1,40,47]

MANAGEMENT STRATEGIES

Once elder abuse or neglect has been identified, the clinician must first and foremost ensure the safety of the older adult while respecting patient autonomy. Development of the management plan is dependent upon the answers to two questions. First, does the patient have decision-making capacity? Second, does the patient agree to the proposed intervention?

If the patient has decision-making capacity and accepts the need for intervention, then a safe plan should be made. In the case of imminent danger, separation from the abuser may require hospital admission, safe house placement, or obtaining a protective order from the court. In less urgent cases, but where neglected injuries or medical problems exist, hospitalization may also be justified. If none of the above situations exist, then the interventions should be tailored to the specific problems identified. For example, if the burden of the older person's chronic illnesses is causing stress in the caregiver, arranging for home health care, visiting nurses, or respite services may significantly improve matters. Referral of the caregivers to chronic disease support groups may also be helpful. Unfortunately, when psychosocial problems of the abuser, such as alcohol or drug abuse or mental illness, are contributing factors, standard interventions are not as effective and separating the party's living environments may be necessary. It is critical in all cases to counsel the older adult about the incidence of elder abuse, its episodic nature, and the tendency for the abuse to increase in both frequency and severity with time. The geriatric patient should be informed that the clinician will remain a source of help, and treatment plan effectiveness should be monitored by the health care provider along with Adult Protective Services.

The most troubling situation for the health care provider arises when a competent victim of elder abuse insists on remaining in the abusive environment. Experiences of this type may cause great stress in the health care provider as well.[7] These patients often are afraid of losing their independence if they leave their current life situation. They may also have been subjected to chronic psychological abuse because of threats to institutionalize the patient by their primary

TABLE 3

CLINICAL PROCEDURES FOR THE DETECTION OF ABUSE OF AN ELDERLY PATIENT*

History
- Interview the patient and the suspected abuser separately and alone
- Make direct inquiries about physical violence, restraints, or neglect
- Request precise details about nature, frequency, and severity of events
- Assess the patient's functional status (independence, activities of daily living)
- Inquire who is the designated caregiver if impairment in activities of daily living is present
- Assess recent psychosocial factors (e.g., bereavement and financial stress)
- Elicit caregiver's understanding of patient's illness (e.g., care needs and prognosis)

Behavioral observation
- Withdrawal
- Infantilizing of patient by caregiver
- Caregiver who insists on providing the history

General appearance
- Hygiene
- Cleanliness and appropriateness of dress

Skin and mucous membranes
- Skin turgor or other signs of dehydration
- Multiple skin lesions in various stages of evolution
- Bruises or decubitus ulcers
- Evaluate how skin lesions have been cared for

Head and neck
- Traumatic alopecia (distinguishable from male-pattern alopecia on the basis of distribution)
- Scalp hematomas
- Lacerations or abrasions

Trunk
- Bruises or welts; the shape may suggest an implement (e.g., iron or belt)
- Genitourinary tract
- Rectal bleeding or vaginal bleeding
- Decubitus ulcers or infestations

Extremities
- Wrist or ankle lesions suggesting the use of restraints
- Immersion burn ("stocking-glove" distribution)

Musculoskeletal system
- Examine for occult fracture or pain
- Observe gait

Neurological-psychiatric status
- Conduct a thorough evaluation to assess faculties
- Depressive symptoms or anxiety
- Other psychiatric symptoms, including delusions and hallucinations
- Formal mental-status testing (e.g., Mini-Mental State Examination or Mental Status Questionnaire)
- Cognitive impairment suggesting delirium or dementia has a role in assessing decision-making capacity

Imaging and laboratory results
- As indicated from the clinical evaluation
- Albumin, blood urea nitrogen, and creatinine levels, toxicological screening (assess caregiver's compliance with medical regimen)

Social and financial
- Inquire about other members of the social network available to assist the elderly person and about financial resources; this information is crucial in considering interventions that include alternative living arrangements and home services

---

*Reproduced with permission from Lachs MS, Pillemer K: Abuse and neglect of elderly persons. *N Engl J Med* 332:437-443, 1995.[20]

caregiver. Unfortunately, these patients have in reality already lost their independence. If these patients cannot be helped with other interventions and no alternative living situations are available or acceptable to the patient, then their quality of life paradoxically may be improved if they can be persuaded to accept placement in long-term care facilities.[20] If the decision-making capability is retained and cognition is not impaired, then the patient's autonomy must be respected. Often, all that can be done is to try to educate the patient about the risks of remaining in the abusive situation and to emphasize that the patient need not remain in that environment. The health care provider should initiate any interventions the patient will accept, develop a follow-up plan, and counsel the patient that the physician remains a source of help.

If the patient does not retain decision-making capacity, the clinician must document not only the findings that suggest elder abuse but also examples evidencing impaired decision-making capacity. These patients must be provided a safe harbor with the assistance of Adult Protective Services, and legal proceedings usually are necessary to appoint a guardian or conservator to act in the patient's interest and make decisions regarding living arrangements, health care, and finances. In extreme cases, protective orders may need to be obtained from the court as well.

ELDER ABUSE REPORTING REQUIREMENTS

Although all 50 states have enacted legislation to protect vulnerable adults, mandatory reporting laws requiring health care workers to report suspected elder abuse to designated state agencies have now been enacted in only 42 states.[10] Although an unannounced visit to the older adult's home usually results from such a report, it has not been possible to show that states with these laws have a more effective process than states without such laws.[10] Although some of this noncorrelation may be due to differences in definitions of elder abuse in various state laws, an increased public awareness of the problem may be more important than reporting requirements in identifying cases of elder abuse.

Health care providers often are concerned by the term "mandatory reporting," fearing that it implies the need for irrefutable proof of neglect or abuse and will result in a punitive investigatory home visit. While a review of the 42 individual state laws is beyond the scope of this chapter, the clinician should be reassured that neither fear need be true. Under many of the laws, only a suspicion of elder abuse is necessary for filing a report and no irrefutable proof is necessary. Indeed, many (but not all) mandatory reporting states provide immunity to reporters who act in good faith and the clinicians may remain anonymous.[1,38] On the other hand, failure to correctly diagnose or report cases of elder abuse may expose clinicians to liability.[1] One can view the home visit not as punitive or threatening but as a way to observe the patient in his or her living environment and to gather information that otherwise would not be available. This view may be helpful when dealing with an older adult who requests that the clinician not report the abuse. Instead of calling the home visit an investigation, it can be termed an attempt to determine the patient's unmet needs and to identify community services that might remediate these needs.

Elder abuse is one piece of the spectrum of violence in the United States. Although there is more public awareness about child abuse and spouse abuse, with the increasing incidence of elder abuse and the "graying of America," the problem will only assume longer and larger proportions. It is therefore, incumbent on all health care providers to have some knowledge of how to recognize, diagnose, and initiate treatment for this disease.

REFERENCES

1. American Medical Association: **American Medical Association Diagnostic and Treatment Guidelines on Elder Abuse and Neglect.** Chicago, Ill: American Medical Association, 1992
2. Bristone E, Collins J: Family mediated abuse of non-institutionalized frail elderly men and women in British Columbia. **J Elder Abuse Neglect** 1:45, 1989
3. Burston GR: Granny-battering. **Br Med J** 3:592, 1975 (Letter)
4. Canadian Task Force on the Periodic Health Examination. Periodic health examination, 1994 update: 4. Secondary prevention of elder abuse and mistreatment. **Can Med Assoc J** 151:1413-1420, 1994

5. Clark CB: Geriatric abuse—out of the closet. **J Tenn Med Assoc 77:**470-471, 1984

6. Coyne AC, Reichman WE, Berbig LJ: The relationship between dementia and elder abuse. **Am J Psychiatry 150:**643-646, 1993

7. Curtin K: Intervention in elder abuse: a swift blade, or a dull-edged saw? **Can Med Assoc J 152:** 1121-1123, 1995

8. Folstein MF, Folstein SE, McHugh PR: "Mini-Mental State." A practical method for grading the cognitive state of patients for the clinician. **J Psychiatr Res 12:** 189-198, 1975

9. Frost MH, Wilette K: Risk for abuse/neglect: Documentation of assessment data and diagnoses. **J Gerontol Nurs 20:**37-45, 1994

10. General Accounting Office: **Elder Abuse: Effectiveness of Reporting Laws and Other Factors**. Washington, DC: US Government Printing Office, 1991 (HRD-91-74)

11. Grafstrom M, Nordberg A, Winblad B: Abuse is in the eye of the beholder. Report by family members about abuse of demented persons in home care. A total population-based study. **Scand J Soc Med 21:** 247-255, 1993

12. Greenberg EM: Violence and the older adult: the role of the acute care nurse practitioner. **Crit Care Nurs Q 19:**76-84, 1996

13. Hazzard WR: Elder abuse: definitions and implications for medical education. **Acad Med 70:**979-981, 1995

14. Hoepfer M: Becoming an advocate for the elderly. **Pa Med 98:**24-26, 1995

15. Homer AC, Gillcard AC: Abuse of elderly people by their caregivers. **Br Med J 301:**1359-1362, 1990

16. Hydle I: Abuse and neglect of the elderly—a Nordic perspective report from a Nordic research project. **Scand J Soc Med 21:**126-128, 1993

17. Jones J, Dougherty J, Schelble D: Emergency department protocol for the diagnosis and evaluation of geriatric abuse. **Ann Emerg Med 17:**1006-1015, 1988

18. Jones JS: Geriatric abuse and neglect, in Bosker G, Schwartz TR, Jones JS (eds): **Geriatric Emergency Medicine**. St Louis, Mo: CV Mosby, 1990, pp 533-542

19. Lachs MS, Fulmer T: Recognizing elder abuse and neglect. **Clin Geriatr Med 9:**665-681, 1993

20. Lachs MS, Pillemer K: Abuse and neglect of elderly persons. **N Engl J Med 332:**437-443, 1995

21. Lett JE: Abuse of the elderly. **J Fla Med Assoc 82:** 675-678, 1995

22. Mackel CL, Sheehy CM, Badger TA: The challenge of detection and management of alcohol abuse among elders. **Clin Nurse Spec 8:**128-135, 1994

23. Moon A, Williams O: Perceptions of elder abuse and help-seeking patterns among African-American, Caucasian American, and Korean-American elderly women. **Gerontologist 33:**386-395, 1993

24. Nelson HW, Huber R, Walter KL: The relationship between volunteer long-term care ombudsmen and regulatory nursing home actions. **Gerontologist 35:** 509-514, 1995

25. Ogg J, Bennett G: Elder abuse in Britain. **Br Med J 305:**988-989, 1992

26. O'Malley TA, Everitt DE, O'Malley HC, et al: Identifying and preventing family-mediated abuse and neglect of elderly persons. **Ann Intern Med 98:** 998-1005, 1983

27. Palincsar J, Cobb DC: The physician's role in detecting and reporting elder abuse. **J Legal Med 3:** 413-441, 1982

28. Paris BCE, Meier DE, Goldstein T, et al: Elder abuse and neglect: how to recognize warning signs and intervene. **Geriatrics 50**(4):47-51, 1995

29. Paveza GJ, Cohen D, Eisdorfer C, et al: Severe family violence and Alzheimer's disease: prevalence and risk factors. **Gerontologist 32:**493-497, 1992

30. Pfeiffer E: A short portable mental status questionnaire for the assessment of organic brain deficit in elderly patients. **J Am Geriatr Soc 23:**433-441, 1975

31. Phillips LR: Abuse and neglect of the frail elderly at home: an exploration of theoretical relationships. **J Adv Nursing 8:**379-392, 1983

32. Pillemer K: The dangers of dependency: new findings on domestic violence against the elderly. **Social Problems 33:**146, 1985

33. Pillemer K, Finkelhor D: Causes of elder abuse: caregiver stress versus problem relatives. **Am J Orthopsychiatry 59:**179-187, 1989

34. Pillemer K, Finkelhor D: The prevalence of elder abuse: a random sample survey. **Gerontologist 28:** 51-57, 1988

35. Pillemer K, Hudson B: A model abuse prevention program for nursing assistants. **Gerontologist 33:** 128-131, 1993

36. Pillemer K, Suitor JJ: Violence and violent feelings: what causes them among family caregivers? **J Gerontol 47:**S165-S172, 1992

37. Podkieks E: National survey on abuse of the elderly in Canada. **J Elder Abuse Neglect 4:**5, 1992

38. Pollick M: Abuse of the elderly: a review. **Holistic Nursing Practices 7:**43, 1993

39. Rathbone-McCuan E, Voyles D: Case detection of abused elderly parents. **Am J Psychiatry 139:**189, 1992

40. Reis M, Nahmiash D: When seniors are abused: an intervention model. **Gerontologist 35:**666-671, 1995

41. Rosenblatt DE, Cho KH, Durance PW: Reporting mistreatment of older adults: the role of physicians. **J Am Geriatr Soc 44:**65-70, 1996

42. Saveman BI, Hallberg IR, Norberg A, et al: Patterns of abuse of the elderly in their own homes as reported by district nurses. **Scand J Prim Health Care 11:** 111-116, 1993

43. Steiner RP, Vansickle K, Lippmann SB: Domestic violence. Do you know when and how to intervene? **Postgrad Med 100:**103-106, 111-114, 116, 1996

44. US House of Representatives Select Committee on Aging: **Elder Abuse: A National Disgrace**. Washington DC: US Government Printing Office, 1985 (Report by the Subcommittee on Health and Long Term Care Committee, Publication 99-502)

45. Vida S: An update on elder abuse and neglect. **Can J Psychiatry 39 (Suppl 1):**S34-S40, 1994

46. Wolf RS: Perpetrators of elder abuse, in Ammerman RT, Hersenn EDS (eds): **Treatment of Family Violence: A Source Book**. New York, NY: John Wiley & Sons, 1990, 310 pp

47. Wolf RS, Pillemer K: What's new in elder abuse programming? Four bright ideas. **Gerontologist 34:** 126-129, 1994

CHAPTER 12

VIOLENCE, PART A: AN OVERVIEW

HOWARD H. KAUFMAN, MD

Violence leading to injury, either of unintentional or intentional origin (i.e., due to physical agents, namely accident, suicide, and homicide), results in a subset of patients of legal interest. The agents of violence include mechanical energy, heat, electricity, and chemicals. It has been pointed out that the subject of violence can be covered in many ways besides intent and agent, including population at risk (e.g., age, sex, and race), type of injury (e.g., head, spine, and sexual assault), activity/setting (e.g., work, home, recreation, and type of vehicle), type of community by size or geographic location, and relation of the individual in interpersonal violence (e.g., child, spouse, and elder). In the United States, one out of four people seeks medical help for injuries each year, over two million are hospitalized, and about 150,000 die. The causes of injuries with varying severity are indicated in Figure 1.

Of note is that the Centers for Disease Control (CDC) was assigned injuries as a major focus in 1977 after it was determined that three of the five leading causes of premature death were accident, suicide, and homicide. Injuries gradually became the central locus for federal activities which are now centered in the National Center for Injury Prevention and Control (established in 1992) for nonoccupational injuries and in the National Institute for Occupa-

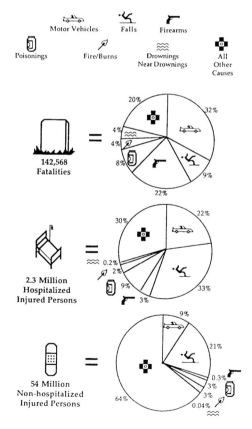

Figure 1: Leading causes of injury in fatalities, hospitalized injured persons, and nonhospitalized injured persons in the United States. (Reproduced from *Cost of Injury in the United States: A Report to Congress.*[39])

tional Safety and Health for occupational injuries. A short review of the history leading to the present coordinated federal effort is available from the CDC.

There is a vast amount of information available concerning injuries to humans, including the epidemiology of injury, theories regarding why they occur, plans aimed at prevention of injuries, and ideas concerning what further data are required to better understand injuries. A main repository for data is the National Center for Health Statistics in the CDC. Important summaries of this information are published in the *Morbidity and Mortality Weekly Report*, and data of general interest are published secondarily in the *Journal of the American Medical Association*. The Fatal Accident Reporting System of the Department of Transportation is another important source. There is also the Uniform Crime Reporting System of the Federal Bureau of Investigation, the National Crime Survey of the Bureau of Justice,[38,40] as well as National Health Interview Survey, the National Hospital Discharge Survey, the National Accident Sampling System, the National Electronic Injury Surveillance System, the National Survey of Catastrophic Sports Injury, and the Survey of Occupational Injuries and Illnesses. An excellent summary of this and other information is *The Injury Fact Book*.[2] The current problems in data collection have been reviewed.[38,42]

A comprehensive review of the literature is impossible here, but a few books which are of particular import and are a comprehensive source of information are listed in the Appendix to this chapter. Most of these books reflect the growing federal commitment to this problem. A great deal of information is available about child abuse, including childhood sexual abuse,[10,12, 13,17,30] violence against women, including rape and intimate partner violence (and notably against pregnant women),[9,12] and elder abuse.[43] Socioeconomic problems are clearly a major cause, with the poor and minorities being affected disproportionately, particularly the young in those groups. Neurological and psychiatric disease may predispose to violence.[15] Alcohol and guns are contributing factors, as is exposure to violence on television and in movies.[1,7,8,11,18, 25,27,31,44]

The magnitude of this problem is reflected

by the numbers of deaths, the total numbers of individuals affected, the years of potential life lost, and the costs both direct and indirect. Those trying to help also may be affected. Among those who may be injured in the line of duty are law enforcement officers as well as physicians.[14,19,37]

INJURIES AND DEATHS

The data available from the CDC reveal that accidents, suicide, and homicide are among the leading 10 causes of death in the United States (Table 1). Accidents result in 5.8% of deaths (3.1% motor-vehicle accidents and 2.7% other accidents, especially falls). Violence or injury to oneself or others is also common: suicides constitute 2.2% of deaths, and homicides 2.0%. When taken together, these three represent the third most common cause of death (10.0%), claiming 217,561 lives in 1992. In terms of all injuries in 1986, 74% were due to mechanical energy, including 31% to motor vehicles, 22% to firearms, and 9% to falls.[2] It must be noted that injuries are the leading cause of loss of life in persons under the age of 44, and thus a terrible problem in terms of lost potential and productivity for the individual, the family, and society (Figure 2). The death rates due to injury are even higher among the elderly (Figure 3), although even more die of other causes.

Simple secondary analyses, looking at gender and age, reveal how important the problem is in each group, and we can consider the reasons and therefore ways to prevent these injuries. For example, one-half of deaths in children are due to unintentional injuries and half of these are due to motor-vehicle accidents. Many deaths are related to the inability of children to appreciate or avoid harm. Youths and members of minorities are at particular risk for death due to violence.[32] Deaths in adolescent and young adult males are frequently related to risk-taking behavior and the use of alcohol. Deaths in the elderly are often related to physical problems which impair the ability to recognize, avoid, and withstand trauma.

A large percentage of murders involve crimes of passion against friends and acquaintances. Many murders and suicides are related to alco-

TABLE 1

Ten Leading Causes of Death in the United States*

	Rate/100,000	Number	Percent
Heart disease	144.3		
Cancer	133.1		
Brain disease	26.2		
Chronic lung disease	19.9		
Accidents	29.5	126,186	5.8
Motor vehicle	15.8	67,444	3.1
Other	13.7	58,742	2.7
Pneumonia and influenza	12.7		
Diabetes	11.9		
Human immunodefiency virus	11.6		
Suicide	11.1	47,863	2.2
Homicide	10.5	43,512	2.0
Total Accidents, Suicide, and Homicide		217,561	10.0

* Data from 1992. Total number of deaths 2,175,613.

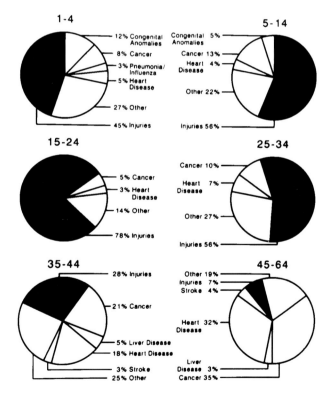

Figure 2: Percentage of deaths due to injury and other causes by age in the United States, 1987. (Reproduced with permission from Baker SP, O'Neill B, Ginsburg MJ, et al: *The Injury Fact Book.* 2nd ed. New York, NY: Oxford University Press, 1992)

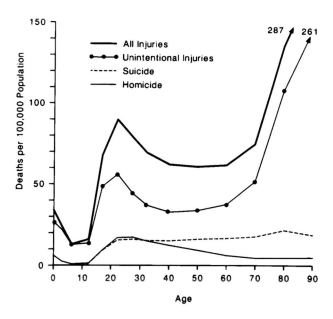

Figure 3: Number of deaths in a population of 100,000 due to various manners of injury by age in the United States, 1986. (Reproduced with permission from Baker SP, O'Neill B, Ginsburg MJ, et al: *The Injury Fact Book.* 2nd ed. New York, NY: Oxford University Press, 1992)

hol and firearms. Alcohol is a contributing factor in over one-half of motor-vehicle accidents. Firearms are involved in more than 60% of suicides and more than 60% of homicides.

Nonfatal Injuries

For every death, there are many nonfatal injuries. Nonfatal assaults and suicide attempts may outnumber homicides and suicides by a ratio of 100 to 1. For a variety of reasons, far less is known about the number of nonfatal injuries. First, there is often no defined threshold to determine when an injury becomes significant, and many minor injuries (even those causing some problems) are never reported. In fact, a particularly stoic individual may not visit a physician and may continue to work or participate in sports after a fairly significant injury. On the other hand, other individuals may exaggerate the impact of a trivial injury and are the bane of state workers' compensation programs. Also, the individual may not recognize the significance of an injury (as in the case of a minor closed head injury) or may be unwilling to report an injury because of shame or fright (as in the case of rape or assault) or because of self-interest (as in the case of assault by a parent). If the law is not specific, police have discretion about whether or not to file a report. Random surveys most likely do not capture all injuries. Problems encountered in obtaining information about domestic assaults, bias crimes, sexual assaults, and assaults on children have also been detailed.[38]

Many interesting statistics are available. In 1987, injuries led to 114 million physician contacts (second highest cause) and 2.8 million hospitalizations, almost one-tenth of acute care admissions (fourth highest cause). The most common injury leading to hospital admission is hip fracture (254,000 a year). In 1989, there were four to five million injuries in motor-vehicle accidents, of which 500,000 resulted in hospital admission.[2] In 1990, of 19 million crimes, about six million involved violence, although in only one-half was medical care required; 4% led to a hospital stay and >1% resulted in death. Of the 1.3 million crimes committed against individuals each year, almost one-fourth involve firearms. In 1985, there were 236,000 nonfatal firearm injuries, of which 65,000 resulted in hospital admission. For every completed suicide, there are 25 suicide attempts (750,000 a year).[41] Each year, one out of every 50 workers suffers a back injury. In 1990, occupational injuries resulted in 2.9 million work days lost.[45] Football, basketball, and baseball each result in over 400,000 emergency room visits a year.

Domestic violence involves wives, children, and siblings. Between 4% and 10% of spouses undergo abuse each year. One-half of all those beaten are injured significantly, and one-half of these seek medical care. Violence against women leads to 39,000 physician visits, 39,000 emergency room visits, 21,000 hospitalizations, and 100,000 hospital days a year.[28] There are 87,000 rapes reported each year. In the mid-1980s there were approximately 1,584,700 cases of child abuse and neglect and 155,900 cases of child sexual abuse each year. Serious harm occurs annually to more than 160,000 children.[38] Over one million elderly (>65 years) are subject to abuse each year. Schools are dangerous—with an average of one-quarter of students in grades 9 through 12 carrying guns and one-quarter being involved in a fight each year.

COSTS OF VIOLENCE

Another index of the magnitude of violence is its cost. The total cost includes the direct cost of both acute and long-term care, as well as the indirect cost of lost productivity. In a report produced for the United States Congress in 1989, the total "lifetime cost" of all injuries that occurred in 1985 was estimated at $158 billion. This included $2.6 billion for emergency room care and $2.5 billion for nursing home care. Motor-vehicle injuries led to costs of $48 billion, while the total lifetime cost of falls was $37 billion. Lifetime costs due to death from all injuries were four times greater than those for cancer and six times greater than those for cardiovascular disease, the latter being problems of older people.[39] The annual cost of intentional violence to oneself or others has been estimated at $60 billion. Suicides, both attempted and completed, were believed to have an annual cost of $3.19 billion in 1989. The cost of gunshot wounds in 1988 was estimated at $14.4 billion,[28]

TABLE 2
YEARS OF POTENTIAL LIFE LOST BEFORE AGE 65 YEARS*

	Percent all YPLL-65	Number
Unintentional injury	17.8	2,150,815
Malignant neoplasms	15.2	
Intentional injury	12.6	1,522,487
Heart disease	11.2	
Congenital anomalies	5.3	
Other	<15	

* Data from 1990. Total number of injuries 12,083,228.

although many estimate this cost to be many times higher. Given the inflation in the general economy and the even higher inflation in medical costs, obviously these costs would be much higher today.

One estimate of costs in the 1990s for nonfatal crimes to an individual includes $16,500 for assault, $19,200 for robbery, and $54,100 for rape.[38] High-risk behavior is associated with the occurrence of traumatic injury, and both occur in people who do not have health insurance and whose care is paid for disproportionally by public funds.[29]

One way of looking at the cost of injuries is to examine the years of potential life lost for people aged less than 65 years (YPLL-65), the usual working years. In 1989 and 1990, unintentional injury (17.8%) was the leading cause of YPLL-65 and intentional injury (12.6%) was the third leading cause.[6] Together they constitute 30.4% of years of life lost (Table 2). Of note, almost 30% of all deaths occurred in those less than 65 years old.

TRENDS

Suicide rates are rising, although only slightly, and the increase has been seen among the young (especially black males) and among elderly males; suicides via firearms account for the increase.[22] The number of deaths due to injury have decreased and could be even lower if preventative measures such as the use of seat-

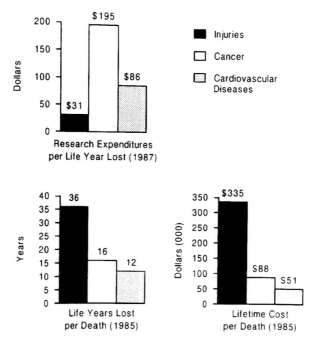

Figure 4: Amount of research expenditures (1987), the number of life years lost (1985), and the lifetime cost (1985) per death due to injury, cancer, and cardiovascular diseases. (Reproduced with permission from Baker SP, O'Neill B, Ginsburg MJ, et al: *The Injury Fact Book.* 2nd ed. New York, NY: Oxford University Press, 1992)

belts and the installation of airbags into automobiles were universal.[24]

In 1994, the number of violent crimes reported dropped by 4%.[26] The incidence of homicide decreased by 12% in the first six months of 1995,[33] a particularly striking finding in several American cities such as New York, Chicago, New Orleans, Washington, St. Louis, and Seattle. Some have attributed the decrease to strict enforcement of gun control laws. However, for some subgroups, especially young males, there has been an increase in the number of violent crimes, probably due to the diffusion of guns and drugs. Such murders are often connected to gang-related activities and are carried out with semiautomatic hand guns, as has been the case in such locales as Los Angeles.[4,21] More deaths occur from firearms than because of motor-vehicle accidents in eight states and the District of Columbia; if this trend continues, this will be true for the entire nation by 2001.[23]

RESEARCH AND FUNDING

A report published in 1989 indicated that the total federal research expenditures directed at injuries in 1985 were $160 million. This sum is inadequate and is not in proportion to the impact that injuries have on years of life lost per death and lifetime costs per death (Figure 4).

Haddon has suggested 10 basic strategies to prevent injuries:[38]

1. Prevent the creation of the hazard.
2. Reduce the amount of the hazard.
3. Prevent the release of the hazard.
4. Modify the rate or special distribution of the hazard.
5. Separate people in time or space from the hazard.
6. Interpose a material as a barrier to the hazard.
7. Modify the basic qualities of the hazard.
8. Make the person more resistant.

9. Prevent further damage.
10. Stabilize, repair, and rehabilitate the injured person.

The National Research Council of the National Academy of Science has discussed the expenditures of money dedicated to research on violence, noting its small amount ($20 million in 1989), the diffusion among various agencies, and the difficulties in coordination; brief funding periods are also of concern.[38] The report suggested the need to increase funding of research toward the understanding of how individuals develop a propensity for violence, the circumstances that are conducive to violent events, and the social processes that foster violence. Their report proposes that short-term and long-term efforts include the following:

1. Problem-solving initiatives in six specific areas:
   a) biological and psychological development;
   b) improve local environments;
   c) disrupt illegal markets for drugs and firearms;
   d) alter the nature and use of drugs and firearms;
   e) sociological interventions (e.g., gangs, bias, and problem communities); and
   f) decrease partner abuse.
2. Improve statistical information systems.
3. New and integrated research on the macrosocial, psychosocial, and neurobiological causes of violence, including:
   a) effect of different weapons on crime;
   b) medications to treat violence; and
   c) violence by custodians against wards.
4. A pilot multicommunity prospective program to collect information about and test prevention strategies using a birth cohort and a cohort of 8-year-old children.

PHYSICIAN RESPONSIBILITIES

The physician must recognize an injury, particularly an intentional one. This requires training and a high incidence of suspicion. A number of articles review the historical and physical evidence of various types of violence.[9,12,13,20,30,34,43]

Treatment, particularly in severe injury, requires specialized centers, whose effectiveness is well demonstrated[35,42] although improvements in care are still possible.[3] After treating the injury, the physician must try to prevent it from happening again. For certain classes of people, the response is prescribed. It is mandatory in all states to report abuse of children and of elderly or disabled persons to protective services or law enforcement agencies,[5] although this also requires long-term intervention to be effective.[16] However, incidents involving competent adults (unless weapons are involved) generally should not be reported because of the ethical and legal principles of confidentiality and informed consent which in a practical sense are required in order to encourage the patient to trust and therefore communicate with the physician.[9] But the physician must secure that trust and try to convince the patient to take proper action for self protection.

Issues concerning recording data and preserving evidence will be dealt with elsewhere. Briefly, all relevant information about the incident must be elicited and recorded. Evidence (e.g., clothing or surgical specimens) must be properly obtained, preserved, and kept in a chain of custody so that it can be produced later. One must also be prepared to testify about the evidence if required.

PREVENTION

Obviously, the major thrust should be prevention. It is encouraging that since 1979, death due to all accidents has decreased by 31.5% (motor-vehicle accidents 31.9% decrease, other accidents 30.1% decrease) and death due to suicides has decreased by 5.1%. (However, death due to homicide has increased by 2.9%.) In fact, since 1930 death due to motor-vehicle accidents has decreased more than 80% if one considers the rate per mile driven[2] (Figure 5). This has been attributed to an approach encompassing multiple risk factors, including improved road design, improved car design, driver education, raising the legal drinking age for alcohol, lowering speed limits, and imposing seatbelt laws, as well as enforcement of all laws. The salutary effect of this multifactorial approach has been used as a model for designing solutions to the

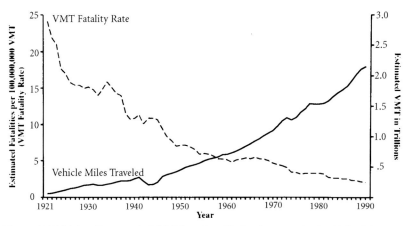

Figure 5: Vehicle miles traveled (VMT) and traffic fatality rates in the United States, 1921-1990. (Reproduced from *Injury Control in the 1990s: A National Plan for Action.*[45])

problems of suicide and homicide.

The need to focus on suicide and homicide is clear, as is highlighted in the foreword of a recent American Medical Association publication on violence:

> A picture of American society is emerging, and it is at once both horrifying and numbing. So much so that we have been unable to stop it. We have become a society at war with itself, a nation at the mercy of a savage beast–violence. . . .
>
> In an attempt to increase public and professional attention to violence, the editors of *JAMA, American Medical News,* and the American Medical Association's nine specialty journals published numerous articles on violence between January and June 1992. The best of these articles . . . are collected in this compendium. . . .
>
> A pervasive, deceptive force, such violence destroys the basic, human foundation of our society and is best characterized with numbers:
> • Homicide is the third leading cause of death among 15-24 year olds and the leading cause of death among 15-24 year old black males. The homicide rates for children and adolescents have more than doubled in the last 30 years.
> • More than 1.5 million individuals in our country are victims of assault each year, and more than 650,000 women are victims of rape.
> • 1.8 million women are beaten by their male partners each year, and 8% to 11% of pregnant women report being physically assaulted

> during pregnancy.
> • Two to four million of our children were abused or neglected in 1991, and more than 1 million elderly were mistreated last year.
>
> . . . The situation is unacceptable. Prior solutions have not succeeded. New approaches are required.
>
> We must demand unprecedented support for additional research into the causes, prevention, and treatments, for both victims and perpetrators, of all forms of violence. We need to recognize and treat violence as more than just a social aberrancy—it is a social disease. We need to educate everyone—physicians, nurses, other health professionals, students, politicians, and the public at large—about what is now known and what can now be done to address this emergency.[28]

Because violence is a health problem, because physicians know about this problem, and because we have a professional responsibility to society as a whole, physicians should also be motivated to become activists and leaders in the movement to prevent violence.[36,41]

REFERENCES

1. Adelson L: The gun and the sanctity of human life; or the bullet as pathogen. **Arch Surg 127:**659-664, 1992
2. Baker SP, O'Neill B, Ginsburg MJ, et al: **The Injury Fact Book.** 2nd ed. New York, NY: Oxford University Press, 1992, 344 pp
3. Bazzoli GJ, Madura KJ, Cooper GF, et al: Progress in the development of trauma systems in the United

States. Results of a national survey. **JAMA 273:** 395-401, 1995

4. Blumstein A: Violence by young people: why the deadly nexus? **Natl Inst Justice J.** Aug 1995, pp 2-9

5. Brewer RA, Jones JS: Reporting elder abuse: limitations of statutes. **Ann Emerg Med 18:**1217-1221, 1989

6. Centers for Disease Control: Current trends: years of potential life lost before ages 65 and 85—United States, 1989–1990. **JAMA 267:**2727, 1992

7. Centerwall BS: Television and violence. The scale of the problem and where to go from here. **JAMA 267:** 3059-3063, 1992

8. Centerwall BS: TV: the message is mayhem. **1995 Medical and Health Annual. Encyclopedia Brittanica.** Chicago, Ill: Encyclopedia Brittanica, 1994, pp 94-99

9. Council on Ethical and Judicial Affairs, American Medical Association: Physicians and domestic violence. Ethical considerations. **JAMA 267:**3190-3193, 1992

10. Council on Scientific Affairs, American Medical Association: Adolescents as Victims of Family Violence. **JAMA 270:**1850-1856, 1993

11. Council on Scientific Affairs, American Medical Association: Assault weapons as a public health hazard in the United States. **JAMA 267:**3067-3070, 1992

12. Council on Scientific Affairs, American Medical Association: Violence against women. Relevance for medical practitioners. **JAMA 267:**3184-3189, 1992

13. Dubowitz H, Black M, Harrington D: The diagnosis of child sexual abuse. **AJDC 146:**688-693, 1992

14. Eichelman BS, Hartwig AC: **Patient Violence and the Clinician.** Washington, DC: American Psychiatric Press, 1995

15. Elliott FA: Violence. The neurologic contribution: an overview. **Arch Neurol 49:**595-603, 1992

16. Faller KC: Unanticipated problems in the United States child protection system. **Child Abuse Negl 9:** 63-69, 1985

17. Fulginiti VA: Violence and children in the United States. **AJDC 146:**671-672, 1992 (Editorial)

18. Gellert GA: Violence: America's deadliest epidemic. **1995 Medical and Health Annual. Encyclopedia Brittanica.** Chicago, Ill: Encyclopedia Brittanica, 1994, pp 70-73

19. Goodman RA, Jenkins L, Mercy JA: Workplace-related homicide among health care workers in the United States, 1980 through 1990. **JAMA 272:** 1686-1688, 1994

20. Hampton HL: Care of the woman who has been raped. **N Engl J Med 332:**234-237, 1995

21. Hutson HR, Anglin D, Kyriacou DN, et al: The epidemic of gang-related homicides in Los Angeles County from 1979 through 1994. **JAMA 274:** 1031-1036, 1995

22. Kachur SP, Potter LB, James SP, et al: **Suicide in the United States 1980-1992.** Atlanta, Ga: National Center for Injury Prevention and Control, 1995, 50 pp

23. Kent C: Fate hinges on money, politics. CDC injury prevention center caught up in controversy over gun control. **Am Med News.** June 26, 1995, pp 3, 24, 25, 27

24. Kent C: Report: seat belts, helmets save lives and health costs. **Am Med News.** Mar 4, 1996

25. Koop CE, Lundberg GD: Violence in America. A public health emergency. Time to bite the bullet back.

JAMA 267:3075-3076, 1992

26. Law, crime and law enforcement: Crime. **1996 Book of the Year. Encyclopedia Brittanica.** Chicago, Ill: Encyclopedia Brittanica, 1996, p 213

27. Loftin C, McDowall D, Wiersema B, et al: Effects of restrictive licensing of handguns on homicide and suicide in the District of Columbia. **N Engl J Med 325:**1615-1620, 1991

28. Lundberg GD, Young RK, Flanagin A, et al (eds): **Violence. A Compendium for JAMA, American Medical News, and the Specialty Journals of the American Medical Association.** Chicago, Ill: American Medical Association, 1992, 434 pp

29. Mackersie RC, Davis JW, Hoyt DB, et al: High-risk behavior and the public burden for funding the costs of acute injury. **Arch Surg 130:**844-851, 1995

30. Marcus DM, Albert DM: Recognizing child abuse. **Arch Ophthalmol 110:**766-768, 1992

31. Marzuk PM, Leon AC, Tardiff K, et al: The effect of access to lethal methods of injury on suicide rates. **Arch Gen Psychiatry 49:**451-458, 1992

32. Mason J, Proctor R: Reducing youth violence—the physician's role. **JAMA 267:**3003, 1992

33. Mathis D: Murders drop 12%, sharpest fall in 35 years. **USA TODAY.** Dec 18 1995, p 1A

34. Moy JA, Sanchez MR: The cutaneous manifestations of violence and poverty. **Arch Dermatol 128:**829-839, 1992

35. Norwood S, Fernandez L, Roettger R: The early effects of implementing ACS level II criteria on transfer and survival rates at a rurally-based community hospital. 54th Annual Meeting of the American Association for the Surgery of Trauma, San Diego, Calif. Sept 29-Oct 1, 1994

36. Novello AC, Shosky J, Froehlke R: A medical response to violence. **JAMA 267:**3007, 1992

37. Paola F, Malik T, Qureshi A: Violence against physicians. **J Gen Intern Med 9:**503-506, 1994

38. Reiss AJ Jr, Roth JA (eds): **Understanding and Preventing Violence.** Washington, DC: National Academy Press, 1993

39. Rice DP, MacKenzie EJ, and Associates: **Cost of Injury in the United States: A Report to Congress.** San Francisco, Calif: Institute for Health and Aging, University of California and Injury Prevention Center, The Johns Hopkins University, 1989

40. Rosenberg M, Fenley MA: **Violence in America. A Public Health Approach.** New York, NY: Oxford University Press, 1991

41. Rosenberg ML, O'Carroll PW, Powell KE: Let's be clear. Violence is a public health problem. **JAMA 267:** 3071-3072, 1992

42. Sampalis JS, Tamim H, Lavoie A, et al: Trauma center designation: initial impact on trauma related mortality. 54th Annual Meeting of the American Association for the Surgery of Trauma, San Diego, Calif. Sept 29-Oct 1, 1994

43. Skelly FJ: When the golden years are tarnished. **Am Med News 35:**159-160, 1992

44. Teret SP, Wintemute GJ, Beolenson PL: The firearm fatality reporting system. A proposal. **JAMA 267:** 3073-3074, 1992

45. Waxweiler RJ, Rosenberg ML, Fenley MA (coordinators): **Injury Control in the 1990s: A National Plan for Action.** Des Plaines, Ill: Association for the Advancement of Automotive Medicine, 1993

APPENDIX

COMPREHENSIVE SOURCES OF INFORMATION
CONCERNING INJURIES AND VIOLENCE

Committee on Trauma Research: **Injury in America**. Washington, DC: National Academy Press, 1985, 164 pp. (From the National Academy of Sciences. The beginning of the modern effort in injury prevention. Injury, both intentional and unintentional, is a major unaddressed public health issue. Need coordinated program administered by one federal agency.)

Committee to Review the Status and Progress of the Injury Control Program at the Centers for Disease Control: **Injury Control: A Review of the Status and Progress of the Injury Control Program at the Centers for Disease Control.** Washington, DC: National Academic Press, 1988, 73 pp. (From National Academy of Sciences. Review of the first two years of activities. Suggested improvements, increased funding, need for specific center.)

Lundberg GD, Young RK, Flanagin A, et al (eds): **Violence. A Compendium for JAMA, American Medical News, and the Specialty Journals of the American Medical Association.** Chicago, Ill: American Medical Association, 1992, 434 pp. (Best of articles published January to June in AMA journals. Excellent and extensive primary source material.)

McGinnis JM, Richmond JB, Brandt EN Jr, et al: Health progress in the United States. Results of the 1990 objectives for the nation. **JAMA 268**:2545-2552, 1992. (By several former and current senior federal officials. Discussion of monitoring of the 1979 blueprint, 226 objectives with reference to interim reports and how they varied from hoped-for results. Discussion of development of **Healthy People 2000** with 300 objectives in 22 areas including alcohol, violent and abusive behavior, unintentional injuries, and occupational safety and health.)

National Committee for Injury Prevention and Control: **Injury Prevention: Meeting the Challenge.** New York, NY: Oxford University Press, 1989, 303 pp. (A voluntary committee of 31 experts funded by federal support. Published as a supplement to the **American Journal of Preventive Medicine**. A discussion of how to detect and analyze a problem, how to develop a prevention program, and how to best care for injured people. Specific recommendations for different types of problems. Includes discussion of current knowledge, how to use it to prevent injuries, and what new data are needed.)

Reiss AJ Jr, Roth JA (eds): **Understanding and Preventing Violence**. Washington, DC: National Academy Press, 1993. (From the National Research Council of the National Academy of Sciences. Comprehensive.)

Rice DP, MacKenzie EJ, and Associates: **Cost of Injury in the United States: A Report to Congress.** San Francisco, Calif: Institute for Health and Aging, University of California and Injury Prevention Center. The Johns Hopkins University, 1989, 282 pp. (A follow-up of **Injury in America** and **Injury Control: A Review of the Status and Progress of the Injury Control Program at the Centers for Disease Control.** A description of the incidence and cost of injuries, sources of payment, possible savings from prevention programs, willingness to pay for this, need for data, and research needed in treatment and rehabilitation.)

Rosenberg M, Fenley MA: **Violence in America. A Public Health Approach.** New York, NY: Oxford University Press, 1991. (By a senior Centers for Disease Control official. Overview of assault, rape, child abuse, spousal abuse, elder abuse, suicide. Need for multidisciplinary and public health approach to control.)

APPENDIX (cont'd)

COMPREHENSIVE SOURCES OF INFORMATION
CONCERNING INJURIES AND VIOLENCE

US Health and Human Services, Public Health Service: **Healthy People. The Surgeon General's Report on Health Promotion and Disease Prevention**. Washington, DC: US Department of Health and Human Services, 1979. (The beginning of a national health strategy to prevent unnecessary health problems.)

US Health and Human Services, Public Health Service: **Healthy People 2000. National Health Promotion and Disease Prevention Objectives**. Washington, DC: US Government Printing Office, 1992, 153 pp. (22 priority areas for health states, risk reduction, services, and protection for the decade. 300 national organizations, all state health departments, the Institute of Medicine, and a total of 10,000 people contributed to this report.)

US Public Health Service: **Promoting Health/Preventing Disease: Objectives for the Nation**. Washington, DC: US Department of Health and Human Services, 1980. (A proposal for the next 10 years. 15 priorities, 220 objectives; many deal with violence.)

Waxweiler RJ, Rosenberg ML, Fenley MA (coordinators): **Injury Control in the 1990s: A National Plan for Action**. Des Plaines, Ill: Association for the Advancement of Automotive Medicine, 1993, 62 pp. (From the Third National Injury Control Conference. Contributions by many public and private organizations including several federal agencies. Linked to **Healthy People 2000** objectives. 22 recommendations for the next 10 years. Emphasis on improved data collection, research, promotion of known effective interventions.)

CHAPTER 12

Violence, Part B: Assault and Homicide

Howard H. Kaufman, MD

Interpersonal violence, namely assault and its most extreme outcome, homicide, is pervasive in our society. On the average day, 65 people die and 6,000 people are injured by interpersonal violence.[9] Annual costs at the end of the 1980s were $34 billion for care and support and $145 billion for lost quality of life.[9]

There are four legal categories of nonfatal assaultive violence: simple assault, aggravated assault, robbery, and rape. Figures regarding these crimes are not comprehensive, and estimates vary from year to year. It was said that in 1986, of 6.6 million victims of violent crimes, 80% were involved in assaults and 18% in robberies (32% of the victims were injured). An additional 2% were rape victims, all of whom were considered injured. Of all victims, 8% were hospitalized. Violence led to billions of dollars in costs, including direct losses and losses in productivity (millions of days of useful life lost each year) and non-monetary losses such as emotional distress.[10] Also in 1986, approximately 20,000 homicides occurred.[14] The figures for other years are not too different. For example, in 1990 the relative incidence of violent crimes included simple assault in 50%, aggravated assault in 30%, robbery in 20%, rape in 2%, and homicide in 0.4%. Injury occurred in 20% of simple assaults and in 13% of aggravated assaults. Homicide occurred in 0.8% of assaults with injury, 0.2% of robberies, and 0.2% of rapes.[13] The highest incidence of offenders and victims occurs in poverty-stricken persons between the ages of 12 and 24 years.[9]

From 1992 to 1994, the number of crimes decreased each year. In 1994, the incidence of robberies was down 5% and murders down 6%. Murders of those aged 25 years and over were down 25% over about a decade. However, murders for this period were up 65% for those aged 18-24 years and up 165% for those aged 14-17 years, with the excess being completely contributed by the use of guns and to drug use by nonwhites.[1] With increasing numbers of teenagers expected in the population, these numbers may rise further since teenagers contribute disproportionately to interpersonal violence.[3]

One issue of interest is violence in the workplace, where health care and social service workers are at particular risk. Of one million assaults each year in the workplace, two-thirds involve this group of eight million people. On the other hand, only 20 deaths in the total 1,071 killed at work are attributed to this group. The Occupational Safety and Health Act of 1970 mandated that all employers have a general duty to provide their employees with a workplace free from recognized hazards likely to cause death or serious physical harm. The Occupational Safety and Health Administration has recently issued

TABLE 1

FAMILY VIOLENCE, 1989: VICTIMIZATION RATES BY VICTIM-OFFENDER RELATIONSHIP AND TYPE OF ASSAULT*

Characteristic	Population	Aggravated Assault				Simple Assault			
		Relatives	Well Known	Casual Acquaintances	Strangers	Relatives	Well Known	Casual Acquaintances	Strangers
Sex									
Male	96,875,920	0.3	2.2	1.2	7.4	0.5	3.1	3.0	10.3
Female	104,499,700	0.7	1.2	0.6	2.0	2.6	3.6	1.7	4.1
Race									
White	172,071,010	0.5	1.6	0.9	4.5	1.7	3.4	2.3	7.3
Black	23,378,200	0.4[a]	2.5	1.3	4.9	1.0	3.4	2.5	5.1
Other	5,926,410	0.4[a]	1.6[a]	0[a]	5.0	2.0[a]	2.9	0.7[a]	9.3
Age (years)									
12-15	13,256,460	0.5[a]	4.4	1.6	6.5	1.7	11.2	9.7	14.4
16-19	14,235,270	0.6[a]	4.9	2.6	13.3	1.8	10.7	7.0	17.2
20-24	18,084,190	1.1	3.1	1.8	9.9	3.9	5.6	4.1	15.7
25-34	43,335,460	0.7	1.7	1.2	5.6	2.6	3.4	2.1	9.1
35-49	50,293,180	0.6	1.2	0.5	3.5	1.5	1.9	1.1	4.6
50-64	32,774,300	0.1[a]	0.4[a]	0.2[a]	1.2	0.4[a]	0.7	0.3[a]	2.1
65 and over	29,396,730	0[a]	0.2[a]	0.2[a]	0.6	0.2[a]	0.2[a]	0.1[a]	0.4[a]
Marital status[b]									
Married	110,124,950	0.3	0.8	0.5	2.7	0.8	1.1	1.0	3.5
Widowed	13,407,180	0[a]	0.1[a]	0.6[a]	0.4[a]	0.1[a]	0.4[a]	0.3[a]	0.4[a]
Divorced or separated	18,786,270	2.3	2.5	2.0	5.7	8.6	5.0	1.4	10.4
Never married	58,618,550	0.3	3.5	1.4	8.8	1.2	7.7	5.5	14.2
Family income (annual)[c]									
Less than $7,500	20,425,690	0.7[a]	3.8	1.6	5.5	3.8	6.7	3.1	9.0
$7,500-$9,999	8,374,160	1.0[a]	2.7	0.8[a]	4.0	1.7[a]	6.2	2.5	5.3
$10,000-$14,999	19,790,200	0.6[a]	1.8	1.0	4.8	3.2	3.7	2.5	8.0
$15,000-$24,999	35,690,810	0.5	2.1	1.0	5.1	1.6	4.2	2.7	6.8
$25,000-$29,999	15,302,260	0.4[a]	1.4	1.1	4.5	1.3	3.8	2.2	7.3
$30,000-$49,999	45,673,340	0.4	0.7	0.6	4.2	1.0	2.2	2.0	7.4
$50,000 or more	28,905,330	0.3[a]	1.1	0.6	3.9	0.6	1.3	2.1	5.9

* Rate per 1,000 persons age 12 and over. Reproduced with permission from *Understanding and Preventing Violence*[13] by the National Academy of Sciences. Courtesy of the National Academy Press, Washington, DC.

[a] Estimate is based on about 10 or fewer sample cases.

[b] Excludes data on persons whose marital status was not ascertained.

[c] Excludes data on persons whose family income was not ascertained.

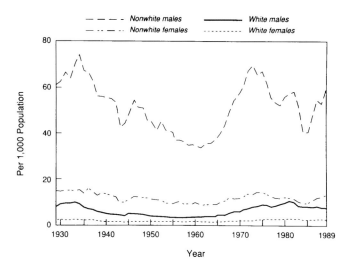

Figure 1: Age-adjusted homicide rates by gender and race in the United States, 1929-1989. (Reproduced with permission from *Understanding and Preventing Violence*[13] by the National Academy of Sciences. Courtesy of the National Academy Press, Washington, DC)

guidelines for controlling violence in the workplace (OSHA 3148-1996).[12]

Data for homicides can be subdivided according to the relationship between victim and offender and the circumstances. Fifteen percent of homicides are intrafamily, 40% involve friends or acquaintances, and 13% involve strangers; in 32%, the relationship is not known (where the relation is not known, it is believed that the parties usually are strangers). About 65% of murders are related to arguments and only 19% to felonies. Murders in families most frequently involve spouses and occur in the home. Murders where the parties are acquainted with each other typically occur in private residences, on the street or in bars, and involve handguns. Murder by strangers most often is associated with robbery and involves firearms. Guns are the agent in 60% of murders, and handguns in three-fourths of these.[11,14]

Fairly detailed statistics about assault have been generated (Table 1). Analysis of race and sex reveals that young nonwhite males, namely blacks and to some extent Hispanics, are at particular risk, and this risk is increasing (Figures 1, 2 and 3). Females are at risk for child sexual abuse, nonfatal rapes, and assaults by intimates. Six percent of severe assaults occur in private homes, and two-thirds are repetitive.

The new National Incident-Based Reporting System of the Federal Bureau of Investigation (FBI) should provide much more comprehensive data on a national level and complement special studies done to date.[15-17] The components that can contribute to violent behavior include biological, psychological, and sociological (cultural, structural, interactionist, and economic) factors. Biological factors range from sex hormones to brain injury. Psychological factors include developmental influences from family and acquaintances. Cultural factors involve influences from a person's wider social group, including glorification of violence on television and in movies and a belief in male dominance and racial discrimination, and are exacerbated by gang activities. Structural factors encompass poverty and lack of opportunity. Interactionist factors involve the evolution of a particular situation as it escalates to violence; the disinhibiting effects of alcohol and drugs are interactionist factors, as is the availability of firearms. The economic factor is profitability of the activity where the anticipated gains outweigh the risks, as in trafficking in guns and drugs, prostitution, and loan sharking.[2,4,5,11,13,14,19]

Experts in the field of violence agree that prevention is the key to reducing the incidence and that this requires a public health approach. It is necessary to gather information and analyze it and then target the problems that lead to vio-

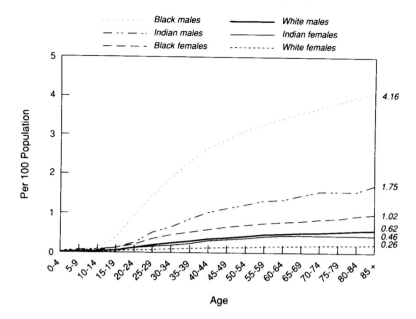

Figure 2: Cumulative homicide rate in 5-year intervals by gender and race in the United States, 1987. (Reproduced with permission from *Understanding and Preventing Violence*[13] by the National Academy of Sciences. Courtesy of the National Academy Press, Washington, DC)

TABLE 2

Comparison of Violence Measurement Systems*

System Characteristic	National Crime Survey	Uniform Crime Reports	National Mortality Statistics
Source	Sample of U.S. households	Incident reports of participating police agencies	Death certificates
Domain	Nonfatal violent victimizations of persons aged 12+	Violent crimes known to police including homicides and violence during crimes against organizations	Homicides
Unit of Count	Most serious victimization during event	Most serious crime during event	Deaths
Timing	Events occurring in 6-month reference period	Collected contemporaneously	Collected contemporaneously
	Published annually with 10- to 12-month lag	Published annually	Published annually, with 2-year time lag
Sources of Discretion/ Error	Respondent recall, construction as victimization, and choice to recount	Victim/witness decision to report to police and discretionary police detection	Medical examiner judgment
	Interviewer judgment	Police determination that crime occurred	
	Agency rules for counting	Counting rules	

* Reproduced with permission from *Understanding and Preventing Violence*[13] by the National Academy of Sciences. Courtesy of the National Academy Press, Washington, DC.

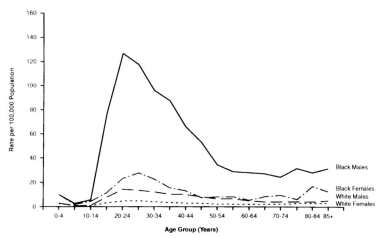

Figure 3: Homicide rates by age, gender, and race in the United States, 1988. (Reproduced from *Injury Control in the 1990s: A National Plan for Action.*[19])

lence. Trials of corrective activities must be instituted and then evaluated and refined. This will require better understanding of the above factors and efforts, ranging from identifying children at risk for injury from violent behavior by adults and improving child rearing to transforming subcultures and society as a whole, an immense undertaking but one justified by the pervasiveness and impact of violence in our society. Specific target levels for decreases in various categories of violence and abusive behavior were proposed in *Healthy People 2000.*[18] The importance of recognizing violence, particularly family violence, and the need for physicians to understand the complexity of the problem were identified during a consensus conference concerning the education of medical students to identify, treat, and help prevent family violence; papers from this conference were published in the November 1995 issue of *Academic Medicine.*

A critical first step is the development of adequate data. Currently, the main sources of information are:

1. The Uniform Reporting System (URS) of the FBI, a voluntary system of 16,000 sources covering 96% of the population. Its reports are available 9-10 months after the end of the year. However, it cannot capture all crimes, many of which are not recorded by the police

or are never reported by the victim, especially because of fear or shame, particularly when the crime occurs within a family. Indeed, four times as many victims are reported by hospitals as are captured in this survey, and in several times more, the victims are either not injured or are not injured seriously enough to go to a hospital. This report is entitled *Crime in the United States* and is published annually.

2. The National Crime Survey (NCS) of the Department of Justice, based on information from 100,000 people in 49,000 households. This survey probably underestimates the extent of victimization because people may not perceive assaults as crimes, may not remember them, or may not report them out of fear or shame (the surveys are not conducted privately). Summaries of the surveys are published annually as *Criminal Victimization in the United States.*

3. The National Center for Health Statistics (NCHS) mortality data, summarizing data from death certificates, which is limited in content. These data are somewhat more detailed than the above, but are not availaable until 2-3 years after the end of the year (Table 2).[14]

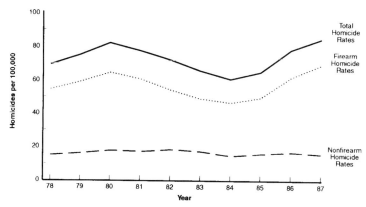

Figure 4: Homicide rates among black males aged 15-24 years, by weapon used in the U.S., 1978-1987. (Reproduced from *Injury Control in the 1990s: A National Plan for Action.*[19])

4. State and local criminal justice and vital statistic systems, child abuse registries, and trauma registries.

5. Violence surveillance by the Centers for Disease Control (CDC), including: surveillance and surveys of nonfatal injuries in the areas of behaviors and risk factors, all injuries, and firearm injuries; surveillance for family and intimate violence; and risk characteristics of injury-related mortality.[8]

There is much more to be done to develop universal and detailed data bases.[19]

Although more analysis of detailed information is needed, there is already sufficient information about age, sex, socioeconomic status, and race of the victims and perpetrators to provide ideas for interventions for discrete subsets of people at many points in the causal chain, and many have been suggested.[13,19] Certain groups are clearly at particular risk and should be targeted. Poor, young, black males in inner cities are at highest risk to be victims and to become offenders.[13,18] Both socioeconomic and cultural factors are likely responsible.[5] Specific aims were built into the numerical objectives of *Healthy People 2000.*[18] Unfortunately, not all are being accomplished.[6,7]

A report published by the CDC-sponsored Third National Injury Control Conference, 1991, suggested that there is an acute need for a "coordinated approach and structure for planning and implementing a comprehensive vio-

lence prevention effort."[19] It suggested four areas of emphasis: 1) firearm injuries, 2) influence of alcohol and drugs, 3) adverse childhood experiences, and 4) treatable mental disorders.

Specific types of violence such as child abuse, spouse abuse, elder abuse, and rape are considered in other parts of this book. Gun control is considered separately since firearms are the instrument of many homicides (and suicides) and appear to be responsible for the increasing incidence of homicide (and suicide) (Figure 4). The literature can be accessed through the National Criminal Justice Service of the U.S. Department of Justice (telephone: 800-851-3420). The American Medical Association has prepared a series of pamphlets which contain background material, information about diagnosis and care, and discussions about legal issues, as well as a directory of other similar materials (Table 3).

REFERENCES

1. Blumstein A, Heinz HJ III: Youth violence, guns and the illicit-drug industry, in Block C, Block R (eds): **Trends, Risks, and Interventions in Lethal Violence: Proceedings of The Third Annual Spring Symposium of the Homicide Research Working Group.** Washington, DC: US Department of Justice, 1995, pp 3-15
2. Buka S, Earls F: Early determinants of delinquency and violence. **Health Affairs** 12:46-64, 1993
3. Butterfield F: Crime trends downward but outlook uncertain. **New York Times.** May 28, 1995
4. Fagan J: Interactions among drugs, alcohol, and vio-

TABLE 3

PAMPHLETS ON INTERPERSONAL VIOLENCE AVAILABLE FROM THE
AMERICAN MEDICAL ASSOCIATION

Diagnostic and Treatment Guidelines in Child Physical Abuse and Neglect. 1994, 26 pp

Diagnostic and Treatment Guidelines in Child Sexual Abuse. 1994, 36 pp

Diagnostic and Treatment Guidelines in Domestic Violence. 1994, 19 pp

Diagnostic and Treatment Guidelines in Elder Abuse and Neglect. 1992, 42 pp

Diagnostic and Treatment Guidelines in Mental Health Effects of Family Violence. 1995, 35 pp

Domestic Violence. A Director of Protocols for Health Care Providers. 1993, 27 pp

Strategies for the Treatment and Prevention of Sexual Assault. 1995, 38 pp

lence. **Health Affairs 12:**65-79, 1993

5. Hawkins DF: Inequality, culture, and interpersonal violence. **Health Affairs 12:**80-95, 1993

6. McGinnis JM, Lee PR: Healthy people 2000 at mid decade. **JAMA 273:**1123-1129, 1995

7. McGinnis JM, Richmond JB, Brandt EN Jr, et al: Health progress in the United States. Results of the 1990 objectives for the nation. **JAMA 268:**2545-2552, 1992

8. Mercy JA: Overview and examples of CDC's violence surveillance activities. Overview of the importance of violence surveillance, in Block C, Block R (eds): **Trends, Risks, and Interventions in Lethal Violence: Proceedings of The Third Annual Spring Symposium of the Homicide Research Working Group.** Washington, DC: US Department of Justice, 1995, pp 321-333

9. Mercy JA, Rosenberg ML, Powell KE, et al: Public health policy for preventing violence. **Health Affairs 12:**7-29, 1993

10. Miller TR, Cohen MA, Rossman SB: Victim costs of violent crime and resulting injuries. **Health Affairs 12:**186-197, 1993

11. National Committee for Injury Prevention and Control: **Injury Prevention: Meeting the Challenge.** New York, NY: Oxford University Press, 1989

12. Page L: First federal guidelines issued on workplace violence. **Am Med News.** Apr 8, 1996, p 5

13. Reiss AJ Jr, Roth JA (eds): **Understanding and Preventing Violence.** Washington, DC: National Academy Press, 1993

14. Rosenberg ML, Fenley MA: **Violence in America. A**

Public Health Approach. New York, NY: Oxford University Press, 1991

15. Saltzman LE: Brief comment on our ability to compare lethal and non-lethal violence in the domestic context, in Block C, Block R (eds): **Trends, Risks, and Interventions in Lethal Violence: Proceedings of The Third Annual Spring Symposium of the Homicide Research Working Group.** Washington, DC: US Department of Justice, 1995, pp 179-180

16. Saltzman LE: Brief comments on the use of NIBRS for family and intimate violence data analysis, in Block C, Block R (eds): **Trends, Risks, and Interventions in Lethal Violence: Proceedings of The Third Annual Spring Symposium of the Homicide Research Working Group.** Washington, DC: US Department of Justice, 1995, p 317

17. Snyder HN: NIBRS and the study of juvenile crime and victimization, in Block C, Block R (eds): **Trends, Risks, and Interventions in Lethal Violence: Proceedings of The Third Annual Spring Symposium of the Homicide Research Working Group.** Washington, DC: US Department of Justice, 1995, pp 309-315

18. US Department of Health and Human Services, Public Health Service: **Healthy People 2000. National Health Promotion and Disease Prevention Objectives.** Washington, DC: US Government Printing Office, 1990

19. US Department of Health and Human Services, Public Health Service: **Injury Control in the 1990s: A National Injury Control Conference. Setting the National Agenda for Injury Control in the 1990s.** Washington, DC: US Government Printing Office, 1991

CHAPTER 12

VIOLENCE, PART C: SEXUAL ASSAULT

MARK GIBSON, MD, AND JOYCE MCCONNELL, JD, LLM

The term "rape," in the past, has implied forced, nonspousal sexual intercourse involving penetration of the vagina by an assailant's penis. Excluded from such a classical definition were other forms of sexual violation or perpetration by a spouse. In the past decade, rape laws have been reformed with repeal of spousal exemption clauses and inclusion of a wide variety of forms of sexual violation. Additional reforms have protected the victim from inquiry as to her personal sexual history. Collectively these reforms have served to recognize the autonomy of women and protect them from losing this autonomy because of marriage or past lifestyle or behaviors.

Rape occurs all too frequently. In 1995, there were 354,670 victims of a rape or sexual assault. In the last 2 years, more than 787,000 women have been the victim of rapes or sexual assault.[7] Rape statistics are affected by a high degree of underreporting. It is estimated that only one-quarter to somewhat more than one-third of rapes are reported to the legal system. The Federal Bureau of Investigation estimates that 72 of every 100,000 females in the United States were raped last year.[5] The reasons for underreporting include fear of reprisal and shame, particularly since two-thirds of rapes are perpetrated by an acquaintance, husband, or boyfriend.[6]

The role of the physician in caring for the rape victim is three-fold: legal/forensic; medical care; and psychological recovery.

Understanding these objectives aids the physician in determining the nature of the post-rape history and examination. To avoid compounding the sense of unwanted intrusion and devaluation experienced by the victim, an evaluation should involve a quiet, secure environment; gentle, objective, and nonjudgmental treatment; the constant presence of an advocate/support person; and freedom from the burden of long waits and procedural mazes often characteristic of emergency departments. In addition, if at all possible, examination of the rape victim with collection of materials should take place in a setting where strict forensic protocol is possible.

The admission of evidence that documents rape is crucial to the prosecution of the perpetrator, and begins with a physician's history, physical examination, and collection of specimens that confirm rape and provide clues as to the identity of the assailant. The consent of the rape victim for the history and examination should be meticulously documented, and this documentation may be required for admission of the evidence during legal proceedings.[3]

From a legal perspective, the medical history given by the patient is hearsay, and the physician is permitted to testify about the history only to the extent the information was pertinent to medical treatment. Circumstances leading to the assault, any background in the relationship between the assailant and the victim, the behaviors of the assailant and victim, or the content of any communication between assailant and victim are not relevant to the medical examination for rape. In fact, the physician is not trained in the obtaining of such facts for legal purposes. If information in the medical history differs from data collected by legal authorities, this may detract from the prosecution's case should the assailant be tried. On the other hand, specific information that will guide the physical examination and collection of forensic materials is important, and documentation of this information is a responsibility of the physician. A record should be made regarding whether and in what manner force may have been used and whether and where intermission and ejaculation may have occurred.[4]

The emotional condition of the victim may or may not reflect the intensity of physical and psychological trauma associated with the attack. A calm or glib presentation may result from trauma-related dissociation, a distraught individual may have sketchy recall, and alcohol or other substances may impair the history. The physician should be circumspect in recording the victim's presentation in view of the potentially misleading inferences that may be drawn since the record will constitute legal evidence. All statements made by the victim to the physician, even if not admissible under the hearsay exception for information related to medical treatment, can be used to impeach (i.e., contradict) the testimony of the victim at trial.

Forensic materials collected include the victim's clothing in their entirety. The victim should be given hospital scrubs or freshly laundered clothing (often provided by rape victim assistance groups) for later wear. The physical examination should document genital and non-genital injury that indicates the use of force in subduing the victim or accomplishing sexual violation. Photographs may improve the documentation of injury and assist in prosecution;

these should specifically be mentioned in the consent to examine.

The gathering of forensic material is facilitated by the standard use of a "rape kit," available in most emergency departments, that includes implements for gathering and transport of specimens and affords a means to establish clear documentation in the chain of evidence. One should collect samples of the victim's blood, saliva, and pubic hair for antigenic, enzymatic, and other characterization for correlation with any materials presumed to have come from the assailant. Oral and vaginal fluids are examined cytologically and biochemically for evidence of sperm/semen and possible antigenic and biochemical characterization. Pubic hair combings are used to identify material that might lead to characterization of the assailant. All materials gathered should be entered into a strictly observed process for maintenance of an unassailable chain of evidence. Eventually, this material should be transferred to a member of the law enforcement system, and this must be documented by signature.

Medical care of the rape victim includes treatment of injuries sustained as a result of the assault, attention to psychological trauma and its aftermath, prevention of unwanted pregnancy, and screening and treatment for sexually transmitted diseases. The victim of rape has experienced not only physical, but profound psychological trauma.[1,2] The rape trauma syndrome includes an early phase consisting of acute responses to trauma and a later phase of attempted adjustment. Long-term sequelae may adversely affect personal relationships and activities of daily life.

In most communities, support organizations are available to counsel and support rape victims, and referrals to these organizations should be made as necessary for professional treatment. Such organizations usually are available 24 hours a day to attend the victim beginning when she reaches the medical system, support her through the history and examination, and see to her safety and security afterward. Such resources are of great value to patients, both acutely and in the weeks and months that follow, and also as an aid to the accomplishment of complete and systematic medical and forensic investigation.

Prevention of unwanted pregnancy requires attention to the patient's contraceptive and menstrual history. Emergency contraceptive regimens are indicated whenever there is a likelihood that there is a risk of conception, and even with such measures, baseline and follow-up pregnancy screening 2 to 3 weeks after the assault by testing for human chorionic gonadotropin should be performed.

Screening for infection includes cultures for gonorrhea and chlamydia, as well as baseline and appropriately timed follow-up serology for hepatitis B, syphilis, and HIV. Dark-field examination for spirochetes and cultures for herpes simplex virus should be undertaken whenever clinically suspicious lesions are present. Prophylaxis for gonorrhea and chlamydial infection is generally recommended, consisting presently of ceftriaxone as a single injection followed by a 10-day course of doxycycline.

References

1. Burgess AW, Holmstrom LL: Rape trauma syndrome. **Am J Psychiatry 131:**981, 1974
2. Burgess AW, Holmstrom LL: The rape victim in the emergency ward. **Am J Nurs 73:**1740, 1973
3. Dupre AR, Hampton HL, Morrison H, et al: Sexual assault. **Obstet Gynecol Surv 48:**640-648, 1993
4. Hochbaum SR: The evaluation and treatment of the sexual assault patient. **Emerg Clin North Am 5:**601, 1987
5. US Department of Justice, Bureau of Justice Statistics: **National Crime Victimization Survey, Criminal Victimization No. 319. Criminal Victimizations and Victimization Rates: 1993 and 1994.** 1996
6. US Department of Justice, Bureau of Justice Statistics: **Violence Against Women.** 1994
7. US Deparment of Justice, Federal Bureau of Investigation. **Uniform Crime Reports, Vol 23.** 1996

CHAPTER 12

Violence, Part D: Suicide

James M. Stevenson, MD

Suicide is a self-inflicted, self-intended cessation of life. It is an act carried out to remove oneself from an unbearable situation and is characterized by helplessness and hopelessness. It is the result of the convergence of three factors: the individual's genetic make-up and personality, the general situation, and the specific problems leading to the act. The majority of deaths are by violent means, (such as self-inflicted gunshot wounds, hanging, and jumping).[14] Lethal overdose by prescribed medication (usually tricyclic antidepressants) alone or in combination with alcohol ingestion is also common.

Suicide is the eighth leading cause of death over all age groups. The rate of suicide in the United States has averaged 12.5 per 100,000 during the past century. This is the current rate,[5] although this rate has varied from 17.4 in the 1930s to 9.8 in 1957. Since 1950, the rate of suicide has decreased in the population aged over 45 years, while the rate has increased in the 15- to 35-year-old group, and is now the third leading cause of death in this age group. There has been a dramatic increase in adolescent suicide, from four per 100,000 in 1950 to 13.2 per 100,000 in 1988. Overall, black Americans complete suicide at one-half the rate of European Americans. Suicide rates of Native Americans are 1.7 times higher than in the nation as a whole. Male suicide rates consistently exceed female rates across races by a ratio of 3:1 to 4:1.[2] Worldwide, countries populated by a majority of people of northern European extraction (including the U.S.) have the highest suicide rates. The adolescent suicide rates in several European countries exceed even that of the U.S.[14] In addition, the under-reporting of the incidence of suicide is considerable, especially in cases of intentional single motor-vehicle accidents and "accidental" medication overdoses.

Risk Factors

Suicide is a complex phenomenon. Society requires responsible behavior which is dependent on the individual's ability to process information rationally. For a few, the act of suicide may result from exercising the right of free choice. However, suicidal behavior is the most serious consequence of many psychiatric disorders. When discovered, the potential danger from the act requires immediate attention.[14] In addition, forms of suicidal thinking exist as a chronic feature in the personal organization of some individuals.[10] An immediate state requires an emergent response; a chronic condition requires long-term support and management. Prediction of outcome in either instance is not always possible; the best treatment will not obviate suicide in some individuals.

Significant risk factors for suicide include being divorced or widowed and/or living alone. Statistics indicate that 50% of suicide victims are unemployed, which supports studies linking suicidality to individual economics.[8] Perhaps the best overall predictor of a completed suicide is a previous attempt at suicide. However, women, who comprise 70% of all suicide attempts, account for less than 25% of those individuals who succeed in taking their own lives. Generally, females attempt suicide by less violent means, such as drug overdose or wrist slashing.

Of the 1% of the population that dies by suicide, 95% suffer a diagnosable psychiatric illness.[1] The majority of the remaining 5% suffer from chronic medical problems. Patients suffering from affective disorders have a 25 times greater risk for suicide and represent upward of 75% of the completed suicides. There is a 15% lifetime risk for completed suicide among those who suffer from affective and recurrent affective illnesses. Twenty-five percent of all suicide victims are alcoholics, and as many as 20% of suicide victims are legally intoxicated at the time of death.[11] One in five alcoholics makes an attempt on his or her life, a 60-120 times greater lifetime risk than the general population. One half of all alcoholics who commit suicide suffer from a major depression at the time of death. Ten percent of schizophrenics die by suicide, generally within the first 2-4 years of the precipitation of their schizophrenia. This is especially true of young male schizophrenics and is thought to be associated with depression as the schizophrenia progresses to a state of chronicity. Three additional psychiatric conditions place victims at particular risk for suicide: organic mental state, borderline personality disorder, and antisocial personality disorder.

Genetics and biological predisposition are additional risk factors for suicidal behavior and have recently been defined more clearly. Several excellent clinical studies[12] reveal a significantly increased incidence of suicidal behavior in the families of the victims of suicide, with more than 80% of these families diagnosed with either an affective disorder or recurrent affective disorder. One study suggested that a family with a history of violent suicidal acts is a strong predictor of active suicidal behavior among patients suffering a major depressive illness.[9] Studies of twins strongly suggest genetics as a factor in suicidal behavior, with consistent significantly higher concordance rates for suicide in monozygotic twins as compared to dizygotic twin pairs.[13] A 100-year retrospective study of suicide victims in an Amish population revealed three-fourths of the victims clustered in just four families, all of whom had heavy gene loading for affective disorder.[4] However, not all families with a heavy genetic predisposition to affective illness and depression displayed suicidal behaviors. This perhaps indicates that the genetic propensity to affective illness alone is not enough for suicidal behavior to become manifest.

The Danish Adoption Studies[6] offer the strongest evidence for genetic factors in suicide. Significant rates of suicide were found in the biological relatives of twins who were adopted at birth and later died by suicide. Matched control groups of adoptees showed no suicidal behavior among their biological relatives. A further study of these patients revealed affective illness of a predominantly reactive nature, indicating depression that may be precipitated by a particular crisis and raising the issue of impulsivity as an important factor in some suicides.[6]

Recent life events may also precipitate suicidal behavior. It is important to evaluate the interpersonal and social milieu of the victim. Many studies have demonstrated the adverse effect of stressful events and situations on both mental and physical health.[5] Thus, many suicide victims have experienced stressful events, particularly the loss of loved ones, changes in living circumstances, and work problems, compared to nonsuicidal normal peers. Current research addresses the role of social support systems as deterrents to suicide during stressful periods. Evidence indicates a trend toward weaker support systems among those who attempt suicide compared to those who do not.

Populations at both ends of the age spectrum require special attention when examining the phenomenon of suicide. Studies of the suicide rate among the elderly have attempted to predict unique characteristics in that age group that contribute to high suicidality. These characteristics differ from younger victims in that financial issues are less prominent and widowhood is more likely.[3] Interestingly, the percentage of those elderly living alone is comparable

(36%) to the younger age group (42%) who commit suicide, and they appear to be no more socially isolated. Not surprisingly, they list current physical illness as a major stressor in their lives. Typically, they are less likely to have attempted suicide and less likely to have ever discussed their suicidal thinking with others.

Unlike the elderly, adolescent suicide victims frequently mention suicidal thinking prior to making attempts on their lives. This is especially true of young females, who are four times more likely to attempt suicide than their adolescent male peers. Consumption of drugs and/or alcohol is more likely among adolescent suicide victims, and they are less likely to have received professional intervention than other populations. Recent literature indicates that adolescents at highest risk for suicidal behaviors are those who experience chronic or acute situational stressors involving social loss, a blow to self-esteem, or anger.[7]

ASSESSMENT

The assessment of suicidal potential in a person requires an intensive physical and psychiatric evaluation with special focus on risk factors. The proportion of completed suicides with a concurrent diagnosis of depression ranges up to 80%.[1] Generally speaking, this clinical diagnostic entity has been well recognized in the patient prior to any six active attempts at suicide. This is not always the case, however, since some attempts follow only a few days of mood change or are a sudden, impulsive act resulting from a rapid mood shift or psychotic thought. Upward of 80% of patients who have completed suicide have communicated to others their intent to commit the act.[14]

There has been established a fairly consistent rate of completed suicide in people with depression, alcoholism, schizophrenia, and a history of previous suicide attempts. This rate ranges from 10% to 15% in each of those groups over an entire lifetime. For the clinician, focus on this phenomenon is often a daily occurrence. As a consequence, accurate assessment should include a complete mental status examination of each patient in crisis to encompass an especially careful examination of thought processes, vegetative signs of depression, and suicidal ideation. The latter is of ultimate importance and should be approached resolutely, although in a manner designed to create a supportive relationship between the patient and physician. Specific questions to ask include the following:

1. Have you ever had thoughts of suicide in the past?
2. Have you ever attempted suicide?
3. Are you currently experiencing thoughts of suicide?
4. Do you have a plan for committing suicide?
5. If so, what is your plan for suicide?

Approaching the issue of suicide in a slow and deliberate manner may assist in establishing a trusting relationship with the patient and therefore allow a more truthful interchange. Clipped, decisive, and rapid-fire questioning can result in the withholding of key and true feelings on the part of the patient, who may perceive the questions of the physician as coming from yet one more inquisitor in his or her own life.

In the progression to the suicidal act that begins with the thought, the patient at greatest risk is the one who has designed a plan that appears workable. Nevertheless, caution should be taken not to dismiss suicidal ideation alone as being without dangerous implications.

TREATMENT

Patients for whom an evaluation indicates an actively suicidal intent should be hospitalized under the care of a psychiatrist. Depending on the level of cooperation of the patient in the clinician's own care, and secondary to the clinical judgment of the psychiatrist, commitment proceedings may be required. Commitment laws and procedure vary by state but are designed to protect the patient's rights. Hearings take place to determine "probable cause" for detainment and/or treatment and involve the clinicians and court-appointed officers, including a chief hearing officer. Hearings are initiated generally by family members or others closely involved with the patient. Immediate endangerment to self or others is an acceptable basis for such proceedings in nearly all states, with rare local exceptions. Either voluntary or involuntary hospitalization ensures treatment implementation and the opportunity for a resolution of suicidality in the patient. If suicidal thinking is a documented part of the patient's record and the act of suicide occurs without proper intervention, the clinician may be liable, depending on additional circumstances.

Although antidepressant medications are important in the treatment of depression, they are also among the most potentially lethal chemical agents available. Careful consideration is required prior to using antidepressants to treat a patient who has a previous history of suicide attempt by overdose. The rationing of antidepressants to an outpatient with depression and at risk for suicide is recommended; however, their use in a hospitalized population is more controlled and therefore less hazardous. Some patients will require electroconvulsive therapy to disrupt a debilitating depressive process, especially one marked with resistance to antidepressant medication and with the presence of persistent suicidal thinking. Treatment after discharge from the hospital should include immediate outpatient follow-up with frequent visits continuing until the full benefits of medication, supportive or insight therapy, and family and environmental changes have occurred sufficiently to remove the suicide risk. When possible, involvement of the family is most helpful in support of both the patient and the clinician.

One recent paper suggests that the more chronic form of suicidal thinking responds best to a less directive and less medication-oriented treatment approach. This "continuing therapy" model of treatment is believed to be more supportive of the chronic character-disturbed patients and emphasizes ongoing therapy principles in treatment. Emphasis in this approach is placed not so much on suicide prevention as in working to redevelop the aspects of the patient's personality that render the individual susceptible to a suicidal inclination.[10]

REFERENCES

1. Barraclough B, Bunch J, Nelson B, et al: A hundred cases of suicide: clinical aspects. **Br J Psychiatry 125:** 355-373, 1974
2. Buzan RD, Weissberg MP: Suicide: risk factors and prevention in medical practice. **Annu Rev Med 43:** 37-46, 1993
3. Carney SS, Rich CL, Burke PA, et al: Suicide over 60: the San Diego study. **J Am Geriatr Soc 42:**174-180, 1994
4. Egeland JA, Sussex JN: Suicide and family loading for affective disorders. **JAMA 254:**915-918, 1985
5. Heikkinen M, Aro H, Lonnqvist J: Recent life events, social support and suicide. **Acta Psychiatr Scand Suppl 377:**65-72, 1994
6. Ketz S: Genetic factors in suicide, in Roy A (ed): **Suicide.** Baltimore, Md: Williams & Wilkins, 1986
7. Ladely SJ, Puskar KR: Adolescent suicide: behaviors, risk factors, and psychiatric nursing interventions. **Issues Mental Health Nurs 15:**497-504, 1994
8. Lester D, Yang B: Social and economic correlates of the elderly suicide rate. **Suicide Life Threat Behav 22:** 36-47, 1992
9. Linkowski P, de Maertelaer V, Mendlewicz J: Suicidal behaviour in major depressive illness. **Acta Psychiatr Scand 72:**233-38, 1985
10. Pulakos J: Two models of suicide treatment: evaluation and recommendations. **Am J Psychother 47:** 603-612, 1993
11. Robins L, Kolbok P: Epidemiologic studies in suicide, in Frances A, Holer RE (eds): **American Psychiatric Press Review of Psychiatry.** Washington, DC: American Psychiatric Associated Press, 1988, Vol 7, pp 289-306
12. Roy A: Family history of suicide. **Arch Gen Psychiatry 40:**971-974, 1983
13. Roy A, Segal NL, Centerwall BS, et al: Suicide in twins. **Arch Gen Psychiatry 48:**29-32, 1991
14. Stevenson JM: Suicide, in Talbott J, Yudofsky S, Hales R (eds): **Textbook of Psychiatry.** Washington, DC: American Psychiatric Associated Press, 1987

CHAPTER 12

Violence, Part E: Observation and Description of Trauma

James L. Frost, MD

Many physicians regularly see patients who have sustained traumatic injuries. These injuries may be from an accident, such as a motor-vehicle collision or a fall; they may be injuries inflicted by another person with a blunt hard object such as a club or hammer, with a knife, or with a gun; or they may be self-inflicted. The physician should locate, describe, and document the injuries. The description of the wound(s) becomes a vital part of the patient's medical record for medical purposes and also for legal-forensic purposes if needed. Evidence, which is the injury or wound, is best seen and documented when it is the freshest. As wounds heal, their appearances change. What was present immediately after the injury was received becomes altered. What was present initially as evidence may be gone. When the patient is first seen and treated, the complete and true story as to what took place may not be known. So adequate observations need to be made at the onset.

When the injury has been inflicted by another person or received in an accident, there may well be subsequent criminal proceedings, possibly civil proceedings, or both. If the injury was self-inflicted, criminal proceedings are precluded but there may be insurance and other civil considerations.

Every blow to the body that produces an injury leaves behind evidence. That evidence may be valuable in determining what object or instrument produced the injury or injuries, and aid in evaluating how the injuries occurred.

The clinician's effort should be toward accurate and complete documentation. Interpretation is not the treating physician's role. Even though many injuries are seen and treated, the clinician may not have the training and experience in the forensic aspects of blunt force injury, sharp force injury, and injuries due to firearms. Inaccurate information may be given by a clinician who may not, for example, have training or experience in interpreting what wounds are gunshot entrance wounds and what are exit wounds or in estimating the range of gunshot wounds.

Investigating police can call upon their jurisdiction's medical examiner, coroner, or forensic pathologist for a more expert interpretation of what the clinician described. That is what their work regularly involves. As a matter of course the medical examiner, coroner, and forensic pathologist perform examinations and documentation of wounds when they are fatal. However, many wounds are not fatal and are seen only by clinicians. In some jurisdictions, the forensic pathologist can be called upon to examine and describe wounds of living patients, which is called clinical forensic pathology.

The following remarks are applicable to types of wounds that are not immediately or almost immediately fatal and which are treated in a hospital. Obviously, there must be documentation of these wounds which would be done by the treating physician.

OBSERVATION AND DOCUMENTATION

Since cleaning a wound may remove evidence, wounds should be examined and observations made before they are cleaned. However, it may be necessary to clean the wound to see the injury in full detail, and this will be done in the course of treating the wound.

The number of wounds observed should be recorded. Each wound should be described. Its location is given along with some parameters—not just right or left side of the head or of the anterior chest or of the abdomen—but where on the right or left side of the head or chest or abdomen and the distance and direction from some structure such as the ear or a nipple or umbilicus, and so many inches below the top of the head and right or left of whichever midline (anterior or posterior) is closest.

A drawing of the wound(s) could be made in the medical record as part of the admission physical examination. The date and time of that entry should be recorded and the note should have a legible signature.

Photographing is an ideal way to document a wound. A camera is especially useful to document injuries in sexual assault victims, child abuse cases, and elder abuse cases. It is, thus, a very valuable investment for the hospital. I prefer an automatic/programmed 35-mm camera with a special lens for close-up work. Flash will be needed. A programmed camera is very simple to use and provides good pictures. Use color print film so that there is a negative from which many prints and even enlargements can be made. Color negative C-41 processed film is recommended because it can be processed locally, often in a day or so, and does not need to be mailed away for developing. I prefer film of 200

DIN film speed. Instant print Polaroid-type pictures allow for rapid review, but often, in my experience, lack adequate sharp definition; in addition, there would not be a color negative.

A few pictures of good quality are sufficient. Both overview and close-up detailed pictures should be made. Therefore, rolls of film with 20 exposures or fewer (if your hospital's or medical school's photography laboratory or biomedical illustration service rolls your film) are suggested. With a shorter roll, the film can be developed and pictures available sooner. If a short roll is used for each patient, there will be less waste of unexposed film.

A very useful feature of some automatic cameras is the recording of the date and/or hour the picture was taken in the emulsion of the film, so that it is in the print (the "quartz date," or QD, feature). An identifying name or number such as the patient's hospital/medical record number in the picture as well as a date and time is also extremely helpful for documentation. A scale in the picture is also helpful.

A set of pictures should be placed in the medical record. If the police are given a set of pictures and/or the negatives, a signed and dated evidence receipt should be obtained and placed in the medical record. It is important to keep a set of pictures and a duplicate evidence receipt secured in the office or department file where they are always available.

THE INJURIES

The features of the following general categories of wounds will be described: 1) blunt force injury; 2) sharp force injury; 3) gunshot wounds; 4) asphyxial injury; 5) thermal injury; and 6) chemical injury.

The track of a wound is the sequence of structures, tissues, and organs through which the missile or knife or other penetrating object has passed from the entrance wound to where it has made the deepest penetration in the body or to an exit wound. The path of a wound refers to the angle and direction of the track in the body such as: front to back, right to left, and slightly above downward. They refer to the patient's anatomy, not that of the describing physician.

Blunt Force Injury

Blunt force injuries include contusions (bruises), abrasions, and lacerations (tears) of the skin—in order of the force required to produce them.

Contusions

Valuable forensic information includes the location of bruises on the body and their color, size, shape, or pattern as well as the number of bruises, and this information should be recorded. As discussed above, location should be described in relation to anatomical landmarks. Injury location may give information as to the direction from which the blows came. The size and shape of contusions may provide information regarding the type of weapon used. Their color may give information about the age of the injury. The number of bruises can indicate the number of blows sustained. Contusions to the scalp may be obscured by the hair. At the autopsy, the forensic pathologist will shave the scalp in the area of wounds (of all kinds) to observe and record wound details. The clinician is not at liberty to do this on the living patient, however. If it is necessary to shave the scalp to close a laceration or operate intracranially, then the wounds are better visualized.

Abrasions

Abrasions are a scraping loss of epidermis and dermis, and sometimes even deeper tissues. A friction component is involved, as well as force. The same features noted about contusions should be noted about abrasions: location on the body, color, size, shape, pattern, and the number of them. Also, any foreign material on or in the abrasion should be noted and removed for evidence. This material may be matched to the object causing the abrasion and/or the place where the abrasion was received. Proper chain of custody must be maintained (vide infra).

Lacerations

Lacerations require still more force. They are tears of the skin or scalp and deeper tissues, extending to various depths. Their edges are irregular or jagged, there may be an abrasion along one or both sides of the edges of the laceration, and they will show bridging of strands of

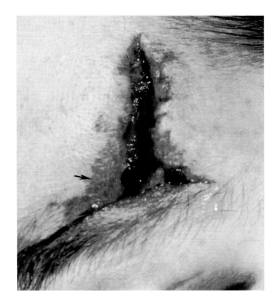

Figure 1: Laceration showing irregular edges and abrasion *(arrow)* at the edges.

connective tissue or small blood vessels in their depths (Figure 1). The location on the body, size, shape or pattern, and the number of lacerations need to be documented. Any foreign material found during cleaning and closing of a laceration should be preserved. If recovered, a small piece of wood or metal broken off of a weapon and embedded in the wound may be matched to a defect (its place of origin) on a suspected weapon, thus putting that weapon at the scene of the crime. Again, it is necessary to maintain proper chain of custody of such evidence materials (vide infra).

Sharp Force Injury

Sharp force injuries are produced by sharp cutting objects, including knives and razors as well as bayonets, swords, hatchets, axes, machetes, and semi-sharp weapons such as mattocks. Screwdrivers, scissors, and icepicks are also included. These produce incised wounds or cuts (which are longer than they are deep) and stab wounds (which are deeper than they are long).

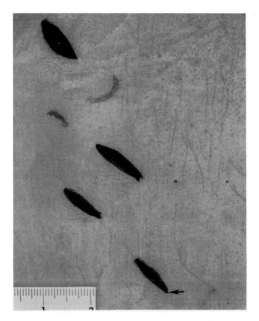

Figure 2: Stab wound with one end sharp *(arrow)*.

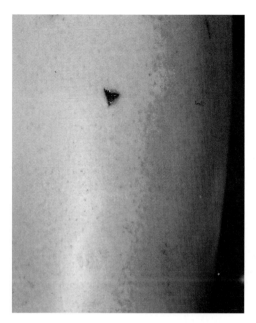

Figure 3: Triangular stab wound due to penetration with triangular blade.

Location on the body, size of the wound hole, shape, angle on the skin surface, direction into the body, and depth, as well as the number of wounds should be recorded. Location on the body, angle (e.g., vertical, horizontal, or diagonal), direction or angle of penetration, and length of the wound track (depth of penetration) can be utilized to determine the direction from which the weapon came as well as whether incised wounds or stab wounds were produced by an assailant or could have been self-inflicted. The size and shape of the wound are utilized to give information about the size and shape of the blade. The length and shape of the entrance wound in the skin, possibly the width of the wound, and whether it is blunt or rounded at one end and sharp at the other end (blade sharp on one side) (Figure 2) or pointed at both ends (blade sharp on both sides) can provide information about the blade. A triangular blade leaves a triangular hole (Figure 3). An icepick or marlin spike or awl leaves a round hole. However, a serrated blade, such as a steak knife, will not leave a hole with a serrated border. If a serrated blade is scraped across the skin surface, the serration of the blade can produce a pattern of parallel linear scratches (abrasions). Sometimes, stab wound edges do not stay together but gap widely apart

or open due to skin tension (or cleavage) lines, thus giving the wound a different and inaccurate appearance and size (Figure 4); when seen, this can be overcome by opposing the edges of the hole more closely with one's finger and then measuring. When photographing, the opposed edges can be brought together and held in the nongaping position by a piece of clear self-sticking tape (Figure 5). Scissors, if the blades are open or separated at the time of injury, will leave pairs of stab wounds, and the wound holes will resemble the cross-section shape of the blades.

Semi-sharp weapons, such as a mattock and sometimes a dull hatchet or ax or machete, and screwdrivers and scissors will leave an abrasion on the edges of the wound. An abrasion will not be present on the wound produced by a sharp blade. However, an abrasion and/or contusion around a wound hole could be produced by the hilt of a knife, indicating that the knife penetrated its full length to the hilt during injury.

If a wound is surgically explored, the track of the wound with the sequence of organs it penetrated can be determined. Such exploration gives a better indication of the angle/direction (path) of the wound into or through the body, and it also gives the depth of the wound from

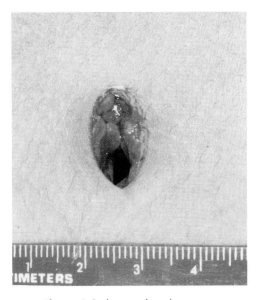

Figure 4: Stab wound gaping open.

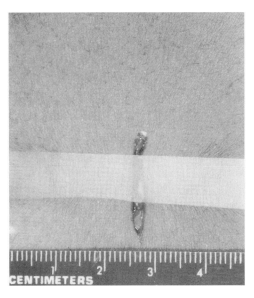

Figure 5: Stab wound with edges pulled together with tape.

the entrance wound at the skin surface, which can be used to estimate the length of the blade used to cause the wound.

Cuts or stab wounds on the back or sides of the hands, wrists, and forearms, or on the palm of the hand and on the flexor surfaces of the fingers, are referred to as "defense wounds" and may occur as the victim attempts to ward off injury (Figure 6). These must be looked for and documented, even when there are larger or deeper serious wounds to the head, neck, or trunk of the body.

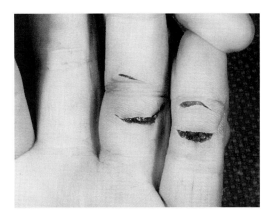

Figure 6: Defense wounds on palm of hand.

Gunshot Wounds

Gunshot wounds are produced by missiles fired from handguns (revolvers and autoloading or "automatic" pistols) and long guns (rifles and shotguns). The commonly encountered handguns and rifles have rifling grooves in the barrel, hence the name rifle, which imparts a spin to the bullet as it travels down the barrel that acts to stabilize the bullet in its flight after it leaves the barrel. The shotgun has a smooth-bore barrel. The missiles fired by weapons with rifled barrels are distinctly different from those fired by shotguns, and therefore so are some features of the wounds.

Wounds Produced by Handguns and Rifles

Handgun and rifle ammunition varies in caliber (inside diameter of the barrel) from 0.22 inches (.22 caliber) to 0.45 inches (.45 caliber). Bullets are entirely of a lead alloy, or may be a core of lead alloy with a harder metal coating called a "jacket" made of copper alloy, steel, or aluminum. The jacket may cover all or part of the core. Bullets from handguns as compared to bullets from high-muzzle velocity rifles are dif-

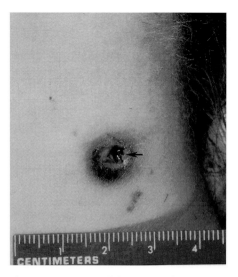

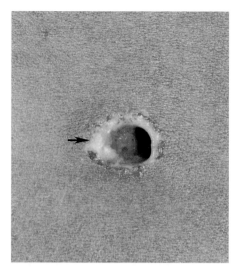

Figure 7: Entrance of distant gunshot wound at right angle to skin surface with concentric marginal abrasion *(arrow)*. The dark area is hemorrhage.

Figure 8: Entrance of distant gunshot wound with eccentric marginal abrasion *(arrow)*.

ferent in size and shape.

Features of the entrance wound give information about the distance from the muzzle of the gun to the patient (range of fire) and the angle at which the bullet struck the body (direction of fire). Entrance wounds and exit wounds differ in many features; grazing wounds are different from both. These features are described below.

Entrance Wounds. Entrance wounds are characterized by an abrasion of the skin around the edge of the wound hole (Figure 7). This is the marginal abrasion and is caused by the pressure of the missile against the skin which is stretched before it breaks and is penetrated by the bullet. The marginal abrasion is generally red to pink, but can be close to white; when it dries it may become very dark red, even red-black to almost black. This dark color can be confused with powder residue. The marginal abrasion will be uniform in width around the wound opening if the bullet strikes the skin at a right angle (Figure 7), but it will be eccentric and wider on one side if it strikes the skin at an oblique angle (Figure 8).

Entrance wound holes will be round if the bullet strikes the skin surface at a right angle

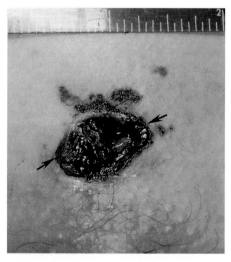

Figure 9: Entrance gunshot wound with irregular shape and irregular width marginal abrasion *(arrows)*. Measure is in inches.

(Figure 7) and oval if it strikes at an oblique angle (Figure 8). If the bullet has struck an intermediary object or target between the gun and the subject and becomes unstable in its flight, the entrance wound may be irregular in shape and the marginal abrasion may be of varying width around the wound hole (Figure 9). If the entrance wound is over the skull and

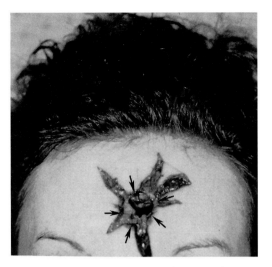

Figure 10: Contact entrance gunshot wound, star-shaped, over skull. Marginal abrasion *(arrows)* is between the lacerations.

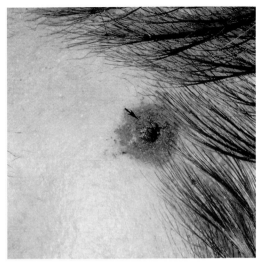

Figure 11: Tight contact gunshot entrance wound with soot (the blackened area) *(arrow)* surrounding the entrance hole.

the gun is fired in contact with the skin, the entrance wound may be "star-shaped" with lacerations of the skin radiating outward from the entrance hole; a marginal abrasion will be present at the gathered edges of the stellate wound around the wound hole where the bullet penetrated (Figure 10).

Entrance wounds generally are smaller than exit wounds, although not always so. A bullet that has struck an intermediary target and become unstable in its flight may produce an entrance wound hole larger than otherwise, and such entrance wounds can be larger than an exit wound. This must be recognized to avoid misidentifying and reversing entrance and exit wounds. Thus, a person may be said to have been shot in the back when indeed they were shot in the front.

The caliber of the bullet cannot be accurately estimated from the size of the wound hole and this should not be attempted.

Exit Wounds. Exit wounds are irregular in shape and size and usually are larger than entrance wounds. With one exception, exit wounds do not have marginal abrasions. That exception is when the skin around the exit wound is supported or shored up either by tight-fitting parts of the clothing (e.g., brassiere strap or tight

waistband or belt) or was supported by being up against a wall or door. In this situation, the skin is pushed out ahead of the bullet and stretched as the bullet exits the body and is abraded against the supported clothing around the exit hole.

Tissues in the body, such as pieces of bone, may be pushed ahead of the bullet and put into flight as secondary missiles and thus may contribute to the exit wound being larger and more irregular than the entrance wound, also sometimes causing an additional exit wound or wounds. An exit wound on the head can be stellate or star-shaped.

Grazing Wounds. A grazing gunshot wound involves the skin and even the underlying subcutaneous fat (Figure 12). It has the appearance of a large abrasion, and is generally oval to oblong. There will be a marginal abrasion, widest at the ends. It may have short diagonal radiating splits/tears/lacerations extending out from its sides which may indicate the direction of missile travel. If the gun was fired at contact, close range, or intermediate range, there will be soot, powder, and/or stippling, depending on the range.

Wound Range and Soot and Powder. In addition to the bullet, when a gun is fired, soot

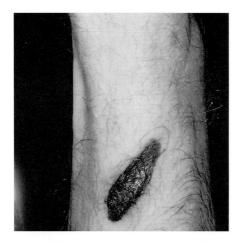

Figure 12: Grazing gunshot wound.

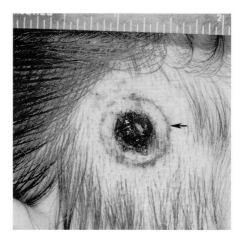

Figure 13: Contact gunshot wound with circular muzzle mark *(arrow)* around and peripheral to the entrance hole. Measure is in inches.

(smoke) and powder come out of the barrel and travel down range. The soot travels only a very short distance beyond the muzzle of the gun. Powder grains, which are unburned, partially burned or burning, are tiny, lightweight missiles that travel a short distance but further than the soot. The greater the distance of the gun muzzle from the skin or clothing, the larger the area over which soot and especially powder are spread. On the other hand, the intensity of their deposition decreases as the distance from the muzzle to the skin or clothing increases. Therefore, the closer the muzzle of the gun to the skin or clothing, the smaller and more intense the area of soot and powder deposition, and the further away, the larger and less intense the area of deposition on the skin or clothing. Grains of powder can strike the skin with enough force to cause small red to red-brown abrasions of the skin surface. These abrasions are called powder stippling (or powder burns or tattooing). Therefore, the presence of soot and powder or just powder and powder stippling, the size of the area of soot and powder deposition, and the intensity of this deposition can be used to estimate the distance from the muzzle of the gun to the person shot.

There are four categories of range: contact, close range, intermediate range, and distant. In a contact wound, if the muzzle of the gun is in tight contact with the skin, soot will be on the edges of the wound hole, but almost all the

smoke and powder enters the wound (Figure 11). They may be seen by the naked eye in the wound track and in microscopic studies of the tissues of the proximal part of the wound track. If the muzzle is in tight contact, there may also be contusions (bruises) and/or abrasions on the skin around the wound opening in the shape of the contour of the muzzle (Figure 13). These could be in continuity with the marginal abrasion and could include the shape of a front sight, or could be a thin partially or completely encircling contusion and/or abrasion parallel to the edge of the entrance hole and separated a short distance from the marginal abrasion. This is a muzzle mark. It is caused by the gases that have traveled down the barrel entering the wound track into the subcutaneous fat and around the wound track and forcing the skin outward against the muzzle of the gun with resultant contusion-abrasion by this contact with the muzzle. On the other hand, if the muzzle is only in loose contact with the skin, there will be a round to oval area around the wound opening where there is much black soot and powder deposited, which may obscure the marginal abrasion, and no muzzle mark. In a close-range wound, where the muzzle is approximately 1"-2" away, soot and powder reach the skin, producing a black area of soot and powder deposition around the wound hole (Figure 14). If the muzzle is further away, at approximately 4"-7", only powder will reach the skin, produc-

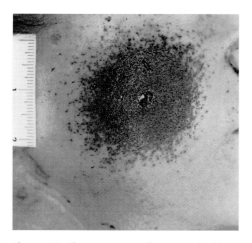

Figure 14: Close-range gunshot wound with intense soot and stippling around the entrance hole. Measure is in inches.

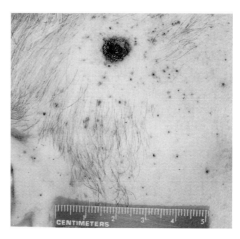

Figure 15: Intermediate-range gunshot wound with surrounding stippling.

ing a red to red-brown area of powder stippling around the wound hole. If the muzzle is still further away, the area of powder stippling will increase in size and the intensity of stippling will decrease because the grains of powder are more dispersed and less powder reaches the skin. Stippling can occur at muzzle distances of up to 42" in experimental firings. If there is stippling but no soot deposition, the wound is referred to as an intermediate-range wound (Figure 15). If no powder reaches the skin and there is no stippling, the wound is referred to as a distant wound (Figure 7). There is a gradual transition from the changes of a tight-contact wound to a loose-contact wound to a close-range wound to an intermediate-range wound to a distant wound.

Soot and powder at a wound can be reduced in amount and even removed entirely by the cleaning of a wound. The abrasions of powder stippling cannot be wiped off or washed away. It is thus necessary to document and photograph the wound before it is cleaned. Then blood and serum on and around the wound need to be cleaned off, taking care to disturb soot and powder as little as possible. Hair around and obscuring a wound may need to be removed (cut or shaved) to reveal the wound in all its detail for description and photographing. The size of the area of soot and stippling needs to be described and measured. The largest diameter of that area should be measured and a second diameter

opposite by 90° should be measured.

If the shot enters the body through clothing, the clothing will impede the soot and powder which will be deposited on them. If the clothing is very dark or very bloody, the soot and powder may not be seen by the naked eye, but it can be detected in the forensic laboratory. In a contact wound, there may be little soot and powder on the outer surface of the outer layer of clothing, but there may be much soot and powder deposited on the inner surface of the clothing. Thus clothing may give information that may not be obtained from examination of the skin around the wound. It is, therefore, of utmost importance that clothing be preserved for the investigating police or the medical examiner. If clothing is bloody, it needs to be hung to dry or it soon will become very foul-smelling and moldy.

When a bullet passes through the barrel, it will pick up dirt, powder, oil, and lubricants from the barrel, and when it passes through clothing, those materials will be wiped off the bullet by the clothing at the edges of the bullet hole. This "dirt wipe" or ring of dirt will be a thin black rim around the bullet hole on the clothing over an entrance wound. It is not seen on the skin. If seen at a wound, it should not be confused with soot deposition of a contact or close-range wound, and it may help in distinguishing an entrance wound from an exit wound on the clothing.

Collecting Forensic Evidence. The following data about a wound should be noted:

1. The location of the entrance wound and exit wound, if present.
   a) location in general descriptive terms.
   b) location in relation to an anatomical location and measured distance from it, or measured distance from the top of the head and measurement distance from the appropriate midline (anterior or posterior).
2. The shape and size of the entrance and exit wounds.
3. The presence, shape, and width of a marginal abrasion.
4. The presence of gunpowder residues (e.g., soot, powder, or stippling).

The recovered bullet or its pieces also provides evidence. The bullet may be intact and nondeformed or may be deformed. It may fragment/disintegrate. The bullet jacket may separate from the core. The missile and its condition may be seen on radiological examination and/or at surgery. Care should be taken in grasping missiles with forceps or clamps so as not to add new marks or obscure the rifling marks on the sides of the base of the bullet. The rifling marks are vital for matching the evidence bullet with a test-fired bullet from a gun suspected to be the one used in the shooting. It is said in forensic pathology that you should not grab a bullet or fragment with anything sharper than your fingers. Bullet fragments can provide valuable information such as its metal composition, whether it was jacketed, its size/caliber and weight, shape, and manufacturer. These analyses and the matching of bullets to barrels are done in the criminalistics laboratory by a firearms/tool mark examiner.

All bullets and fragments are, thus, valuable forensic evidence. From the place and time of recovery until they are turned over to investigating police, the chain of custody must be maintained. To do this, the bullet and/or pieces (missiles) must be placed in a labeled container with a secure top. The physician recovering the missiles must take charge of them and ensure that they cannot be tampered with until they are turned over to surgical pathology. A receipt must be obtained following delivery of evidence or the missiles may be signed over on a multiple signature chain of custody record. The surgical pathology department should describe them and return them to the same labeled, closed container. They must be maintained in a locked secure place until investigating police take possession of them. Upon release to police, surgical pathology must maintain a signed chain of custody record and, in turn, obtain a signed receipt from the police or keep a copy of the chain of custody record. Each hospital must have a procedure for maintaining an unbroken chain of custody. The procedures must be available in writing and also must be in the pathology laboratory's written procedures.

Handgun wounds can produce skull fractures which vary in extent, but the skull will usually maintain its normal shape. Intracranial wounds can cause orbital ecchymoses, which are due to orbital hemorrhage associated with fractures of the thin orbital plates of the frontal bone. A high-muzzle velocity rifle or a shotgun (with pellet or rifled slug loads), particularly if fired in contact with the skull or in the mouth or beneath the chin, will produce massive destruction of the skull with very marked distortion. Such wounds are rapidly fatal at the scene and are not generally seen by a treating physician.

X-rays may show a shower of small to tiny missile fragments of a disintegrated or fragmented bullet along the wound track in an area that enlarges going away from the entrance. This pattern points back to the entrance.

A bullet that has penetrated certain bones may leave evidence at the entering and exiting sites indicating the direction of travel. The skull and the hip bones are where this is regularly found. These bones have a layer of dense bone, then a layer of soft bone-diploe or marrow space, and then another layer of dense bone. As the bullet enters the skull, fracturing the bone at the point of penetration, the bones are fractured so that a bevel is formed around the internal side of the wound hole ("internal bevel"). The bullet leaves the skull and fracturing produces a bevel on the external side of the bone ("external bevel"). The bevels alone track the bullet from the hole with the internal bevel to the hole with the external bevel.

Missile injury found in the course of surgical

exploration should be described in the operative notes. Wound tracks produced by high-muzzle velocity bullets from hunting rifles and military type weapons may cause more destruction along their tracks than large-caliber handgun bullets which are of lower muzzle velocity. The high-muzzle velocity bullet produces a much larger temporary cavity as it goes through the tissues.

Wounds Produced by Shotguns

Entrance wounds produced by the missiles fired by shotguns have certain basic features similar to those due to handguns and rifles. The differences are due to the different type of missiles fired by shotguns.

Two types of missiles are fired from shotguns: pellets and rifled slugs. Pellets are round, usually of lead alloy but sometimes steel, and vary from 0.05" in diameter (No. 12 shot) to 0.15" (No. 2 shot). Pellets larger than No. 2 are called buckshot and vary from 0.24" in diameter (No. 4 buckshot) to 0.36" (No. 000 buckshot). Also in a shotgun shell are wads and gas seals. These can be made of plastic and are either one or two pieces, or made of cardboard and/or fiber material and are more than one piece (usually two pieces). There may be a separate plastic "collar" around the pellets in the upper part of the shotgun shell, or this "collar" may be part of a one piece wad/gas seal/shot collar combined. The rifled slug is a large, lead alloy, low-muzzle velocity missile. It has raised ridges at angles on the sides (giving it the name "rifled" slug) to impart some spinning along its long axis as it traverses down the barrel to aid in stabilizing the slug in flight after it leaves the barrel. In its shell will be one or two disc-shaped gas seals and wads, either of plastic, cardboard, or fiber material. These waddings will travel down and out the barrel as missiles when the gun is fired. Depending on the range from which the gun was fired, wadding could enter the wound, hit the skin near the wound and cause an abrasion, or veer off the straight course of the pellets or slug and not hit the victim but be somewhere at the scene of the shooting.

Pellets. The pellets fired from a shotgun shell will spread out fairly uniformly as they leave the muzzle and travel down range. Their path and

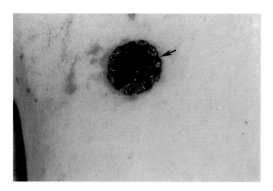

Figure 16: Shotgun wound with scalloping *(arrow)* at the edges.

spread can be described as being a cone, with the point of the cone at the muzzle and the enlarging area of the cone representing the pellets as they spread out progressively while traveling away (down range) from the shotgun.

At contact range or close range, the entrance wound will be round (the barrel at right angles to the skin) to oval (the barrel at an oblique angle to the skin surface) and have a generally smooth edge, a marginal abrasion, and soot on the margin. A contact wound could have a muzzle mark. The pellets here are all in one conglomerate mass. The wads and gas seals will enter the wound track. If the muzzle is a short distance further away, the hole in the skin produced by the pellets may begin to show small rounded indentations/irregularities at the edge of the hole ("scalloping") (Figure 16). This is due to the mass of the pellets beginning to disperse a little. There will continue to be a marginal abrasion. As the range increases, the wound hole may increase in size and the scalloping become very pronounced. This is due to the mass of pellets dispersing more as they travel down range. There will still be a margin abrasion. As the range continues to increase, the mass of pellets will disperse more and there will be a major entrance wound that may now be irregular in shape and still have a marginal abrasion; also, there will be varying numbers of separate individual pellet entrance holes (satellite holes), each with a marginal abrasion (Figure 17). At a still greater range, the pellet mass will be completely dispersed and there will be many entrance wounds due to individual pel-

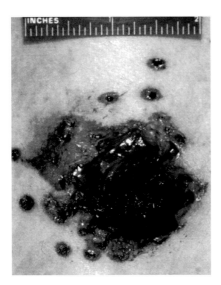

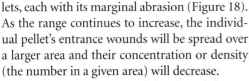

Figure 17: Shotgun wound with large hole and surrounding satellite pellet holes.

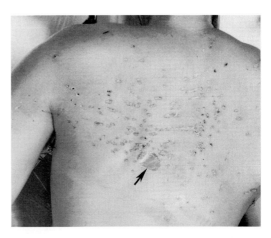

Figure 18: Distant shotgun wound with wad abrasion *(arrow)* at lower edge of area of pellet penetrations.

lets, each with its marginal abrasion (Figure 18). As the range continues to increase, the individual pellet's entrance wounds will be spread over a larger area and their concentration or density (the number in a given area) will decrease.

It is important to record the size of the entrance hole, the marginal abrasion, if there is scalloping, satellite pellet entrances or dispersion of the pellets, and the overall size of the spread of all of the pellet entrances in the two major opposite axes. These dimensions can be compared with the spread of the pellets in a test-fired pattern to aid in determining the distance from which the gun was fired.

The concentricity or eccentricity of the margin abrasion(s) will give information as to whether the pellets struck the skin at right angles to its surface or at a tangential (oblique) angle. Soot, powder and soot, and just powder stippling will be present on the skin at and around the wound depending on the range (contact, loose contact, close range, intermediate range, and distant range) as in the case of wounds produced by handguns and rifles. These features need to be documented and the same measurements made. A feature of shotgun shells loaded with buckshot is a white granulated polyethylene or polypropylene buffer or filler between the pellets. This material will

travel out the barrel and down range as light small missiles and may be seen on the clothing or on the skin. If seen, its presence and, if possible, the size of the area in which it is found should be recorded.

Some pellets should be recovered for firearms identification purposes; about a dozen are usually adequate, and preferably ones not deformed. Any wads or gas seals found at surgery should be recovered. Their location in the wound track should be recorded.

A feature unique to shotgun wounds by pellet loads can be abrasions produced by the waddings. These abrasions are produced by the leaves/petals of the shot collar portions of a plastic shotgun wad. There are usually four of these petals. As the wad leaves the barrel as a missile, the air resistance may spread the collar petals out at right angles to the long axis of the wad and they may protrude like propellers. These will not be seen in contact or loose-contact wounds, but may be present when the range is such that the pellet load is beginning to spread apart a little. When this occurs and the spread-out configuration enters the wound hole following the pellets, the petals may strike the skin around the entrance hole producing these abrasions. These may be in the form of rectangular-shaped abrasions extending outward from the entrance hole, with quite sharp discrete borders, often four in number (Figure 19),

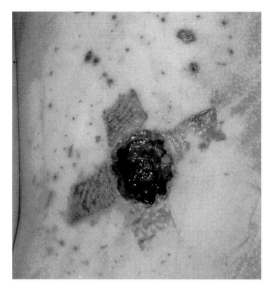

Figure 19: Shotgun wound with abrasions by the leaves/petals of the wad.

paired up two opposite each other across the wound hole, evenly spaced around the wound hole. The number of petal abrasions may range from one to four, because not all of the petals have folded out or back and/or because the wadding has tilted in its travel between muzzle and skin and all the petals do not strike the skin evenly. When wadding abrasions are present, the wadding is following the pellet load straight down range. As the range increases, the waddings will be slowed and diverted in any direction by the air resistance they encounter and may veer off a straight down range path and strike the skin adjacent to the entrance wound hole or in the area struck by the spread-out pellet load, producing abrasions in various shapes, depending on the shape of the wadding and what part of it hits the skin. They can be round, oval, linear, or irregular in shape (Figure 18). The wad will not penetrate the skin as a missile by itself. If wadding is found in the wound track, it got there by entering through the entrance hole produced by the pellets. In addition, these wads are radiolucent.

Pellet load wounds directly into the trunk of the body most often are penetrating wounds (i.e., the pellets do not exit). Bruises and pellets may also be found palpable in or beneath the skin on the chest or abdomen on the opposite side of the body from the entrance wound. If the direction of the shot is tangential to the trunk or is directly to the neck or an extremity (so the pellets only traverse a small distance in the body), the pellet may exit. The area of exit will be very jagged and irregular with extensive destruction of tissue.

Rifled Slugs. The entrance wounds produced by rifled slugs have features like those of the bullet of handguns and rifles: marginal abrasion, ring of dirt, as well as soot, powder, and stippling depending on the range. However, they may be larger wounds, depending on the gauge of the shotgun shell. Rifled slugs are available in shotgun gauges 0.410 to 12. Wounds to the trunk or upper leg will most likely be penetrating. There is greater likelihood of the missile exiting (being a perforating wound) if the wound is quite tangential to the trunk or enters directly to a small part of an extremity. An exit wound will have features similar to those of bullet exit wounds, but may be larger due to the larger size of the rifled slug. These missiles may shed pieces of the metal if they hit bone. The wads and gas seals of rifled slug shells are round discs of cardboard, fiber material, or plastic. They will behave similarly to the wadding of shotgun pellet loads but will not produce the characteristic abrasions around the entrance wound produced by leaves of the shot collar of a plastic wad of a pellet load. These wads are radiolucent. It is important to preserve any pieces of the wadding or gas seal found during treatment. It also is important to recover the slug itself and all pieces of it for firearms identification studies.

Defense Wounds. Some gunshot wounds are "defense" wounds due to warding off a gun or "protecting" oneself by putting a hand or an arm between oneself and the gun. The bullet producing such a defense wound of an upper extremity will very likely go through the hand or wrist or arm (be a perforating wound) and enter another part of the body (re-enter the body).

Asphyxial Injury

Depending on how produced, asphyxial injury may show: 1) a ligature mark on the neck; 2) contusions and/or abrasions due to fingers and fingernails pressing on and/or scraping the skin of the anterior and lateral neck; 3) pressure marks or contusions or abrasions on the lips; and 4) petechial hemorrhages on the palpebral conjunctivae and globes of the eyes and the skin of the face particularly around the eyes.

Thermal Injury (Burns)

Burns can be caused by hot liquids accidentally spilled or purposely poured on the victim, fires, matches, cigarettes, and hot objects such as a clothes iron or stove burner plate. These can occur almost anywhere on the body and range in severity from first degree to fourth degree. Fourth-degree burns are those with charring, complete destruction of the skin and underlying tissues (including bone). The location, size and shape, and degree of the burn need to be documented. The pattern of the burn is very important. Pattern refers to the area involved or exposed such as a hand (glove pattern), foot-ankle (sock pattern), or buttocks-perineum-contiguous lower anterior abdomen and proximal upper legs (diaper distribution). The shape of the burn might be the shape of an object such as a clothes iron. Cigarette burns are characteristically round and the size (diameter) of the cigarette, and may be multiple. The type of burn defined by size, shape, or pattern may give excellent clues as to how the burn was incurred, where in the household, and with what object. The burns may be fresh, healing, or old and/or scarred. There may be more than one and of different ages or stages of healing. It is important to consider whether the injury matches the story as to how the burn(s) occurred.

Good color photographic documentation is critical when documenting burns. Photographs should be taken from various angles and include overall/overview pictures for the distribution/area involved and close-up pictures for detail of the burn.

In addition, if there is suspicion that the fire may have been produced with a flammable substance, or there is a suggestive odor, or if the event is already under investigation, there is a need to obtain an appropriate specimen. Police, fire department, or fire marshal's office may need to be notified. Clothing or a piece of the clothing or a wiping or swabbing of skin surface on which the odor is noted may be wanted. The specimens are best stored in a new or unused metal paint-type can with tightly sealable lids available from the fire department or their arson investigator. Other containers are problematic. Plastic containers may be acted upon or dissolved by the volatile substance and are not suitable containers. A glass test tube could be used, but there is the concern that the substance could react with the rubber or plastic stopper of the tube.

Chemical Injury

Chemical injury is a complex topic because of the great diversity of substances to which there could be exposures as well as the diversity of situations in which there could be exposure, including accidents, assaults, and suicides in the home, industrial work places, transportation, agriculture, outdoors and wilderness settings, and terrorist attack. It includes the field of toxicology. Acid or alkaline substances thrown on people cause chemical burns of the exposed skin of the face, including the eyes, and hands. Strong acids or alkali-soaked clothing can result in burns in which the substances reach the skin under the clothing. Identification of the acid or alkali substance is followed by decontamination with removal of exposed clothing and neutralization/removal of the substance on skin and eyes. If a specimen of the offending liquid can be obtained from the skin surface or clothing, it should be preserved as documentation. Chemical analysis of it may be able to match it to the same substance found in a suspect's possession.

In the industrial setting, there is the potential for exposure to an almost inexhaustibly long list of substances. In agriculture, there is potential for exposure to a large variety of pesticides, fungicides, herbicides, and fertilizers. In both of these workplaces, as well as in transportation (i.e. rail, highway accidents), prompt information from the scene is vital concerning what took place and what chemical exposure occurred.

Ethyl alcohol is the most abused drug consumed in the United States. Hospital laboratories are equipped to promptly provide blood alcohol concentration levels. These are usually serum alcohol levels which are slightly higher than whole blood alcohol levels on the same specimen, but whole blood levels are the levels referred to in statutes on driving under the influence.

Drug abuse is the second most common chemical injury that the medical examiner or coroner encounters. These can be prescribed drugs or drugs available "on the street." The substance may be inhaled, injected, or ingested. If inhaled, it may be identified by swabs of the nasal passages sent to the toxicology laboratory. If injected into a vein with a clean sharp needle, the initial needle puncture will be tiny but may have a drop of fresh or dried blood over the puncture to help identify it. Very often, dirty needles are used, resulting in inflammation and scarring of the injection sites which will be spread along the course of a vein. These are usually readily visible and also are knobby to palpation. They are referred to as needle tracks or scarred veins (Figure 20). Their usual locations are on the flexor surfaces of the forearms and the distal upper arms, antecubital fossae, and anteromedial surfaces of the lower legs into the ankles and feet. Other injection sites include the inframammary fold in females, between the toes, and sometimes beneath the nails where nail polish can hide them. Sites of subcutaneous drug injection, so called "skin popping" site, can become infected, resulting in a small abscess (often round), which can resemble a cigarette burn site as it heals. Hospital clinical pathology laboratories are able to perform panels of drug screens on blood or urine or send the specimen out to a reference laboratory. In addition, a toxicology laboratory can analyze an excised injection site for drugs.

An occurrence well recognized in forensic pathology is that of transporting illicit drugs by

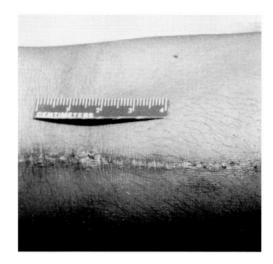

Figure 20: Needle tracks or scarred veins visible on the skin.

swallowing packets (formed from balloons, condoms, or the fingers of Latex surgical gloves) that are filled with the drugs, such as heroin and cocaine, and tied shut. This is known as "body packing" or "body carrying." At their destination, usually across an international border, the filled packets are recovered when they have passed through the gastrointestinal tract and out in the feces. All is well unless one or more breaks, and then the carrier is exposed to a lethal amount of the drug being transported. Such a patient, previously healthy, may present with progressive lethargy or relatively rapid onset of lethargy to unconsciousness and death for no apparent cause. While the packets are radiolucent, they may be outlined by the contrast with the surrounding intestinal contents on an x-ray of the abdomen.

APPENDIX

Sources For Additional Information Relating to These Topics

Auerbach PS: **Wilderness Medicine—Management of Wilderness and Environmental Emergencies.** 3rd ed. St Louis, Mo: Mosby-Year Book, 1995

DiMaio VJM: **Gunshot Wounds—Practical Aspects of Firearms, Ballistics and Forensic Techniques.** New York, NY: Elsevier Scientific, 1985

Ellenhorn MJ, Barcelous DG: **Medical Toxicology—Diagnosis and Treatment of Human Poisoning.** New York, NY: Elsevier Scientific, 1988

Rosen P, Barkin RM (eds): **Emergency Medicine—Concepts and Clinical Practice.** 3rd ed. St Louis, Mo: Mosby-Year Book, 1992

Spitz WU (ed): **Spitz and Fisher's Medicolegal Investigation of Death.** 3rd ed. Springfield, Ill: Charles C Thomas, 1993

QUESTIONS

The Physician's Perspective on Medical Law, Volume I

The following questions have been provided to give physicians the option of testing their comprehension of the material provided in *The Physician's Perspective on Medical Law, Volume I.* The test is to be self-scored. Answers may be found in the back of this book. A Continuing Medical Education (CME) certificate will be mailed upon the return of the enclosed test evaluation/feedback card along with a $25 administrative fee. Telephone 847-692-9500 to order additional evaluation/feedback cards or for more information about other CME products from the American Association of Neurological Surgeons.

After reading this book, a physician should be able to:

- understand the basic structure of the legal system and the rules that govern a physician's participation in legal proceedings.

- understand the legal rules that complement the ethical responsibilities of physicians in their relationships with patients.

- recognize the public health issues that cause the greatest problems in our society and understand the opportunity for physicians, as citizens having special expertise, to take an active role in addressing these problems.

- understand the need to protect both the physician and the patient in interactions with the health care and judicial systems.

CHAPTER 1

BACKGROUND: THE AMERICAN LEGAL SYSTEM

1. The term "common law" refers to:
   (A) the legal rules that existed in medieval England.
   (B) the legal rules applied by courts prior to legislation on a particular subject.
   (C) the legal systems of the United States and other counties which are derived from the English system and rely heavily upon judge-made law.
   (D) any of the above, depending on the context

2. When a court applies the precedent of a decision in a prior case to resolve a current dispute involving different parties, which of the following is *not* an option available to the court?
   (A) The court can follow the rule established by the prior decision under the doctrine of *stare decisis.*
   (B) The court can decline to apply the rule established by the prior decision by overruling that decision.
   (C) The court can decline to apply the rule established by the prior decision by finding the facts of the current dispute are distinguishable from the facts of the prior dispute.
   (D) none of the above: all of these options are available to the court under the common law system

3. Which of the following statements about the power of the federal government is *not* correct?
   (A) The federal government has power to make laws only to the extent granted by the U.S. Constitution.
   (B) The federal government has power to make laws except to the extent that it is limited by the Constitution.
   (C) The Constitution's grant of specific powers to the federal government necessarily includes the implied powers required for their implementation.

   (D) The powers not given to the federal government by the Constitution are reserved to the states or to the people.

4. Which of the following best describes the power of the federal government to regulate intrastate activities?
   (A) The federal government has no power to regulate intrastate activities.
   (B) The federal government has power to regulate intrastate activities under the police power.
   (C) The federal government has power to regulate intrastate activities that have a substantial impact on interstate commerce.
   (D) The federal government has power to regulate intrastate activities except to the extent it is pre-empted by prior state regulations.

5. Which of the following statements about the power of local government is most accurate?
   (A) Both the federal government and local governments derive their powers from grants of authority by the states.
   (B) Just as the federal government derives its authority from the Constitution, local governments derive their authority from grants by the states.
   (C) Just as county governments derive their authority from grants by the states, city governments derive their authority from grants by the counties.
   (D) Just as state governments function as independent sovereigns within the United States, local governments generally function as independent sovereigns within each state.

6. Which of the following statements about appellate jurisdiction in civil cases is most accurate?
   (A) After trial in state court, parties have the right of appeal to a federal district court located in that district.
   (B) After a state trial court decision has been appealed to the highest state court, the next appeal is to the federal district court located in that state.

(C) After a state trial court decision has been appealed to the highest state court, the next appeal is to the federal circuit court of appeals for that state.

(D) After a state trial court decision has been appealed to the highest state court, the next appeal is a request for review by the U.S. Supreme Court.

7. The federal circuit courts of appeal hear appeals from which courts?
   (A) state trial courts
   (B) state appellate courts
   (C) federal district courts
   (D) all of the above

8. The decision in *Marbury v. Madison* established which fundamental aspect of the American legal system?
   (A) judicial review
   (B) dual sovereignty
   (C) separation of powers
   (D) the adversary system of justice

9. To what extent are citizens protected against state infringement of rights established in the Bill of Rights?
   (A) The Bill of Rights establishes rights that protect citizens against actions by both the federal government and state governments.
   (B) The Bill of Rights establishes rights that protect citizens against actions by state governments but not against actions by the federal government.
   (C) The Bill of Rights establishes rights that protect citizens against actions by the federal government, while state constitutions provide the sole protection against actions by state governments.
   (D) The Bill of Rights establish rights that protect citizens against actions by the federal government, and most of these protections are applicable against state governments under the Due Process Clause of the Fourteenth Amendment.

10. Which of the following is *not* a characteristic of the adversary system of dispute resolution?
    (A) reliance on the judge as a neutral umpire
    (B) reliance on pretrial proceedings to narrow the issues for trial
    (C) the tendency of parties to slant their presentations of evidence
    (D) reliance on an active judiciary to decide what issues to raise and what witnesses to call

CHAPTER 2

THE PHYSICIAN AND THE
LEGAL SYSTEM

1. In addition to the risk of malpractice actions, physicians should understand that they can become involved in legal proceedings whenever one of their patients is:
   (A) the victim in a criminal prosecution.
   (B) the defendant in a criminal prosecution.
   (C) a claimant seeking state or federal benefits based on temporary or permanent disability.
   (D) a plaintiff in civil litigation seeking compensation for personal injuries allegedly caused by other persons.
   (E) all of the above

2. Which one of the following statements about the physician's obligation to participate in legal proceedings is *least* accurate?
   (A) All parties to civil and criminal proceedings have the right to compel attendance at trial of a physician who has firsthand knowledge of relevant facts.
   (B) The physician has an ethical obligation to assist in the administration of justice and to furnish medical evidence to secure a patient's rights.
   (C) Under some circumstances, a physician might be civilly liable to a patient for refusal to cooperate in legal pro-

ceedings in which the patient is a party.

(D) Unless the patient obtains a subpoena to compel the physician to attend pretrial or trial proceedings, a physician has no legal duty to participate in civil litigation in which a patient is a party.

3. "Spoliation of evidence":
   (A) is the technical name for the crime of destruction of evidence.
   (B) refers to the inevitable destruction of evidence that frequently occurs in the course of rendering care and treatment to a patient.
   (C) refers to tort liability for destruction of evidence which a physician had a duty to preserve in the course of rendering care and treatment to a patient.
   (D) refers to tort liability for violation of a physician's special duty to preserve evidence beyond that necessary for the appropriate care and treatment of a patient.

4. Statutes that require reporting of traumatic injuries or infectious diseases usually provide immunity from civil liability unless the report was:
   (A) disclosed to the wrong person.
   (B) prepared or filed in bad faith.
   (C) prepared negligently or carelessly.
   (D) both inaccurate and seriously prejudicial.
   (E) A or B

5. Which of the following is *least* likely to be subject to statutory reporting requirements?
   (A) child abuse
   (B) elder abuse
   (C) spouse abuse
   (D) gunshot wounds

6. In the absence of statutory reporting requirements, under what circumstances might a physician be held liable for failure to take appropriate actions?
   (A) Failure to warn identifiable individuals who are the target of specific threats by a patient.

(B) Failure to warn identifiable individuals about whom a dangerous patient has expressed anger.

(C) Failure to take appropriate measures to prevent violent acts by a dangerous patient even without specific threats of violence or expressions of anger against identifiable individuals.

(D) any of the above, depending on the jurisdiction

7. Several states have statutes with regard to human immunodeficiency virus (HIV)-infected patients that:
   (A) require nondisclosure and provide immunity from liability to persons at risk for failure to warn them of the risk.
   (B) require disclosure to persons at risk and provide immunity from liability to the patient for breach of confidentiality.
   (C) permit either disclosure or nondisclosure and provide immunity from liability regardless of whether the physician chooses to disclose the information or to maintain confidentiality.
   (D) permit either disclosure or nondisclosure and provide immunity from liability for disclosure but do not provide immunity for failure to warn persons at risk if the physician chooses to maintain confidentiality.

8. The physician-patient privilege:
   (A) applies in all jurisdictions.
   (B) does not apply in all legal proceedings.
   (C) applies to all physicians, regardless of specialty.
   (D) can be waived either by the physician or by the patient.

9. *Ex parte* contacts between a physician and the attorney representing the patient's opponent in litigation is:
   (A) permitted in all states.
   (B) permitted in most states.
   (C) prohibited in all states.
   (D) prohibited in most states.

10. When a physician receives a subpoena for a patient's medical records, the physician should:
   (A) comply with the subpoena and then notify the patient.
   (B) comply with the subpoena without informing the patient.
   (C) before complying with the subpoena, contact the patient so that any questions about the validity and scope of the waiver of confidentiality can be resolved prior to disclosure.
   (D) before complying with the subpoena, contact the court that issued the subpeona to verify its authenticity.

CHAPTER 3

INTERFACE WITH THE LEGAL SYSTEM BEFORE TRIAL

1. As a matter of both legal and medical ethics, it is improper for a physician to accept compensation for participation as an expert witness if the amount of the fee is:
   (A) contingent on the outcome of the lawsuit.
   (B) substantially higher than the hourly rate of the physician's fees for medical consultations.
   (C) calculated on a daily basis, even when the physician spends substantially less than a full day attending a deposition or trial.
   (D) all of the above

2. Pretrial discovery of expert witnesses in civil litigation:
   (A) facilitates settlement of disputes prior to trial.
   (B) contributes to the quality of expert testimony at trial.
   (C) is essential to the adversary process of dispute resolution.
   (D) all of the above

3. Amendments to the Federal Rules of Civil Procedure in 1993 require an expert witness to:

   (A) appear at a deposition, in lieu of the prior practice of having the attorney supply a summary of the expert's anticipated testimony.
   (B) appear at a deposition, in lieu of the prior practice of having the expert prepare a signed report summarizing the anticipated testimony.
   (C) prepare a signed report summarizing the anticipated testimony, in lieu of the prior practice of having the expert appear at a deposition.
   (D) prepare a signed report summarizing the anticipated testimony, in lieu of the prior practice of having the attorney supply a summary of the expert's anticipated testimony.

4. With respect to physicians who have no firsthand knowledge of relevant facts and who have been retained as *expert witnesses* by parties to civil litigation, the 1993 amendments to the Federal Rules of Civil Procedure:
   (A) retain the requirement that the opposing party obtain a court order to take the deposition of such a physician.
   (B) retain the authority for the opposing party to take the deposition of such a physician without obtaining a court order.
   (C) allow the opposing party to take the deposition of such a physician without a court order, in contrast to the prior rule that required the party to obtain a court order to authorize the deposition.
   (D) require the opposing party to obtain a court order to authorize the deposition of such a physician, in contrast to the prior rule that allowed the party to take the deposition without a court order.

5. If a physician has *no* firsthand knowledge of relevant facts and has *not* been retained by either party to the litigation, under what circumstances, if any, will a federal court issue a subpoena compelling the physician to provide information for use in civil litigation?

(A) Under no circumstances can such a physician be compelled to participate involuntarily in civil litigation.

(B) A party can compel such a physician to disclose existing information or previously formed opinions under extraordinary circumstances if the party has a substantial need for the information that cannot be otherwise met without undue hardship and the party agrees to provide the physician with reasonable compensation.

(C) A party can compel such a physician to provide copies of documents or testify at a deposition or trial unless the physician can demonstrate that participation in the proceedings would impose a substantial hardship on the physician or on the physician's patients or associates.

(D) A party can compel such a physician to participate involuntarily in civil litigation so long as the information sought is relevant and will be helpful to resolution of the case, for the right to compel attendance of witnesses at pretrial or trial proceedings is fully applicable to experts, regardless of whether they have firsthand knowledge or have been retained by one of the parties.

6. If a physician has been retained as an *expert consultant* by a party to civil litigation and has no firsthand knowledge of relevant facts, under what circumstances, if any, will a federal court issue a subpoena compelling the party to provide information to the opposing party about facts known or opinions held by the physician?

(A) Under no circumstances can a party be compelled to provide information about a retained expert consultant who is not expected to testify at trial.

(B) The opposing party can compel disclosure of facts known or opinions held by a physician who is a nontestifying expert consultant under exceptional circumstances if it is impractical for the opposing party to obtain this information by other means, such as when a tissue sample was altered or destroyed after an examination by the physician but prior to any examination by the opposing party.

(C) The opposing party can compel disclosure of facts known or opinions held by a physician who is a nontestifying expert consultant unless the party can demonstrate that this would impose a substantial hardship on the physician or on the party who retained the physician.

(D) A party can compel disclosure of facts known or opinions held by a physician who is a nontestifying expert consultant if the information sought is relevant and will be helpful to resolution of the case, for the right to compel attendance of witnesses at pretrial or trial proceedings is fully applicable to experts, regardless of whether they have firsthand knowledge or have been retained by one of the parties.

7. A request to have a case decided by the judge without a trial based on the undisputed facts established during discovery is called:

(A) a petition for *certiorari.*
(B) a motion for a directed verdict.
(C) a motion for summary judgment.
(D) a motion for judgment notwithstanding the verdict.

8. In civil litigation, to what extent, if any, is the plaintiff entitled to be accompanied by an attorney during a medical examination that is conducted by a physician designated by the defendant pursuant to the rules of civil procedure?

(A) The plaintiff's attorney is more likely to be allowed to accompany the plaintiff in state court proceedings than in federal court proceedings.

(B) Most courts allow the plaintiff to be accompanied by an attorney unless the defendant can demonstrate a substantial need for a private examination.

(C) Most courts do not allow the plaintiff

to be accompanied by an attorney unless the plaintiff can demonstrate a
substantial need for the attorney's
presence.

(D) The plaintiff is never allowed to be
accompanied by an attorney at such a
medical examination because the
presence of an attorney could interfere
with the examination.

9. In state criminal proceedings, the victim's
treating physician generally cannot be:
(A) compelled to attend and answer questions at a pretrial deposition.
(B) compelled to meet privately with the
defendant's attorney for an informal
interview.
(C) forbidden from meeting privately with
the defendant's attorney for an informal interview.
(D) all of the above

10. The 1993 amendments to the Federal
Rules of Criminal Procedure now give the
defendant the right to request:
(A) a deposition of the government's
expert witnesses.
(B) a private meeting with the government's expert witnesses to discuss
their anticipated trial testimony.
(C) a written summary of the anticipated
trial testimony of the government's
expert witnesses.
(D) a signed report from the government's
expert witnesses summarizing their
anticipated trial testimony.

CHAPTER 4

TESTIMONY AT TRIAL

1. In comparison with ordinary lay witnesses,
during direct examination the courts are
more likely to allow expert witnesses to:
(A) answer leading questions.
(B) testify in narrative form.
(C) testify to opinions and conclusions.

(D) base their testimony on hearsay as to
which they have no firsthand knowledge.
(E) all of the above

2. Under the Federal Rules of Evidence,
expert testimony is permitted only if it:
(A) would assist the judge or jury.
(B) is necessary for proof of a relevant
fact.
(C) relates to a topic on which lay testimony is unavailable.
(D) relates to matters beyond the ken of
the average lay juror.

3. In order to qualify as an expert, a witness
must have:
(A) acquired expertise through postsec-
ondary education.
(B) at least 3 years of training or practical
experience.
(C) special knowledge, skill, experience,
training, or education.
(D) received a degree or certificate from
an accredited educational institution
or training program.

4. Which of the following most accurately
describes the relationship between *United
States v. Frye* and *Daubert v. Merrell Dow
Pharmaceuticals*?
(A) *Daubert* reaffirmed *Frye* in requiring
that scientific evidence satisfy the
standard of general acceptance within
a relevant scientific community.
(B) *Daubert* overruled *Frye* and requires
that scientific evidence satisfy the
standard of general acceptance within
a relevant scientific community.
(C) *Daubert* overruled *Frye* and prohibits
trial courts from considering whether
scientific evidence satisfies the standard of general acceptance within a
relevant scientific community.
(D) *Daubert* overruled *Frye* and declared
that trial courts should consider general acceptance within a relevant scientific community as one of several
factors for assessing the reliability of
scientific evidence.

5. Under the decision of the U.S. Supreme Court in *Daubert v. Merrell Dow Pharmaceuticals*, which of the following should *not* be a factor in the trial judge's evaluation of the admissibility of expert opinion testimony?
   (A) the reliability of the expert's methodology
   (B) the validity of the expert's reasoning or conclusion.
   (C) the relevance of the opinion to an issue in the case
   (D) whether the opinion was based on facts or data of a type reasonably relied upon by experts in that field
   (E) none of the above; all of these are appropriate factors for the trial judge to consider

6. According to a recent decision of the U.S. Court of Appeals for the Third Circuit in *In re Paoli RR Yard PCB Litigation*, medical testimony based on differential diagnosis in which the testifying physician relied entirely on the patient's medical records, without taking a medical history or performing a physical examination, is:
   (A) inherently unreliable and is inadmissible in all cases.
   (B) presumptively inadmissible, unless the proponent can demonstrate its reliability.
   (C) presumptively admissible, unless the opponent can demonstrate its unreliability.
   (D) admissible in all cases, because physicians regularly request that colleagues offer opinions based on a review of patient medical records.

7. Insofar as a physician's opinion testimony is based upon facts that would not otherwise be admissible into evidence, such as hearsay learned from others:
   (A) the physician is free to disclose those facts if asked about the basis of the opinion during cross-examination.
   (B) the physician is free to disclose those facts during direct examination in order to explain the basis for the opinion.

   (C) a controversy exists as to whether the physician can disclose those facts during direct examination in order to explain the basis for the opinion.
   (D) both A and C are correct

8. When a physician states an opinion with "reasonable medical certainty," the courts will interpret this as a statement that the physician believes the proposition:
   (A) is more likely to be correct than incorrect, as a matter of probability.
   (B) is almost certain to be correct, within the reasonable limits of medical science.
   (C) represents a considered professional opinion, based on accepted medical principles and methodologies.
   (D) A court may apply any of the above interpretations, depending on the jurisdiction.

9. Which of the following best describes the legal perspective on the ethical problems in the preparation for testimony by expert witnesses?
   (A) It is unethical for an expert witness to rehearse testimony prior to trial.
   (B) Witness preparation is permeated by ethical uncertainty about the line between permissible and impermissible conduct in the shaping of testimony to satisfy legal standards and persuade the finder of fact.
   (C) Witness preparation is permeated by legal uncertainty about the line between permissible and impermissible conduct resulting from the competing goals of partisan representation and truth seeking in the adversarial system of justice.
   (D) Witness preparation is essential in order to present expert testimony that is concise, accurate, accessible to lay jurors, and consistent with technical legal rules of evidence and proof.
   (E) B, C, and D

10. In most jurisdictions, the contents of a medical treatise:
    (A) can be read to the jury during direct examination if the witness establishes the reliability of the treatise.
    (B) can be relied upon by a physician as an expert witness but cannot be read to the jury during direct examination because the written statements of the authors are inadmissible hearsay.
    (C) can be read to the jury during cross-examination so long as the witness agrees with the particular passage read by the cross-examiner, the witness admits having relied upon the treatise, the witness concedes the reliability of the treatise, or the cross-examiner is prepared to establish the reliability of the treatise through other witnesses.
    (D) A and C

CHAPTER 5

RELATIONS BETWEEN PATIENTS AND PHYSICIANS IN MEDICAL DECISION-MAKING

1. The current model for the relation between a physician and a patient is:
   (A) a paternalistic model.
   (B) a participatory model.
   (C) both
   (D) neither

2. The patient-physician relationship is governed by:
   (A) contract law.
   (B) tort law.
   (C) both
   (D) neither

3. "Standard of care" refers to all of the following *except*:
   (A) national standard.
   (B) specialty standard.
   (C) local standard.
   (D) established standard.

4. The physician may refuse to see a patient *except* if the patient:
   (A) threatens suit.
   (B) does not pay incurred medical bills.
   (C) does not follow the physician's advice.
   (D) has acquired immunodeficiency syndrome (AIDS).

5. In order for the physician to obtain informed consent, the patient must be given information about:
   (A) the nature of the illness and the proposed therapy in terms of nature, risk, and terms of success expected, and the results of forgoing it.
   (B) alternative therapies.
   (C) both
   (D) neither

6. Mental competency in a patient requires the ability to:
   (A) understand relevant facts.
   (B) make a rational judgment based on the facts.
   (C) make a rational judgment based on the patient's value system.
   (D) all of the above

7. Parent's wishes about stopping care for a child must be followed in all circumstances *except*:
   (A) the patient is comatose.
   (B) the patient is mentally retarded.
   (C) patient care would prolong dying.
   (D) patient care would be futile and inhumane.

8. The definition of mental incompetence includes all but which one of the following?
   (A) patients with brain death
   (B) patients in a permanent vegetative state
   (C) Jehovah's Witnesses
   (D) anencephalics

9. The "futility of care" involves:
   (A) the chance that care will help.
   (B) the quality of improvement that care will provide.
   (C) both
   (D) neither

10. In order for the physician to avoid futile treatment, there should be all of the following *except:*
    (A) guidelines to assist such decisions.
    (B) absolute power for physicians.
    (C) more authority for physicians.
    (D) participation by outside parties.

11. Rationing, or allocation of resources, should include all of the following *except:*
    (A) expert arbitors.
    (B) age of the patient.
    (C) guidelines.
    (D) public debate.

12. There may be warrantless seizure of a blood sample for assessment of blood alcohol level in all of the following *except:*
    (A) in connection with a motor-vehicle accident.
    (B) where there is probable cause.
    (C) when the collection method is acceptable.
    (D) when done for medical diagnosis and care.

13. The physician must notify the medical examiner/coroner in all of the following *except:*
    (A) death by criminal action.
    (B) death by industrial accident.
    (C) death from vehicular accident.
    (D) death between 24 and 48 hours after hospital admission.

CHAPTER 6

DECISIONS AT THE END OF LIFE

1. There has become a focus on decisions at the end of life because:
   (A) technology leads to prolongation of life which may be burdensome.
   (B) technology leads to utilization of scarce resources.
   (C) the use of available resources may involve excessive cost.
   (D) all of the above

2. Mechanisms to deal with decisions at the end of life for people who have lost competence include:
   (A) advance directives.
   (B) designation of power of attorney.
   (C) both
   (D) neither

3. Patients who have never been competent include:
   (A) the fetus.
   (B) the anencephalic.
   (C) a variety of older people.
   (D) all of the above

4. Terminal patients must be given:
   (A) food.
   (B) water.
   (C) pain control.
   (D) futile care.

5. Factors which interact in the decision for suicide include:
   (A) the individual's personality.
   (B) the general situation.
   (C) the specific problem.
   (D) all of the above

6. Physician-assisted death may include:
   (A) the "double-effect" of medication to relieve pain and suffering.
   (B) giving information about suicide.
   (C) helping with suicide.
   (D) all of the above

7. Issues about physician-assisted death:
   (A) have been argued in state courts.
   (B) have been presented to the U.S. Supreme Court.
   (C) both
   (D) neither

8. Issues to be considered in surrogate decision-making include:
   (A) the patient's prior wishes.
   (B) the patient's best interest.
   (C) both
   (D) neither

9. "Do not resuscitate" orders:
   (A) should be discussed with the patient.
   (B) should be followed in the operating room.
   (C) should not be followed in emergency situations.
   (D) all of the above

10. Brain death is currently defined as:
    (A) irreversible cessation of all functions of the entire brain.
    (B) loss of cortical function.
    (C) an illegal concept.
    (D) all of the above

11. The permanent vegetative state:
    (A) involves complete unawareness of the self and environment.
    (B) cannot be determined.
    (C) cannot be used to make treatment decisions.
    (D) all of the above

12. In a patient with anencephaly:
    (A) the diagnosis is straightforward.
    (B) support can be withdrawn.
    (C) families cannot request support.
    (D) all of the above

13. In the case of an impaired infant:
    (A) the family can request that care be withdrawn.
    (B) the parents may require that care be given.
    (C) both
    (D) neither

CHAPTER 7

MENTAL AND EMOTIONAL COMPETENCE

1. When civil competency is being considered:
   (A) uniform standards are applied to all functional capacities.
   (B) financial decision-making capacity is held to a higher standard than is medical decision-making capacity.

   (C) legal standards vary according to the function in question.
   (D) the capacity to make a will is the same as the capacity to enter into a contract.

2. The "reasonable man" standard concerns:
   (A) a patient's emotional capacity to consider treatment options.
   (B) a patient's intellectual capacity to consider treatment options.
   (C) the adequacy of information provided a patient being asked to consent to treatment.
   (D) the mental state of a patient who rejects all treatment.

3. The doctrine of "informed consent" extends from:
   (A) the fiduciary relationship between doctor and patient.
   (B) the *parens patriae* relationship between doctor and patient.
   (C) the "reasonable man" standard.
   (D) an acknowledgment of medical fallibility.

4. In states that provide for nonjudicial emergency commitment to a mental facility, it is virtually always necessary that the patient:
   (A) be documented to have a treatable psychiatric illness.
   (B) first is examined by a physician.
   (C) has harmed himself or someone else.
   (D) represents a threat to self or others.

5. The *Tarasoff v. Board of Regents* decision held that clinicians must:
   (A) detain potentially suicidal patients.
   (B) detain potentially violent patients.
   (C) warn a violent person's intended victim.
   (D) maintain patient confidentiality in all circumstances.

6. The "Dusky test" is used to determine an individual's competence to:
   (A) waive Miranda rights.
   (B) stand trial.
   (C) be held criminally responsible.
   (D) receive sentencing.

7. The M'Naghten test is a competency standard relating to an individual's capacity to:
   (A) waive Miranda rights.
   (B) stand trial.
   (C) be criminally responsible.
   (D) receive sentencing.

CHAPTER 8

REPRODUCTIVE HEALTH, WOMEN, AND THE LAW

1. In the Supreme Court decision in the landmark case of *Griswold vs. The State of Connecticut:*
   (A) contraception by unmarried persons is allowed.
   (B) women are given the right to do as they please regarding contraception.
   (C) married couples gained the right to use family planning methods.
   (D) contraception is permitted for minors.

2. In providing family planning services to minors without parental consent:
   (A) there is a high likelihood that the provider will be prosecuted.
   (B) although parental consent may be required by law, such laws are not constitutional.
   (C) provider discretion may allow application of the generally accepted exceptions to parental consent including the "mature minor" and the "emancipated minor."
   (D) should be done with great care and only under special circumstances.

3. A minor requests an abortion but refuses to speak to her parents about the matter. What is the physician's appropriate response?
   (A) An abortion cannot be provided without legal risk.
   (B) After the first trimester, this presents no obstacle.
   (C) If an abortion provider feels the minor understands the nature of her decision, the physician may proceed to provide the service.

   (D) The minor's situation should be examined for the possibility of obtaining judicial bypass.

4. According to the most recent rulings of the U.S. Supreme Court:
   (A) the requirement for parental notification of abortion for minors is unconstitutional.
   (B) the requirement for spousal notification of abortion is constitutional.
   (C) the state may place requirements on the information provided a woman before obtaining consent for abortion.
   (D) the state may require the publication of the names of women having abortions.

CHAPTER 9

LEGAL ASPECTS OF ALCOHOL AND DRUG TESTING

1. Which of the following is true regarding testing of breath or urine for legal reasons?
   (A) All motorists are considered to have given consent for testing by implication.
   (B) Physicians are frequently called upon to administer such testing.
   (C) In some states, a person may refuse to take such tests.
   (D) Written consent is always required.

2. Regarding blood alcohol and drug testing in patients, which of the following is true?
   (A) Testing may be performed as part of the medical evaluation even if the patient refuses.
   (B) Verbal or written consent is required in all cases.
   (C) Each medical facility has a policy and procedure for alcohol testing which must be strictly followed.
   (D) Chain of custody is not required unless police request the alcohol testing to be done.

3. When a patient injured in a motor-vehicle crash refuses testing:
   (A) implied consent remains valid and the testing should be performed.
   (B) in some states, physicians are called upon to use physical force to obtain such samples.
   (C) the blood test may not be performed.
   (D) the physician should try to talk the patient into having the test.

4. In an unconscious patient:
   (A) blood sampling may be performed under the doctrine of implied consent.
   (B) a physician may be liable for technical battery if blood is removed for testing in an unconscious patient.
   (C) since the patient is unable to consent, testing may never be performed.
   (D) even if acting in good faith in caring for an unconscious patient, a physician who performs blood testing is likely to be found liable for battery.

5. If a law enforcement officer requests information regarding the status of a patient:
   (A) the physician should freely divulge any and all pertinent information to the officer.
   (B) only general information related to the patient's condition should be released.
   (C) the physician should release a copy of the medical record as well as any test results to the police as soon as such information is available.
   (D) state reporting statutes never apply to the acute care setting.

CHAPTER 11A

CHILD ABUSE AND NEGLECT

1. Warning signs of child abuse include all of the following *except:*
   (A) multiple wounds of varying ages.
   (B) a crying, hostile child.
   (C) a delay in seeking treatment.
   (D) multiple "histories" of conflicting nature.
   (E) a discrepancy between history and severity of injury.

2. Documentation of physical injury is necessary when abuse is suspected. The best means for doing this is to:
   (A) draw sketches of the wounds.
   (B) describe the wounds in the medical history and physical examination.
   (C) take Polaroid photographs and tape them in the chart.
   (D) take color and black/white 35-mm photographs with the patient's name and hospital number clearly visible.
   (E) take color 35-mm photographs with date/time, but protect the patient's anonymity.

CHAPTER 11B

SPOUSE ABUSE

1. Spouse abuse:
   (A) occurs primarily in urban settings.
   (B) includes battering, sexual abuse, psychological abuse, social isolation, deprivation, and intimidation of a victim by an intimate partner.
   (C) is usually the result of the batterer's drinking problem.
   (D) occurs only in heterosexual relationships.

2. Concerning the "cycle of violence," which of the following is true?
   (A) The cycle consists of three phases: tension building, acute battering, and honeymoon phase.
   (B) Once the cycle is complete, the abuse rarely recurs.
   (C) In cases where the cycle continues, the frequency and severity of abuse decreases.
   (D) Most women take legal steps for protection after the first episode of abuse.

3. Regarding the history of spouse abuse, which of the following is true?
   (A) Spouse abuse was rare before the 20th century.
   (B) It is still accepted as a way of life in many subcultures in the U.S.
   (C) The first shelters for abused women were established in the 1920s.
   (D) Legislative, social, and therapeutic reform to control spousal abuse began in the 1800s.

4. The impact of spouse abuse can be summarized by which of the following?
   (A) Approximately 12 million women are abused annually in the U.S.
   (B) 20%-30% of all women will be physically assaulted by an intimate partner at some time in their lives.
   (C) The rate of injury to women from battering surpasses that of motor-vehicle crashes, rapes, and muggings combined.
   (D) 50% of the women murdered each year are murdered by a current or former intimate partner.
   (E) all of the above

5. Women who are at greater risk for abuse include:
   (A) mothers of abused children.
   (B) women between the ages of 17 and 28 years.
   (C) pregnant women.
   (D) all of the above

6. Barriers to identifying spouse abuse include:
   (A) a reluctance of the victim to seek help for fear of retaliation by the abuser.
   (B) the lack of outside communication and transportation.
   (C) cultural, ethnic, and/or religious factors.
   (D) the lack of screening by physicians.
   (E) all of the above

7. Screening of females for domestic violence is indicated:
   (A) in all patients.
   (B) only in those with physical injuries.

   (C) only in those who are poorly educated and from a low socioeconomic class.
   (D) only if the patient seems receptive to the screening questions.

8. Typical presentations of spouse abuse include:
   (A) cases where the explanation of how an injury occurred does not fit with the clinical picture.
   (B) cases where there has been a delay in seeking treatment.
   (C) women with injuries incurred during pregnancy.
   (D) cases in which the woman appears frightened, ashamed, or embarrassed.
   (E) all of the above

9. The role of the health care provider in spouse abuse includes:
   (A) providing/ensuring the safety of the patient.
   (B) identifying battered women through screening.
   (C) documenting findings.
   (D) referring the patient to support agencies and shelter services.
   (E) all of the above

CHAPTER 11C

GERIATRIC ABUSE

1. The three segments of the population most prone to domestic abuse are:
   (A) children, gang members, and parents.
   (B) children, spouses, and the elderly.
   (C) spouses, the physically challenged, and the elderly.
   (D) nursing home residents, the mentally ill, and other elderly.
   (E) the elderly, parents, and children.

2. Epidemiological studies show:
   (A) child abuse is more than twice as common as elder abuse.
   (B) elder abuse is less common than spouse abuse.
   (C) elder abuse is only slightly less common than child abuse.

(D) the incidence of elder abuse is at least 25%.

(E) nearly all cases of elder abuse are reported to the proper authorities.

3. Common characteristics of abusers of the elderly include:
(A) violent or antisocial behavior.
(B) alcohol or drug abuse.
(C) financial dependence on the victim.
(D) all of the above
(E) none of the above

4. On examination, presentations suggestive of elder abuse include:
(A) multiple injuries in various stages of healing.
(B) neglected injuries.
(C) fearful or withdrawn behavior.
(D) unexplained malnutrition or dehydration.
(E) all of the above

5. Elderly persons living in nursing homes may be at risk of abuse from which of the following?
(A) nursing home staff
(B) other residents
(C) visitors
(D) all of the above
(E) none of the above

6. Although no consensus definition of elder abuse exists, which of the following are generally accepted types?
(A) physical abuse
(B) psychosocial or emotional abuse
(C) sexual abuse
(D) all of the above
(E) none of the above

7. Health care providers who should be prepared to recognize, diagnose, and initiate treatment for elder abuse include:
(A) emergency department physicians.
(B) visiting (home health care) nurses.
(C) neurosurgeons.
(D) all of the above
(E) none of the above

8. Which of the following statements concerning elder abuse is true?
(A) Failure to correctly diagnosis or report cases of elder abuse may expose clinicians to liability.
(B) Under many of the mandatory reporting laws, irrefutable proof of elder abuse is required.
(C) Few (if any) states with mandatory reporting laws provide immunity to reporters of elder abuse who act in good faith.
(D) All 50 states have now enacted mandatory reporting laws requiring health care workers to report suspected elder abuse.

9. When considering the problem of elder abuse:
(A) the true incidence and prevalence are known.
(B) epidemiological studies suggest an incidence rate of 20%-25%.
(C) only 60% of cases are being reported.
(D) overall, only 4% to 10% of cases of abuse reported to protective service agencies involve the elderly.
(E) of the putative risk factors for elder abuse, only cognitive impairment and shared living arrangements with the abuser find strong support in the literature.

CHAPTER 12B

ASSAULT AND HOMICIDE

1. Interpersonal violence causes:
(A) 65 deaths a day.
(B) 6,000 injuries a day.
(C) almost $200 billion/year for care and suppport and lost quality of life.
(D) all of the above

2. Categories of violent crime include:
(A) simple and aggravated assault.
(B) robbery.
(C) rape.
(D) homicide.
(E) all of the above

3. The highest incidence of victimization involves:
   (A) poverty stricken persons.
   (B) the use of guns.
   (C) the use of drugs.
   (D) nonwhites.

4. It appears that interpersonal crime incidence:
   (A) is increasing.
   (B) is decreasing.
   (C) is staying the same.
   (D) is will decrease further.

5. Homicide tends to involve:
   (A) the family.
   (B) friends.
   (C) both
   (D) neither

6. The following factors are important to violent behavior:
   (A) biological
   (B) psychological
   (C) sociological
   (D) all of the above

7. Control of violence will require:
   (A) more data.
   (B) prevention.
   (C) both
   (D) neither

CHAPTER 12C

Sexual Assault

1. When a rape victim appears calm:
   (A) she will probably not experience rape-trauma syndrome.
   (B) she may be fabricating the rape allegation.
   (C) a contact for support may not be necessary.
   (D) she may be in a dissociative state.
   (E) it should be reported in the physician's emergency department notes.

2. Which one of the following observations should be reported in the physician's examination?
   (A) The physician's impression as to whether the victim "led on" the assailant.
   (B) The physician's assessment as to whether the victim may have been under the influence of alcohol or other drugs.
   (C) The state of dress of the victim.
   (D) All bruises, abrasions, and cuts.
   (E) Tattoos, piercings, and adornments.

3. Forensic specimens:
   (A) should be taken directly to the hospital laboratory.
   (B) should be transferred to law enforcement personnel with a signature documenting the transfer, place, and time.
   (C) may be omitted selectively, depending on the history obtained.
   (D) should be taken regardless of patient consent.
   (E) are not necessary if the victim states no intent to prosecute.

4. Consent for the post-rape examination:
   (A) is not necessary and serves no purpose.
   (B) may be crucial to the admission of evidence.
   (C) should be obtained at all costs.
   (D) need not be witnessed to be valid.
   (E) can be deferred until after the examination if the victim is distraught.

5. The history recorded by the examining physician:
   (A) should be exhaustive.
   (B) should include the events preceding the encounter leading to rape.
   (C) should record the victim's analysis of why the rape occurred.
   (D) may be omitted entirely, as the specimens collected will tell the story.
   (E) is important to guide the physician in observations and collection of evidence that may be used to verify the victim's recollection of events.

CHAPTER 12D

SUICIDE

1. Since 1950, the rate of suicide has increased in which age group?
   (A) 15-35 years
   (B) 45-60 years
   (C) 60-75 years
   (D) over 75 years

2. The highest suicide rate in the U.S. is among:
   (A) black females.
   (B) white males.
   (C) Native Americans.
   (D) Asian Americans.

3. Significant risk factors for suicide include all of the following *except:*
   (A) a previous attempt.
   (B) living alone.
   (C) recent life events.
   (D) the presence of psychiatric illness.

4. All but which one of the following is characteristic of the adolescent suicide victim?
   (A) drug/alcohol consumption
   (B) high academic performance
   (C) prior professional intervention
   (D) situational stress

5. Patients who complete the act of suicide rarely communicate to others their intention to do so.
   (A) true
   (B) false

6. The most significant indicator of potential suicidal intent in a patient is:
   (A) antidepressant blood level.
   (B) withdrawn behavior.
   (C) agitation.
   (D) thoughts of suicide.

7. A 10%-15% rate of suicide over a lifetime is characteristic of which group of patients?
   (A) schizophrenic patients
   (B) patients with depression
   (C) alcoholic patients
   (D) previous attempters of suicide
   (E) all of the above

8. Generally, proof of immediate dangerousness of self or others is sufficient to institute "probable cause" hearings for the suicidal patient.
   (A) true
   (B) false

INDEX

Volumes I and II

Page numbers for figures and tables are followed by *f* and *t,* respectively.
(1) = entry in Volume I
(2) = entry in Volume II

H

"Habit-forming" substances, labeling and distribution of, (2) 282
Haddon, William
  and gun control, (2) 209
  and National Traffic Safety Bureau, (1) 136
  and unintentional injury
    epidemiology of, (1) 134-135
    prevention of, (1) 164-165
Hall, Mark, on medical directives, advisory vs. binding, (2) 310-311
Hamilton, Frank, on malpractice suits in 19th century, (2) 412
Hammurabi, code of
  and licensure history, (2) 294
  and workers' compensation, (2) 390
Handguns, (1) 191, (2) 203, 204-205, 209
  wounds produced by, (1) 191-197
Handicap, workers' compensation definition of, (2) 395
Harrell v. Total Health Care, Inc., and managed care liability, (2) 361
Harvard Medical School
  and malpractice study, (2) 416
  and physician licensure, (2) 295
Hazard, exposure to, and toxic tort litigation, (2) 269-270
HCQIA. *See* Health Care Quality Improvement Act of 1986
Head Injury Foundation, and trauma registry, (2) 350
The Health Benefits of Smoking Cessation, (2) 229
Health care finance, (2) 358-359
Health Care Financing Administration (HCFA)
  and investigational devices, reimbursement for, (2) 290-291
  and Medicare/Medicaid managed care, (2) 359-360
  and patient satisfaction, (2) 324
Health care providers, rights and responsibilities of, under insurance contract, (2) 369-370
Health Care Quality Improvement Act of 1986 (HCQIA), (1) 23, (2) 302-303, 305-306
  effects of, (2) 332-333
  and hospital peer review, (2) 320-323, 328-330, 337, 339
  specific provisions of, (2) 330-332
Health insurance, (1) 23, (2) 369-371
  and confidentiality/disclosure, (2) 370-371
Health law, field of, (1) 19
Health maintenance organizations (HMOs), (2) 355-356. *See also* Managed care organizations (MCOs)
  and cost reductions demands, (2) 335
  and licensing laws, (2) 310-311
  negligence of, and physician liability, (2) 311-314
  and practice parameters, (2) 417
Healthy People 2000, (1) 175, 176
  homicide and suicide rates in, (2) 204

and tobacco use, (2) 235
Hearsay, (1) 16
  depositions as, (1) 41
  and expert testimony, (1) 52, 57, 62
  medical history as, (1) 180
Hedonic damages, in malpractice cases, (2) 411
Heifetz, euthanasia guidelines of, (1) 86
Helmet laws, (1) 137
Hematological death, from radiation exposure, (2) 255
Hierarchy of sources of law, (1) 8-13
High-resolution computed tomography, and toxic tort litigation, (2) 268
Highway and Motor Vehicle Safety Act of 1996, (1) 136
Highway safety, (1) 135-138
Hippocratic Oath, and confidentiality, (1) 30
HIV. *See* Human immunodeficiency virus
HMOs. *See* Health maintenance organizations
Homeopathic Pharmacopoeia of the United States, and drug definition, (2) 282
Home visit, and geriatric abuse, (1) 155, 157
Homicide, (1) 171-177. *See also* Violence
  and guns, (2) 204-206
  incidence of, (1) 160-161, 171, 173*f*-175*f*
  prevention of, (1) 166
Horizontal Merger Guidelines, and hospital mergers, (2) 363-364
Hospitalization, involuntary, (1) 110-113, 114*t*-115*t*
  for alcoholic patients, (2) 225
  for suicidal patients, (1) 185-186
Hospital peer review, (2) 317-343
  and economic credentialing, (2) 333-337
  effectiveness of, (2) 318-333
  improved participation in, (2) 333
  JCAHO accreditation and, (2) 319
  and managed care, (2) 337-343
  as regulatory mechanism, (2) 320-324
  socialization to importance of, (2) 327-328
  state/federal governments and, (2) 319-320, 328-330
Hospitals
  disclosure issues in, (1) 77
  and duty to patients, (2) 325-327
  mergers of, and antitrust law, (2) 363-364
Household safety, (1) 138-139
Human immunodeficiency virus (HIV)
  and Americans With Disabilities Act, (2) 245-250
  and confidentiality, (2) 242-243
  and discrimination cases, (2) 245-250
  fear of contracting, emotional distress from, (2) 245
  health care providers infected with, (2) 247-250
  in health care workplace, (2) 240-250
  legal controversies surrounding, (2) 240-250
  as public health issue, (2) 239-250
  reporting requirements for, (1) 27, (2) 241-242
  and reproductive health of minors, (1) 124
  voluntary vs. mandatory testing for, (2) 240-241

U.S. Medical Licensing Examination (USMLE), (2) 300-301
USMLE. *See* U.S. Medical Licensing Examination
U.S. Nuclear Regulatory Commission (NRC), and radiation guidelines, (2) 253, 256-258, 260, 261*t*
U.S. Pharmacopoeia
and drug definition, (2) 282
and radiation safety, (2) 260
U.S. regulatory agencies, for radiation exposure, (2) 257-258
U.S. Statutes at Large, (1) 12
U.S. Supreme Court, (1) 5-7
U.S. v. Miller, and Second Amendment, (2) 214
U.S. v. Morvant, and HIV-positive patients, duty to treat, (2) 247
Utah Experiment in Patient Injury Compensation (EPIC), (2) 434

V

Vaccine-related injury, litigation regarding, (2) 239
Vegetative state. *See* Permanent vegetative state
Verol v. Blue Cross and Blue Shield of Michigan, and managed care decision-making, (2) 312
Veto power, (1) 4
Viability, of fetus, (1) 96
Violence. *See also* Assault; Homicide; Injuries; Rape; Sexual assault; Suicide; Trauma
and alcohol abuse, (2) 220-221
cost of, (1) 163, 163*t*
data sources for, (1) 168-169
comparison of, (1) 174*t*
against elderly, (1) 151-152
factors contributing to, (1) 173
within families, (1) 172*t*
and gunshot wounds, (2) 205-206
overview of, (1) 159-169
physical trauma, description of, (1) 187-202
and physician responsibilities, (1) 165
prevention of, (1) 165-166, 173-175, (2) 207-208, 208*t*
reporting requirements for, (1) 26-27
research on, (1) 165, (2) 207
and socioeconomic problems, (1) 160
on television, (2) 208
trends in, (1) 163-164
in workplace, (1) 5, 138, 171
Voluntary active euthanasia, (1) 85
Voluntary cooperation, in litigation. *See* Legal compulsion, and trial attendance
Vulnerable populations, injuries to, reporting requirements for, (1) 27

W

Waiting period, for gun purchases, (2) 212, 214
Wanglie, Helga, and futile care case, (1) 73

Warning labels, on tobacco products, (2) 233, 234
WESTLAW computer database, (1) 13
White House Mini-Conference on Emerging Issues in Mental Health and Aging (Feb. 1995), (1) 83
Wickline v. State, and managed care decision-making, (2) 312, 361
Wills, (1) 88
contesting of, and confidentiality override, (1) 77
Wilson v. Blue Cross of Southern California, and managed care liability, (2) 361
Wilson v. Office of Civilian Health and Medical Programs of the Uniformed Services, and managed care decision-making, (2) 313
Witnesses. *See* Expert witnesses; Occurrence witnesses
Witness fee, (1) 36
Women
and alcohol abuse, (2) 219, 220
battered. *See* Spouse abuse
and reproductive health issues, (1) 123-127
and self-defense, using guns, (2) 207
and suicide, (1) 184
Work disability, CDC definition of, (2) 395-396
Workers' compensation, (1) 23, 35, (2) 387-405, 393*t*
and disease vs. injury, (2) 395
and fraud/abuse, (2) 394-395
future of, (2) 401-405
historical overview of, (2) 390-393
problematic issues of, (2) 403-405
problem cases, "red flags" for, (2) 400*t*
and psychiatric illness, (2) 399-400
role of physician in, (2) 387-390, 388*t*-389*t*
terminology regarding, (2) 393-396
vs. Americans With Disabilities Act, (2) 396-397
vs. Family and Medical Leave Act, (2) 397-398
vs. mental stress claims, (2) 398-399
vs. other litigation, (2) 396-400
vs. toxic tort litigation, (2) 263-264
and written medical reports, (1) 39
Workplace smoking ban, (2) 234
Work-Relatedness Criteria Questions, (2) 388, 388*t*
World Health Organization, and alcoholism screening, (2) 224
Wound range, and soot/powder, (1) 193-195
Wounds, (1) 187-202
track vs. path of, (1) 188
"Writ of certiorari," and U.S. Supreme Court, (1) 6-7
Written medical reports, (1) 39-40

Y

Years of potential life lost before 65 (YPLL-65), as measure of injury cost, (1) 163, 163*t*, (2) 203
Youngstown Sheet & Tube Co. v. Sawyer, and judicial review, (1) 7
YPLL-65. *See* Years of potential life lost before 65

ANSWERS TO CME QUESTIONS
The Physician's Perspective on Medical Law, Volume I

Chapter 1
1. D   2. D   3. B   4. C   5. B
6. D   7. C   8. A   9. D   10. D

Chapter 2
1. E   2. D   3. C   4. E   5. C
6. D   7. C   8. B   9. B   10. D

Chapter 3
1. A   2. D   3. D   4. C   5. B
6. B   7. C   8. A   9. D   10. C

Chapter 4
1. E   2. A   3. C   4. D   5. B
6. B   7. D   8. D   9. E   10. D

Chapter 5
1. B   2. C   3. C   4. D   5. C
6. D   7. B   8. C   9. C   10. B
11. B   12. D   13. D

Chapter 6
1. D   2. C   3. D   4. C   5. D
6. D   7. C   8. C   9. A   10. A
11. A   12. B   13. C

Chapter 7
1. C   2. C   3. A   4. D   5. C
6. B   7. C

Chapter 8
1. C   2. C   3. D   4. C

Chapter 9
1. C   2. C   3. C   4. A   5. B

Chapter 11A
1. B   2. D

Chapter 11B
1. B   2. A   3. B   4. E   5. D
6. E   7. A   8. E   9. E

Chapter 11C
1. B   2. C   3. D   4. E   5. D
6. D   7. D   8. A   9. E

Chapter 12B
1. D   2. E   3. B   4. B   5. C
6. D   7. C

Chapter 12C
1. D   2. D   3. B   4. B   5. E

Chapter 12D
1. A   2. C   3. C   4. B   5. B
6. D   7. E   8. A

PREVIOUSLY PUBLISHED BOOKS IN THE *Neurosurgical Topics* SERIES

For order information call (847) 692-9500.

Howard H. Kaufman, MD, is Professor and Chairman of the Department of Neurosurgery at West Virginia University School of Medicine. He received a BA from Yale University and an MD from Columbia University. He did his internship in Minnesota, studied a year at the National Hospital for Nervous Diseases in London, spent 2 years at the National Institutes of Health, and then did a residency at Neurological Institute of Columbia University. He was a member of the faculty of the University of Arizona and the University of Texas at Houston before moving to West Virginia. He has been involved with many legal issues, among them brain death and the permanent vegetative state, organ retrieval, and device regulation. He will be developing a national effort on gun safety for organized neurosurgery.

Jeff L. Lewin, JD, is Professor of Law at the Widener University School of Law in Wilmington, Delaware. The son of a psychiatrist and the grandson of a general practitioner, Professor Lewin broke with family tradition to major in Economics at the University of Michigan and receive a JD from Harvard Law School. After several years of law practice, he joined the faculty of the West Virginia University School of Law. Service on that University's Institutional Review Board for the Protection of Human Research Subjects from 1985 to 1990 rekindled his interest in medicolegal issues, and he began collaborating with Dr. Kaufman on a series of projects that culminated in this book. In addition to works on medicolegal issues, Professor Lewin has published articles on such diverse topics as nuisance law, tort law, environmental law and economics, valuation of criminal gains in cost-benefit analysis, and ownership of coalbed methane. The *Maryland Law Review* is publishing his article on the origins of the phrase "reasonable medical certainty," and he currently is exploring the relationship between this phrase and recent developments in evidence and tort law.

This two-volume set is the first contribution to the series for Dr. Kaufman and Mr. Lewin. Dr. Kaufman has been a chapter author in several previous books in the *Neurosurgical Topics Series*.

Publications Office
Lebanon, New Hampshire

Gay Palazzo
Joanne B. Needham
Katherine Mann

Compositor
Barbara Homeyer

Indexer
Sarah Allen Smith

Reference Editor
Kim DeVillers